The Future of Healing

Exploring the Parallels of
Eastern and Western Medicine

Michael P. Milburn
B.S., M.S., Ph.D., Dip.Ac., D.Ac.

THE CROSSING PRESS
FREEDOM, CALIFORNIA

Copyright © 2001 by Michael P. Milburn
Cover design by Petra Serafim
Chinese calligraphy by Terry Louie
Interior design by Courtnay Perry
Printed in the U.S.A.

First printing, 2001

The publishers wish to thank the following for permission to use copyright material: Paradigm Publications for the illustration on page 54 from *Fundamentals of Chinese Acupuncture*, by Nigel Wiseman et al., © 1991; Shambhala Publications for illustrations on pages 26, 67, 241, 263 reproduced from *Chinese Herbal Medicine* by Daniel Reid, © 1992; Cambridge University Press for the illustration on page 80 and excerpts reprinted from *Science and Civilisation in China*, Vols. 2 and 5, by Joseph Needham, © 1974; NTC/Contemporary Publishing for excerpts reprinted from *The Web that Has No Weaver* by Ted J. Kaptchuk, OMD, © 1985.

For information on bulk purchases or group discounts for this and other Crossing Press titles, please contact our Special Sales Manager at 800/777-1048.
Visit our Web site: **www.crossingpress.com**

Library of Congress Cataloging-in-Publication Data

Milburn, Michael Peter
     The future of healing : exploring the parallels of Eastern and Western medicine / by Michael Peter Milburn.
          p. cm.
     Includes bibliographic references.
     ISBN 1-58091-065-3 (pbk.)
          1. Holistic medicine. 2. Medicine, Chinese. I. Title.

R733.M535 2001
610--dc21

                                                          2001017462

Acknowledgments

I am indebted to my teachers of traditions both East and West, without whose willingness and enthusiasm for the sharing of knowledge this book would never have been written. Grandmaster Sherman Lai, Jing-song Tao, O.M.D., Kai Chen, Ph.D., Colin Paddon, D.Ac., Master Hyunoong Seunim, and Ja Gwang Seunim, among others, opened the door to the East. Professors Jim Davis, Ken Jeffrey, and James Mathews, among others, gave me the privilege of participating in the Western scientific engagement of nature and a sense of its beauty and joys.

An individual is but one wave upon a great ocean, and the wave that produced this book was shaped by others from many directions. The late, great Joseph Needham and the brilliant thinker and scientist Fritjof Capra built a bridge of East-West understanding upon which I could walk. Nobel Laureate Brian Josephson helped a young undergraduate mind open to the broader possibilities of science. Westerners and Easterners too numerous to mention have worked to plant the seeds of Eastern medicine in the West—seeds that have taken root and become healthy, flourishing seedlings. Without their efforts the questions from which this book arose would never have presented themselves in the first place. And without scientists who dare to challenge the dogma of their time, science would not have progressed, let alone emerged in the first place. This book is a celebration of these "frontier" scientists whose efforts will in future bear fruits of surprising texture and taste.

Special thanks to Robert Phripp for many useful discussions, to Norman Temple for reviewing the manuscript, and to Carol Kraft and James Saper for help with research. And finally, without the enthusiasm and effort of my editor Caryle Hirshberg and the Crossing Press staff this book would never have been more than a good idea.

Life is short, the Way is long, and many forsake the Tao.
To All—Past, Present and Future, East and West—
who strive to drink at its source,
To taste and bring forth this Tao beyond space and time,
So All Beings may benefit from the compassion and wisdom
Of the Tao of health and healing.

Table of Contents

Preface

At the dawn of the twentieth century medicine was a pluralistic activity, with a variety of practitioners offering a variety of practices. Yet during the twentieth century one particular approach came to dominate medicine in the industrialized world. This Western scientific medicine—with its lifesaving antibiotics and miraculous organ transplants—has improved the quality and duration of human life. It also rendered its ostensibly superstitious and ineffectual counterparts redundant. Or so it seemed! As the twenty-first century dawns, medicine has once again become a pluralistic activity. Homeopathy, herbs, and acupuncture, among others, have become common and are used by a growing number of people.

This book is the result of a long struggle to make sense of the contradictions and questions that arise from the return to medical pluralism. With the remarkable accomplishments of Western scientific medicine and its cures around every corner, what is behind the dramatic rise of complementary approaches? Of what possible value could the ancient technique of acupuncture be in a world of X-rays and insulin, MRIs, and artificial joints? Is it possible to reconcile a commitment to science with arcane concepts like qi—the mysterious "energy" so central to the theory of Chinese medicine?

I am interested here in Eastern medicine, not just as a repository of knowledge about herbs and acupuncture, but as a system with a complementary framework for understanding "what is wrong" and "what can help." I am interested in more than medicine in the narrow sense of the word, and explore more broadly questions of health and healing. And I am interested in the underlying world views of East and West, and their relationship in the context of health and healing.

I argue that it is possible to maintain a deep respect and admiration for Western scientific medicine while acknowledging limitations that leave room for complementary approaches and scientific medicine's own evolution.

I describe a science that embraces a "spirituality inherent in matter." This is a science well beyond its common conception, but it is one with a thread of continuity through the history of science and one that brings together body, mind, and spirit. It offers a more humble path for humanity, a Way that includes a broadly holistic conception of health and healing. This Tao of health and healing is imbued with compassion and in its richness includes traditions both Eastern and Western.

The problem of an integrated, yet diverse, medicine requires the rigorous examination of what works and what doesn't. But we must also explore deeper questions about health and healing, an exploration toward which I hope this book makes a small contribution.

Michael P. Milburn

Introduction| **Where East Meets West:**
A Cultural Journey in Health and Healing

Karl and Diana struggled with infertility for over a year. Tests revealed the young couple to be in good health. Karl's sperm count was ever-so-slightly below normal, but their physician did not think this was the cause of the problem.

Karl and Diana were referred to a local fertility clinic. Specialists there ordered more tests, but again found nothing that would account for the couple's inability to conceive. The clinic's most experienced physician took on the case, and recommended that Diana try a new fertility drug that held promise for her situation.

Karl was unsure about the idea of using drugs to help them conceive. Diana was steadfast in her opposition to the idea. Her aunt's negative experience with the side effects of drugs while pregnant influenced her decision. She struggled with the thought of simply accepting the possibility of never being able to have children.

A friend at work suggested complementary medicine. While Diana had heard of healing systems such as naturopathy, homeopathy, and acupuncture, she had never thought about them seriously.

Diana called a Chinese medicine specialist recommended by a friend and made an appointment. Her visit was pleasant and surprising. Instead of a brief visit and subsequent tests to which she was accustomed, the practitioner carefully listened to her story and asked her questions about her diet, emotional patterns, and general health. The practitioner studied Diana's tongue, delicately felt the pulses of both wrists, and even pressed the length of her spine looking for tender areas.

The most shocking thing was the diagnosis: too much cold,

especially in the stomach and spleen. Diana was impressed by the fact that this system of medicine has been around for thousands of years and is still widely used today as part of the health care system in China. But it still seemed strange. Karl also visited the clinic for an assessment. He was told he was too hot and his kidneys were a little on the weak side, particularly the yin aspect.

Over the next several months, the young couple drank many cups of herbal tea, brewed from an odd assortment of roots, twigs, berries, and bark, according to instruction. In time, these not-so-pleasant-tasting decoctions even had an odd sort of appeal. They visited the clinic regularly to have their progress monitored and new combinations of herbs prescribed. In the first several weeks, they began to feel different—they experienced a heightened sense of energy, improved digestion, and a deeper, more relaxed sleep.

The practitioner recommended that Diana wait six months or more before trying to get pregnant so that she would become as healthy as possible. After so many unsuccessful months of trying, the couple was not particularly optimistic that it would happen quickly, but three months later Diana was pregnant.

While not all experiences with complementary medicine are this successful, Karl and Diana are just two of a growing number of people exploring a wide variety of "unconventional" approaches to health care. A *New England Journal of Medicine* study published in 1993 found that 34 percent of Americans had used "unconventional" medicine in 1990. People with higher education and incomes made the most frequent use of such therapists, and surprisingly the estimated 425 million visits in that year exceeded the 388 million visits to all United States primary care physicians.[1]

This growing enthusiasm for "unconventional" therapies is surprising considering the remarkable progress that has occurred in the field of medicine. Discovery of the microbial basis of infectious disease and various means of prevention and treatment have dramatically reduced the communicable scourges of civilization. Surgical skills have improved unimaginably: limbs can be reattached, worn out joints replaced with artificial equivalents, and organs transplanted. With so much success, why is there so much interest in "unconventional" health care?

Despite the achievements of Western medicine, and the promise of many more, it is not without limitations.[2] This highly technological, complex system of medicine is a mirror of our society, a mixture of miracle and muddle, promise and peril.

In the movie, *The Meaning of Life*, a team of physicians doted over the spectacular machines in the delivery room, until they suddenly realized something was missing—the patient. The cast's parody highlights a contradiction in modern medicine between an enthusiasm for technology and a disdain for its dehumanizing effects.

In the 1970s, after decades of miraculous success with penicillin and a panoply of antibiotic drugs, physicians were ready to close the book on the problems of infectious disease. Yet this turned out to be premature. Over the years antibiotic use has become widespread and the drugs overused. In time, the bacteria have adapted and antibiotic-resistant strains have evolved, and our belief in antibiotics as a panacea has been weakened.

Dave Dingwall, then Canadian Minister of Health, noted in an October, 1996, speech that prescription drug use in Canada had climbed by 15 percent in the previous year, but added, "This statistic does not allow me to say that we are now a healthier society." [3] The problem is that the promise of more and better drugs has not often translated into better health. As disease patterns have shifted from the acute to the chronic, from infectious to degenerative, progress in dealing with chronic illness has been more limited.

Cracks are appearing in medicine's conceptual foundation as basic assumptions come into question. Success in dealing with chronic disease and complex non-infectious problems like cancer has never come easily, and some researchers have pointed to the need for completely new approaches. Rather than focusing on the discovery of new magic bullets, scientists are realizing that prevention is important. Long-held ideas that have guided Western medicine for centuries are falling by the wayside. The assumption, for example, that mind and body are separate, non-interacting entities is losing support, and research has now turned to the interaction between them.

These changes in medicine are indicative of a broader, more general shift in science and society. Much of the power of science has come from its method of analysis, breaking complex things into small bite-sized pieces. The idea is to understand the parts in order to comprehend the whole. But science has never accomplished this goal: it has been focused on ever smaller parts, on the parts of parts, and parts of parts of parts. Without a vision of the whole, it has often led to knowledge without wisdom.

While research is still dominated by the study of parts, some pioneering scientists have begun to think about wholes. Let us turn to agriculture for some useful illustrations of this shift and for metaphors that can be applied to changes in health and healing. Plant nutrition, for example, is typically viewed in terms of a simple part-based model of three nutrients—potassium, nitrogen, and phosphorus. Creating healthy plants is reduced simply to figuring out the correct ratio of these three elements. (You may have noticed the N:P:K ratio prominently displayed on bags of lawn fertilizer.) Pioneering scientists are now searching for the basis of plant nutrition in a more complex system composed of living and non-living facets, the soil.

Agriculture has for decades focused on using chemicals to kill insect pests and eradicate competing plant species. Many farmers and scientists are now concerned about the ecological consequences of this approach and have turned to the understanding of whole, complex agricultural ecosystems, favoring strategies without chemical agents. While scientists and agricultural experts motivated by the technological approach have been arrogant, dismissing traditional farming systems, a new breed is beginning to explore indigenous wisdom for its many insights into the management of complex agricultural ecosystems. In this view, progress can be achieved by learning traditional ways. Better farming systems can be built by cooperation and mutual exchange between the two systems of thought.

This change in perception is also evident in biology and medicine. Eva Turley, a scientist studying cancer at Toronto's Sick Children's Hospital, feels that medical researchers should be forgiven for failing to solve the problem of cancer.[4] The limitation on success has not come from a lack of effort, but from the overly simplistic model they have used. In this model, a tumor is a thing, separate from the person, that needs to be killed.

Turley and her coworkers are concerned about the limitations of such a model and suggest an alternative way of thinking. Cancer can be viewed not as a thing, but as an abnormal process, a failure of natural regulatory systems that is reversible and intimately linked to the person. Like the agricultural scientists who have turned their gaze to the complexity of living and non-living components that comprise an agricultural ecosystem, these cancer scientists are looking at a larger, more complex system composed of normal and abnormal cells and their environment. This complex system is at the edge of chaos, exquisitely sensitive to small changes so that even the smallest perturbation can lead to either the death or cure of the patient. New cancer therapies must focus on restoring natural regulatory processes, not on killing the cancerous cells.

Like the agricultural scientists who have begun to appreciate traditional farming knowledge, some medical researchers are now beginning to appreciate traditional systems of medicine. Psychiatrist Jacques Bradwejn, for example, is studying traditional Chinese herbal treatments for acute and chronic mental illnesses. Impressed by the wealth of Chinese knowledge on the subject, Bradwejn, Head of the psychobiology and clinical trials unit of the Clarke Institute of Psychiatry in Toronto, sees promise in a "collaboration between these traditional practitioners and their wealth of information and the conventional practitioners in psychiatry."[5]

Ancient Medicine for a Modern World

This shift in the conceptual framework of science is a mirror of social evolution. There is now a trend toward things "holistic." In medicine this is evidenced as enthusiasm for practical exploration of what have come to be called complementary or alternative approaches to health and healing. Therapeutic touch—a technique of passing, without physical contact, the therapist's hands over the patient's body—has spread like wildfire among the nursing community and has even made its way, albeit gingerly, into hospitals. Homeopathy, a centuries-old European approach to healing, is now undergoing a revival. And many people are exploring indigenous and traditional systems of healing.

Chinese medicine is one of the most sophisticated, elaborate, and enduring traditional systems of healing. Traditional Chinese Medicine (TCM), despite being thousands of years old, has survived China's modernization and continues to play a significant role in the health care system in modern China.[6] TCM followed Chinese emigration to North America, always finding a home in centers of ethnic concentration. Today, Chinese herb shops—timeless apothecaries hawking an exotic array of roots, berries and twigs, pills, and potions—remain prominent features of North American Chinatowns.

Over the past several decades, ginseng and acupuncture have become as much part of Western culture as yin and yang. A number of Westerners have traveled to China to study TCM in its entirety, returning to plant the seeds of a Western version of this traditional medicine. Texts have been translated, schools established, and many thousands of patients treated. The seeds have sprouted: TCM has taken root in a new home.

One of the most curious treatments used in TCM is acupuncture. Thread-like needles are inserted in a patient at particular sites along meridians or channels of qi (pronounced *chee*), an "influence" or information signal responsible for the integrative coordination of mind and body. These acupoints are also treated sometimes with heat or pressure. The points themselves are chosen according to a sophisticated combination of theory and utility.

TCM also includes an extensive selection of medicines made of plant, mineral, and animal substances. These "herbs" are prescribed systematically in groups of up to a dozen or more, using well-defined rules and combinations based on centuries and even millennia of empirical experience. While herbal medicine and acupuncture form the mainstay of therapy, other techniques—including special exercises like t'ai chi chuan and qi qong, dietary and lifestyle adjustments, and massage—are also used, depending on the practitioner and circumstance.

TCM is more than a collection of healing techniques. It is a way of seeing, a way of organizing psyche and soma, organism and environment. Oriental medicine does not simply offer novel techniques of healing the sick: its efficacy arises as much from its unique conceptual framework as from its empirical, therapeutic tools. The "clinical gaze," as scholar and doctor of Oriental medicine Ted J. Kaptchuk puts it, of Eastern medicine is set in the dynamic interplay of yin and yang, the web of relations between mind and body, inner environment and outer milieu. Health is a dynamic balance of mind and body, a balance described in terms of qualities (like hot/cold, damp/dry, etc.) rather than quantities (like a 120/80 blood pressure measurement) and subject to clinical intervention.[7]

Complementarity in Medicine

While Eastern medicine is enthusiastically embraced by some people, it remains, from the point of view of scientific medicine, largely unproven. The possibility of empirical serendipity is acknowledged, but the system as a whole is too medieval and even too mystical to be easily compatible with modern science. Acupuncture does seem to stimulate natural biochemicals, making it potentially valuable in the treatment of pain. And some Asian herbs contain valuable pharmaceuticals that can be extracted and incorporated into Western medicine's repertoire of biologically active chemicals.

However, by and large, science and especially medicine believes it has carved out a rational, progressive methodology that supersedes the superstition and ignorance of our ancestors. From these lofty heights, TCM is a vestige, a curious relic most fruitfully studied by historians and anthropologists. Not surprisingly, the study cited previously, looking at the use of "unconventional" medicine in the United States, found that almost three out of every four people who used "unconventional" medicine did not disclose this fact to their "conventional" physician.

Yet despite the predictable difficulties of interaction between the conventional and unconventional, there is movement toward a more pluralistic approach to health and healing. In Europe, for example, of 88,000 practicing acupuncturists, over 60,000 are medical doctors. In Edmonds, Washington, family physician Jennifer Jacobs' pragmatic approach is indicative of changing attitudes: "I do what works best for my patients. There are certainly situations where modern medicine is appropriate and lifesaving, but perhaps the pendulum has swung too far toward technology and standard pharmaceuticals and not enough toward some of the early healing methods that have a track record in many cultures."[8]

Chicago's Grant Hospital has set up a Section of Holistic and Preventative Medicine. This is not a physical division of the hospital, but an effort to integrate alternative medicine into health care, something that was facilitated by an alliance with the Chicago Holistic Center, a novel mix of conventional medical doctors and practitioners of alternative healing arts such as Chinese herbal medicine and homeopathy.[9] Such developments have been spurred by the need to cut the costs of high-tech health care (in many cases alternatives can be cheaper), and simply by public demand for more healthcare choices.

There is also an emerging understanding that alternative approaches to medicine are not really alternative: they are complementary. At the practical level this may mean that more natural, less invasive and safer approaches might be preferable for chronic health concerns, while high tech intervention is the choice in emergency situations. TCM may help with the treatment of chronic eczema, while Western medicine may be essential in treating acute infection. Hospital patients struggling with pain may benefit from a nurse's therapeutic touch. Cancer patients may use Chinese herbs to strengthen their bodies during a course of radiation or chemotherapy. Or heart disease sufferers may find their long-term health optimized by following a program of diet and lifestyle modification while under the care of a heart specialist and making use of the most advanced heart medications.

Complementarity also makes sense at the conceptual level. Reality is like an infinite-sided die. Humans build up models and ways of seeing the die, but each perspective is limited, only able to see the die from a particular angle. You might see the 2, 3, and 6 sides, but miss the 1, 4, and 5. It is natural that there exist different, complementary views. This is why Lao Tzu, the great sage of Taoism, said that "The way that can be spoken of is not the constant way."[10] The Way or Tao, the ultimate reality, is just too great to be encompassed by any single limited conception.

Modern physics too has pointed to the complementary nature of the physical world. It is possible to prepare an experiment carefully to look at electrons, and discover that electrons are particles. It is also possible to look at the electron in another experiment only to find that electrons are not particles, but waves. The physical world, it seems, can be two things at the same time.

TCM and Western medicine are indeed different, complementary ways of seeing. Let us imagine the human physical and mental landscape as a field of strawberries and, as a metaphor of illness, imagine a fungus infestation in the middle of the field. The Western approach would be to study the fungus carefully. It would be classified, measured, investigated in the lab and under the microscope. Specific chemical agents would be developed to effectively eradicate the fungus. While there may be side effects when the anti-fungal agent is applied to the field—it may be toxic to local fauna, for example, and disrupt natural ecological processes—this approach may be the only way to save the strawberries.

The Oriental approach does not focus so much on the fungus itself as on the web of relations characterizing its existence. How wet or dry, hot or cold has the weather been that season, and how does that relate to the infestation? Does the field where the strawberries are affected by fungus get enough sun? Is the field too wet because of a lack of drainage? Perhaps the soil is deficient, with too little organic matter or poor mineral content. All these factors may weaken the plants, making them susceptible to fungus. Corrective measures would follow naturally: deficient soil would require amendments, excessive dampness could be drained by adding sand, problems of cold weather could be dealt with early in the season by using heat-trapping plastic coverings over the rows of strawberries. While a season's crop may be lost, this approach helps to build a healthy crop in following years.

In the case of medicine, consider a child's ear infection. Western-style treatment would likely rely on antibiotics, chemical agents designed to kill the pathogen in question—in this case, not a fungus but a bacteria. TCM, in contrast, would look carefully at the environment that gave rise to the bacterial infection. Perhaps the child's natural resistance was weak and her/his constitution needed to be fortified. Or the child's environment may be too hot and damp, offering a favorable environment for bacterial growth. Herbs or acupuncture would be applied on a case by case basis, for the problem, though there are common general patterns, is unique for each individual.

While the antibiotic may save a life and offer a speedy cure for acute cases, it might prove less beneficial for chronic, recurring infections. By addressing the fundamental conditions of the disorder over the long term, the Oriental model may bring improvements. In this way different healing models offer complementary perspectives and therapeutic possibilities.

Public interest, the need for cost control, and the changing perspectives of health care practitioners are all factors favoring a pluralistic approach to medicine. The notion of complementarity is important and will be a driving force in health care in the short term. The best system of health care is clearly not one of competition between alternatives, but one of integration and the careful, studied application of complementary approaches.

While the complementary relationship between Eastern and Western approaches to health is important for the short term, there is a more interesting possibility for the long term. Western culture is shifting and its science, biology, and medicine are changing. Models and ideas centuries old are evolving in recognition of their limitations and in the face of new problems. As it changes, Western science is developing perspectives that have intriguing parallels with the East. As the West shifts from a fascination with parts to study the interactions of those parts, from narrow notions of cause and effect to the non-linear dynamics of complex systems, this new territory comes closer to that of the East, which centered on patterns, processes, and relationships. Instead of considering the complementary characteristics of East and West, it is now possible to explore emerging parallels between East and West.

Physicist Fritjof Capra was the first to explore East-West parallels in the understanding of physical reality. In his book *The Tao of Physics,* Capra described how in the sixteenth and seventeenth centuries geniuses like Isaac Newton combined atomistic theory borrowed from the Greeks with new mathematical skill to set out a mechanical description of the physical universe. In this model the universe was composed of tiny bits of matter called atoms. The goal was to discover the basic principles behind the movement of these atoms and to link past, present, and future with the predictions of absolute mathematical certainty. The human mind was viewed as an isolated shoal of consciousness in the midst of an infinite mechanical sea.

As physicists probed further, driven by the idea the atoms themselves could be broken into parts, this neat, predictable mechanical world began to dissolve. Electrons were not hard little balls that, when put together with other balls called protons, constituted an atom. Electrons appeared to be waves at times, particles at others, depending on how you chose to look at them. This subatomic world of probability waves was not a world of absolute certainty, but an unpredictable dance of potential and being, pattern and process. The consciousness of the observer could not be so easily separated from what is observed, parts could not be easily defined except in relation to the whole, and mysterious connections appeared between isolated parts of the universe.

Fritjof Capra showed that the world view of the new physics was uncannily parallel to the Eastern conception of the universe. Although the Eastern view emerged from a less analytical and more mystical tradition, it also had a strong empirical foundation. Taoists—followers of a system of thought in China that played a major role in the development of the Eastern world view—escaped the fickleness of civilization for the mountains, observing and reflecting on the natural order of things. Capra points out that while the Taoists had little faith in analytical reasoning, their careful observations of nature, combined with mystical intuition, brought them to "profound insights which are confirmed by modern scientific theories."[11]

Western science was built on the idea that the universe is built of stuff, which for physics meant atoms. With the emergence of modern physics in the late nineteenth and early twentieth centuries, this model of the universe underwent a conceptual shift. As scientists probed further, the stuff of the universe appeared to be more process than substance, and atoms appeared as a dynamic pattern in a universal flux. Such a conception has common ground with the Buddhist notion of the fundamental impermanence of all things and the Chinese view of matter as a dynamic part of a nexus of evolving patterns.

The Evolution of Biology and Medicine

Biology and medicine in the West were also founded on atomistic ideas, and taking things apart to discover their inner workings became the established approach. The human body and innumerable flora and fauna were dissected to obtain detailed anatomical knowledge. With the invention of the microscope, things progressed further. Organs, tissues, and other parts of living systems were found to be composed of cells, the basic units of life. The microscope allowed one of the greatest triumphs, the discovery of bacteria and viruses—single-celled organisms—as a cause of many diseases, particularly the great epidemics of civilization like smallpox and cholera.

These amazing discoveries did not stop here. Cells were found to be composed of molecules and, outfitted with a startling array of new technology, scientists analyzed these biological molecules, studying their structures and functions. Many diseases could be traced to the fact that certain molecules were not behaving as they should. The pinnacle of success came when the code of life hidden in that most fundamental of molecules, the DNA, was cracked.

There is still a powerful momentum driving research and medical practice in the direction of the atomistic idea of taking things apart into their components and searching for answers at the smallest level. This can be seen in the current focus on the gene as a means of therapy. Writing on the future of medicine in *Scientific American*, W. French Anderson, a medical doctor and professor of pediatrics at the University of Southern California School of Medicine, points to three great leaps in medicine: public health measures like sanitation helped mitigate epidemic illnesses; surgery and anesthesia made lifesaving procedures like appendectomy possible; and the development of vaccines and antibiotics aided in the treatment of infectious disease. "Gene therapy will constitute a fourth revolution because delivery of selected genes into a patient's cells can potentially cure or ease the vast majority of disorders," says French, "including many that have so far resisted treatment."[12]

While there is no doubt that useful knowledge will result from further study of genes, it is a leap of faith to consider gene therapy as a panacea. The enthusiasm for making adjustments at this smallest level of life is also now joined by an enthusiasm for a more holistic conception of health and disease. This new model considers the broader context of sickness and disease—the dynamic interplay between the individual and his/her social and natural environment. It seems that, just as in the case of physics, finer and finer tuning of the microscope eventually brings the whole into focus.

The molecular theory of disease—the idea that sickness is caused by molecules not doing what they should—is useful, but at the same time limited. It is always possible to continue the search for the cause of disease and ask what is causing the molecules to misbehave. Our bodies and the molecules of which they are built are intimately linked to our minds and to the greater whole of which the body-mind is a part. The inside is deeply connected to the outside, the microcosm to the macrocosm. The most complete picture of health and the challenge of disease requires an understanding of the organic body in relation to the whole person and the broader social and physical environment.

Larry Dossey, maverick medical doctor and author, points out that the molecular theory of disease causation is so deeply ingrained in medicine that doubting has become a heresy. "It is assumed that in any given disease, if our knowledge is complete, we shall be able to pinpoint how the molecule is misbehaving. That other explanations might exist simply is not ordinarily considered."[13]

While Dossey is quick to point to the wonderful accomplishments of the molecular approach to medicine, he also characterizes it as incomplete. It fails to consider what he calls the human factor, which can play a central role in the dynamic process of health and illness. This human factor—the close connection between mental-emotional facets of our lives such as stress, kindness, and loving relationships and our health—suggests an intimate link between mind and body, a link that has been up to now ignored.

Dossey chronicles some of the fascinating evidence of a mind-body interaction. Techniques like visualization and relaxation affect physiological processes and can be potent factors in the course of a serious illness. Meditation can lower blood cholesterol in people with elevated levels. Job satisfaction and overall happiness are key indicators of survival from heart disease. Three-quarters of the people who have migraine and tension headaches can learn to reduce their symptoms using biofeedback.[14]

There is now considerable interest in the relationship between lifestyle factors, like exercise and eating patterns, and health. The powerful and profound impact of regular exercise has become the subject of medical research. Results show that even the very elderly can benefit from an appropriate exercise regimen. Nutrition has typically received such little attention that physicians often graduate from medical school with minimal or no knowledge of the subject. Yet, as Andrew Nicholson, Director of Preventative Medicine for the Washington-based Physicians' Committee for Responsible Medicine (PCRM), points out: "Today we have accumulated unmistakable evidence demonstrating the links between diet and heart disease, breast, prostate, and colon cancer, diabetes, obesity, osteoporosis, high blood pressure, and the list goes on."[15]

PCRM President Neal Barnard echoes this enthusiasm for the power of food to heal or destroy. Barnard argues it is possible to prevent and treat heart disease with food and, by combining dietary changes with an avoidance of tobacco, "You could prevent probably 70 or 80 percent of cancers, just by those steps alone."[16] The fundamental problem, according to this new breed of physician, is to prevent disease from occurring in the first place.

Statistical studies of cultures that live and eat differently from the West indicate that they get sick in different ways. Dean Ornish, an American medical pioneer, has demonstrated the ability of lifestyle change not simply to prevent but to reverse heart disease, a problem epidemic in industrial society. At his Sausalito, California research institute, Ornish puts patients through a program that, typically at only 1/10 the cost of bypass operation, gets results. The Ornish program combines radical dietary change with exercise, stress reduction, and group support. Many health insurers cover the cost of the program, since as Ornish himself says: "When you compare the cost of an angioplasty to the cost of this program, the insurers are saving $5.55 for every dollar they spend. Moreover, 90 percent of the people recommended for bypass have been able to avoid it."[17]

This emerging approach to medicine centers on the potential of prevention and gravitates towards therapies that are safer and more empowering to the patient than conventional pharmaceutical and surgical therapies which require only passive acceptance. It is based on ideas about health and healing that encompass genes and molecules, together with the broader connections between mental and physical, an individual and his/her environment.

The Meeting of Mind and Body

For thousands of years the Chinese have observed life processes, setting out a description of health and disease in the context of the interaction between humans and their environment. At an early stage these observations coalesced into a system of medicine, a set of tools for restoring and maintaining health with a theoretical structure to guide their application. While Chinese medicine has little common ground with a system of medicine focused almost exclusively on the biochemical and anatomical features of disease, there are parallels with this new medicine that includes mind-body interaction, the study of nutrition and lifestyle, and the primary notion of prevention.

The Chinese never separated the mind from the body, but studied them as mutually interacting facets of a greater whole. Physical therapies affect mental patterns, just as psychological events affect the soma. The herb Radix Polygalae Tenuifoliae, known as *yuan zhi* or "profound will" in Chinese, can calm the mind and help temper pent-up emotions, while the acupuncture point heart 7, the seventh point of the heart channel, known as *shen men* or "spirit gate" in Chinese, can help resolve anxiety and mental disturbance. A repeated pattern of anger can aggravate a liver problem, while weak kidneys can make a person fearful.

The Chinese developed special exercises to harmonize the mind and body and build intrinsic health. Exercises like t'ai chi chuan serve to integrate mind with breathing and movement, affecting one's qi (the "energy" that flows through the acupuncture channels and animates physiological function) and fostering a deep sense of relaxation. These ancient exercises are increasingly popular today, in part because they help buffer the stresses and strains of life in modern civilization.

The longstanding separation of mind and body has been a major obstacle for the Western comprehension of Eastern ideas. The new-found Western realization that mind and body are intimately linked is nothing new in the East. With growing interest in mind-body problems, common ground has emerged, producing parallel insights with implications for the future of health care.

Exercise and Diet As Foundations of Health

In Chinese medicine, lifestyle factors such as diet and the level of physical activity are very important in the prevention of disease. Either too much or too little physical activity can cause injury. Too little makes the body sluggish, the qi and blood stagnant. Too much can tax the system beyond recovery, causing a deficiency of qi. Hua Tuo, China's most famous surgeon who lived in the second century A.D., was an early advocate of regular exercise. According to Hua Tuo, "The body needs exercise, only it must not be to the point of exhaustion, for exercise expels the bad air in the system, promotes free circulation of the blood, and prevents sickness."[18] He likened the body to a door hinge, which in ancient times was made of leather. A used door hinge, like the body, would not rot. With regular use it stayed supple and healthy.

The Chinese studied the relationship between food and health, stressing the importance of healthy eating and elaborating both preventative and curative diets. Sun Si-miao, a renowned physician of the Tang Dynasty, claimed that "a truly good physician first finds out the root cause of the illness. Having found that out, he first tries to cure it by food. Only when food has failed does he prescribe medications."

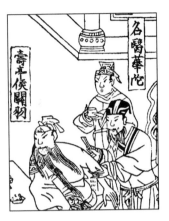

Hua Tuo performing surgery

Sun treated goiter with seaweed and pork thyroid gland, beriberi with a prescription that included rice bran.[19]

While modern Western nutrition centers on understanding the various molecular components of food, such as vitamins and minerals, proteins and carbohydrates, Chinese nutrition looks at the "energetic" and organic actions of food. Western nutrition bases its dietary recommendations on the study of large populations, while Chinese nutrition emphasizes the needs of each individual. Nevertheless, the basic healthy diet that has emerged from Western scientific research in the past decade is strikingly parallel to the pattern of healthy eating recommended by ancient Chinese physicians. Food as medicine is an old idea—temporarily forgotten, but ready to play a prominent role in the future of health and healing.

Prevention: The Root of Medicine

Prevention has come to be a hallmark of the emerging medicine. As the PCRM's Andrew Nicholson notes, there is a shift underway toward focusing on the prevention of disease. Others echo this sentiment. "Until recently, there was little funding for studies of cancer prevention; curing cancer was seen as a quicker fix," claims Grant Steen of the Memphis-based St. Jude Children's Research Hospital.

"Now that we know how effectively an established cancer can resist treatment, prevention is widely perceived as preferable."[20]

The Yellow Emperor who lived some two millennia ago had thoughts on prevention that are parallel to this modern insight: "The sages did not treat those who were already ill; they instructed those who were not yet ill....To administer medicines to diseases which have already developed and to suppress revolts which have already developed are comparable to the behavior of those persons who begin to dig a well after they have become thirsty, and those who begin to cast weapons after they have already engaged in battle. Would these actions not be too late?"[21]

Paradigm Parallels

The parallels between East and West are evident at the paradigm level. The broader conceptual framework of Eastern culture and medicine has always been opposite to that of the West. But with new "systems" approaches in Western science, concepts are emerging that resonate strongly with those of the East.[22]

Western medical and biological science is primarily analytical, responding to the question of how things work by dissecting wholes into parts. This conventional approach, which goes back to René Descartes and the emergence of modern science, is centered on the hope that wholes can be understood by examining their parts in isolation. Yet, from ancient times there has existed a split between the study of substance and the study of form. Science has largely responded to the question of how things work by attempting to discover what things are made of—an emphasis on substance.

At the same time, other "frontier" scientists have emphasized form, pioneering a response to the question of how things work by looking at relationships between the parts, patterns, and processes that mold the whole. This organismic or systems biology, as it has been called, deals with systems and their complex nature. It asserts that wholes are more than simply the sum of their parts, and that it is important to study the complex patterns and principles of organization emergent in living systems.

The Chinese approach to understanding nature, and hence their underlying approach to health and healing, is also a relational one. Like Western science, the Chinese organized their observations of the world around them from a rational and logical base, but, unlike Western science, they favored relational rather than analytical understanding. The Chinese developed what can be considered a form of systems theory, understanding parts in relation to their wholes and looking for organizational principles governing macrocosm and microcosm. The theory and diagnostic approach of Chinese medicine shares many of the fundamental characteristics of the new Western systems approach that represents the cutting edge of science.

Yin and yang, for example, are universal features of natural processes in the philosophy of the East. Yin represents the inward, cold, condensing, and substantial tendency, yang the outward, hot, expansive, and motive aspect. Yin and yang are not elements to be isolated, but inseparable qualities in dynamic equilibrium: "Yin alone cannot arise; yang alone cannot grow. Yin and yang are divisible but inseparable."[23]

In medicine, the kidneys are yin, the bladder yang, blood is yin, qi yang, not as absolute categories, but in context and relation. TCM diagnosis is a differentiation of patterns set in a relational framework. An eye problem, for example, may be seen in the relation between the eyes and the liver and its corresponding meridian network. For example, the herb Fructus Lycii Chinensis—the fruit of the matrimony vine called *gou qi zi* in Chinese—is known for its ability to nourish the blood of the liver and has the special property of treating blurred and poor vision.

The Mystery of "Energy" in Medicine

One of the most intriguing facets of TCM is the technique of acupuncture and the elaborate network of channels and acupoints discovered by the Chinese. Even more mysterious is the qi, the organizing influence coordinating organic function, thought to flow through these channels. Needles, inserted at points selected according to a diagnostic system of pattern recognition, heal by restoring the natural flow of qi.

Heat and pressure can also provide a healing stimulus. Moxibustion is a technique of burning the leaf of the mugwort plant to heat particular acupuncture points. Chinese massage therapy also relies on the theory and physical manipulation of channels and points.

Western science and medicine has until recently ignored acupuncture. The reason for this is clear. There were not even vague correspondences between Chinese concepts such as qi, channels, and points and anything Western. It has been hard from a Western point of view to see acupuncture as anything more than a collection of fanciful theories.

Yet, parallels are emerging between acupuncture and new research into the incredible organization and communication seen in living systems. Scientists have progressed from anatomical to cellular to molecular studies of the living state, but the nature of the exquisite organization of biological structures and functions has remained elusive. While many scientists focus on the chemistry of life, others have begun to ask questions about the organization of these hundreds of chemicals into a patterned whole. While enzymes (protein molecules that stimulate chemical reactions) coordinate with their substrate (the molecules upon which the enzyme acts) like a lock and key, just how does the key find the lock? Or how do thousands of complex processes shape an embryo into a fully developed organism?

Using some of the most modern physical knowledge, such as quantum theory and non-equilibrium thermodynamics, pioneering scientists are beginning to explore how weak electromagnetic signals can influence living systems. A new field of study, called bioelectromagnetics, has emerged. Some pioneers are investigating the ability of weak physical signals to coordinate and regulate physiological activity. The late Herbert Fröhlich, for example, studied the coherence (coordination) of biomolecular systems, and postulated that particular vibrational modes may be responsible for communication and coordination in organ systems.

It is here, in this fascinating biophysical research being carried out around the globe, that we find the beginning of parallels to the ancient Chinese concept of the meridians, points, and qi, a system of regulation and control that can be adjusted to harmonize physiological function. Reminiscent of Fröhlich's vibrational control of organs, for example, is the ancient Taoist exercise of the healing sounds, where particular sounds resonate with major organ-meridian networks to harmonize emotions and preserve health. In acupuncture we already have the elaboration of a non-chemical regulatory system that can be harnessed for healing, and in time as parallels grow the gap between West and East will narrow.[24]

The Future of Health and Healing

Taken together, these fascinating developments point to fundamental shifts in health and healing. As interest in complementary approaches to medicine grows amongst patients and practitioners alike, a more pluralistic health care landscape is emerging. Western medicine is undergoing a shift in its conceptual framework, changing from a focus on sickness to a focus on prevention and wellness. Many of the new developments—interest in mind-body interaction, the development of preventive and curative therapies centered on the relationship between lifestyle and health, and the study of complex systems—show strong parallels to TCM. What all this will mean for the future can only be guessed, but the possibilities are exciting.

It is possible for individuals to feel confident in wellness strategies that involve diet and lifestyle. There are many opportunities for physical and mental fitness programs, both Western techniques of physical training and Chinese disciplines like t'ai chi chuan and qi gong. It is clear that typical North American eating patterns are unhealthy, but the search for a healthy diet is no longer so elusive.

At the social level, a health care system centered on prevention of illness and offering a dynamic and diverse platter of therapies will not only be cheaper but more empowering and safer. High tech surgery will have its place, so too will medical qi gong and acupuncture. Modern drugs will complement ancient herbal therapies understood in the context of contemporary health care needs. As barriers between seemingly contradictory systems of healing are bridged, teams of practitioners can develop integrative approaches to healing with optimal efficacy.

1 | Tuning to the Rhythm of Space and Time: The Theoretical Foundations of Oriental Medicine

By studying the organic patterns of heaven and earth a fool can become a sage. So by watching the times and seasons of natural phenomena we can become true philosophers.

—Li Quan, Yin Fu Jing (735 A.D.)[1]

The Story of Master Shan

Shan had lived on the mountain for as long as anyone could remember. In fact, Shan had *lived* as long as anyone could remember. Despite his appearance, a testament to his advanced age, the old man stood as straight as an arrow. His eyes radiated a youthful brightness that contrasted with his long, gray beard, and his gait was as confident as that of the mountain goats with whom he shared the alpine trails.

Those who traveled from afar to get herbs from the old man simply called him Master. Shan was a skilled herbalist, making regular treks to collect an odd assortment of roots, berries, twigs, and bark from the hills and valleys of his district. On his trips, Master Shan consorted with his many friends, an odd assortment of men and women who varied in character like the herbs in Shan's satchel. After laughing, joking, and catching up on news, discussion among these friends turned to serious subjects: new knowledge about herbs, martial arts, and metaphysics—and of course the weather. While the arts they practiced were based on a long and honorable tradition, there was always much to learn. And there was the thrill of discovery about a new herb, new health exercises, or ideas about the cosmos.

Master Shan kept a stock of some 200 different herbs in his mountain abode, a rather large wood-framed building tucked neatly into a spectacular grove of pines. He would have preferred a smaller home, but there were always several guests, patients eager to see if one of his legendary herbal prescriptions could improve a long-standing ailment and students eager to learn about herbal medicine, qi gong, and martial arts. Despite the inconvenience, Shan enjoyed the challenge and the small income his herbal practice brought and felt it his duty to pass on his acquired knowledge. He had learned in turn from accomplished Masters who had themselves dutifully passed on their knowledge, maintaining a lineage that reached back into the mists of time.

Through his decades of study Master Shan developed an intimacy with the healing plants he used. He knew their properties, when to pick them, and how to combine them. Always keen to unearth new healing techniques, Shan observed the plants eaten by animals when they were sick, carefully testing promising finds on his own person, and exchanging information with other herbalists and village healers.

His skills in diagnostics were honed by years of experience. He would look carefully at his patients, noting the color of their skin, the quality of their voice, and their posture. He might take note of strange odors, stiff shoulders, or a nervous twitch. He would listen attentively to their stories, occasionally interrupting for clarification or detail. He then observed their tongues in a deliberate, almost ritual, way. And an examination was not complete without feeling the pulses at each wrist, a procedure that gave him insight into each patient's struggle between health and disease.

From this information Shan recognized patterns of disturbance, minor or major disruptions in the dynamic equilibrium of mind and body. Sometimes he relied on time-tested formulas—combinations of six or even ten herbs to be boiled and consumed by the patient—

modified to suit a particular case. Other cases required novel formulas, crafted to strengthen natural resistance or drive out pathological factors. The herbs in Shan's formulas reflected a pattern that fit the patient like an axle to a wheel, forming a functional completeness that activated natural healing processes.

Master Shan's own good health and long life was a testament to his skill in the healing arts. He regularly imbibed decoctions of special herbs renowned for their ability to build intrinsic health, and diligently followed a daily regimen of exercises designed to harmonize and strengthen the mind and body. Each morning by the bank of the mountain stream near his home, Shan practiced qi gong, a ritualized breathing exercise and meditation combined with special movements. Entering a state of deep relaxation and tranquility, he placed his consciousness in an area below his navel, creating a warmth that quickly grew and spread throughout his body. This energy tingled and danced along distinct pathways like the foamy stream gushing along the mountainside. Concentration on special points caused the energy to travel to distant regions of the body, healing injuries and improving the health of the organs and tissues through which the energy coursed.

The Clinical Gaze

The origins of Chinese medicine are shrouded in the mists of time. The discoveries of many of its central components—such as the flow of qi in the human body and the channels through which it circulates—date to prehistory and are the subject of legend and speculation. While it is not possible to speak with confidence about the early development of Chinese medicine, it is clear that figures like the fictitious Master Shan played a role.

Scholars—an important part of the highly centralized bureaucracy that ruled China for millennia—craftspeople, and technicians of every sort helped forge China's high culture and technical achievement.[2] Throughout Chinese history there were also men and women, like Master Shan, who wandered the country or lived in secluded mountain ranges, seeking the challenge of metaphysical discourse and studying natural phenomena with an enthusiasm rivaling that of the modern scientist.

While modern scientists and natural philosophers of the East share an enthusiasm for knowledge about the natural world, they do not see the world in the same way. The way people relate and interact with the world around them is shaped by their underlying worldview. Different ways of understanding health and healing arise from different conceptions of reality.

Much of what we "see" around us is shaped by our underlying notions of reality. In an interesting experiment, subjects were presented with playing cards for a brief moment and asked to identify them. Every now and then an odd card, like a black queen of hearts, would be secretly introduced into the sequence. The subjects could rarely "see" such cards; instead, they might identify the card as a queen of spades or clubs, fitting the anomalous card into already formed preconceptions of playing cards.

One Western medical doctor, an authority on skin cancers, talked about a dilemma he faced while waiting in line at the supermarket. He could not help but notice a distinct mole on the neck of a man in the line. The mole looked suspiciously dangerous: its shape and color suggested the man should see his doctor as soon as possible and have the mole examined. It was years of training and clinical experience that caused the doctor to see something suspicious in what would appear to be a harmless mole to others.

Chinese medicine's unique "clinical gaze" can create similar experiences for its practitioners. This gaze is not fixed on specific parts of the body, but on patterns that emerge from a patient's constellation of signs and symptoms. A series of conversations with a neighbor, for example, may merge a collection of facts into a pattern of imbalance, suggesting a particular herbal treatment or acupuncture prescription.

A neighbor's complaints about acute migraine headaches, his thin appearance, agitated state, and often angry mood together with his often swollen, red eyes and his crimson tongue with a dry, yellow coating, suggest a disharmony with the liver. Too much hot and active qi coursing through the liver and meridian could cause migraine headache, problems with the eyes—a sense organ with a recognized connection to the liver—and a proclivity for anger. Of course, a careful and detailed diagnosis of the case would have to be made to confirm these suspicions.

A Contrast of East and West

The complementary clinical gazes of East and West emerge from complementary world views. In the West, the greatest effort has been applied to understanding substance by breaking things down in the search to discover what they are made of. This atomistic orientation traces back to Greek philosophers such as Democritus, who argued that the world was made of atoms, small fundamental units of matter that were quite separate from spirit. This emphasis on substance, and separation of spirit and matter, reappeared with the scientific revolution. Physical scientists such as Isaac Newton mathematically described the motion of matter and, in time, physicists discovered small, seemingly indivisible particles which they aptly called atoms.

In biology, inquiry into the substance of living things began with dissection and anatomy. It then turned to smaller units of life—cells—when the discovery of the microscope opened up a world hitherto hidden by the limitations of human senses. But the cell did not turn out to be the "atom" of life, for cells were made of molecules—collections of the atoms discovered by the physicists—and soon scientists turned to the study of biologically constructed molecules. The greatest triumph came with the study of the gene, the premiere molecule of life containing the blueprint for the protein molecules that lie at the heart of the structures and functions of organisms.

And so Western medicine emerged in its present form. Mental and physical disorders are dealt with by their respective experts as compartmentalized problems. Diseases are considered in terms of their molecular manifestations, and drugs—chemical substances chosen for their effects on biomolecular processes—are a mainstay of therapy. Surgery, the other foundation of therapy, is built on several centuries of anatomical exploration. Today, these therapies have evolved to an impressive level and are joined by a new frontier: the study of the genetic basis of disease. Scientists are now looking at how the blueprint of life can go awry and result in the cascade of molecular events that lie at the root of disease.

In contrast to the West's fascination with substance, the East has been enamored with form. Instead of asking what things are made of, the Chinese were intrigued by the fact that, while everything in the universe is in a constant state of flux, a wide variety of forms maintain a constant, though evolving presence. While Western natural scientists focused on specific chains of cause and effect, the Eastern naturalists noted resonances between events at drastically different scales—macrocosm and microcosm. Europeans studied things and their parts by analysis; Chinese looked at relationships, processes, and patterns from a synthetic perspective.

While change is a fundamental feature of reality for the Chinese, regularity in the flux brings order out of chaos. The Earth turns on its axis, for example, bringing forth a regular cycle of day and night, and every year completes an orbit around the Sun, bringing a regular series of seasonal changes. These macrocosmic cycles have a profound effect on the microcosm. Plants and animals display daily rhythms—flowers open and close, plants absorb oxygen and release carbon dioxide, animals alternate rest and activity—superimposed on annual rhythms of seasonal adaptation.

Even the non-living features of the Earth are subject to the ineluctable patterns of change. Water cycles and weather patterns, intimately linked to living systems, fluctuate seasonally and are dependent on geographical factors that relate in turn to cosmic configuration. The daily heating and cooling of rocks, the wind, the rain, and even living organisms play a role in the weathering of mountains, part of the cycle of geological creation and destruction.

The ancient Chinese proto-scientists would have concurred with the emerging view of the Earth as a superorganism, but added that it is also an organism that pulses to the beat of the larger cosmos. The rhythms and animating force of Gaia are intricately interwoven with the fabric of the universe: the planet along with its organisms are participants in a dance of cosmic scale. This cosmic dance they called the Tao, the Way of the Universe, the Ultimate Reality behind all phenomena from which patterns and regularity arise amidst inexorable change and transformation.

While Western science seeks to discover the "laws" of nature—an idea that had its origins in the belief in an external lawgiver—the Chinese held to the view, described so eloquently by Joseph Needham, that "the harmonious cooperation of all beings arose, not from the orders of a superior authority external to themselves, but from the fact that they were all parts in a hierarchy of wholes forming a cosmic and organic pattern, and what they obeyed were the internal dictates of their own natures."[3] This holistic, organic view of nature implied that every system was part of a larger whole and that there was a way of nature, the Tao, ineluctably acting, not as a causal agent, but so that each actor played a proper role in a spontaneous cosmic dance.

Joseph Needham: Scientist, Philosopher, Historian, and Sinophile (1900–1995)

Joseph Needham was born in 1900, the only son of a doctor. He studied science at Cambridge University, eventually focusing on biochemistry, not in its narrow sense, but in its relation to broader biological problems of embryology and morphology. For this work he was elected a Fellow of the Royal Society.

Needham was not content to confine his interest to one or several scientific problems, nor even to science as a whole. Even his early writings and talks roamed from philosophy and history to culture and politics. Perhaps because of his divergent and ever-inquiring mind Needham soon took on a mammoth task: understanding the science and civilization of China and the relationship between Eastern and Western cultures.

Through close contact with visiting Chinese scientists Needham became intrigued by Chinese science and civilization. At the same time, he had become disillusioned with mechanically based scientific thinking and was an enthusiastic exponent of the organismic philosophy developed to its highest degree by Alfred North Whitehead. Needham recognized the profound resonance between the philosophy of organism in both the East and West and became aware of the many achievements of Chinese science and technology. Gunpowder, printing, and the magnetic compass, for example, all hallmarks of human civilization, were Chinese discoveries.

His knowledge of China led to an appointment in that country during the Second World War, and his travels, discussions, and experiences left him a with a burning question: why, despite the advanced level of Chinese science and civilization, did the scientific and industrial revolutions occur in the West and not the East? Eventually returning to Cambridge, Needham began to write a single volume, *Science and Civilization in China*, to address the question. The single book proved inadequate for the task, and it was expanded into a series that is still in progress.

When he died in 1995, at the age of ninety-four, Needham was still at work at the Needham Research Institute at Cambridge. This scholarly center, named in his honor, is home of the Science and Civilization project and the East Asian History of Science Library there is used by researchers around the world. What started as a single question has turned into an encyclopedic project on the history of science, technology, and medicine in China continued today by scholars climbing that great mountain Needham discovered and began to scale.

Yin and Yang

The cosmic dance of Tao is expressed in the complementary qualities of yin and yang. Yang represents the active tendency, yin the substantive phase. While yang is hot, outward, expansive, yin is cold, inward, contracting, thus balancing yang. Yin and yang are not parts of things that can be considered in isolation, but complements that depend on each other for existence. They are innate tendencies in dynamic equilibrium.

Yin yang

The cycle of night and day, darkness and light, for example, can be described by the interdependent dynamic equilibrium of yin and yang. While the period of darkness is yin relative to daylight which is yang, there is not an abrupt transition between two absolute qualities, but a continuous wavelike evolution. As the sun sets and a period of quiescence begins, yin is still gaining and yang in decline. Yin does not reach its peak until the middle of the night, when yang is at its lowest point. Yet there is still yang within yin, for from midnight to sunrise yang gains strength against a waning yin. As the sun rises, yang continues to grow, reaching a peak at midday when the sun is highest in the sky. Finally, the cycle returns to its beginning as yang loses its strength and the yin within yang regains vitality.

Through yin and yang the Tao manifests itself in all things, from the daily rotation of planet Earth to the rise and fall of civilizations, from the gentle opening and closing of a lily to the economic cycle of boom and bust in industrial cultures. As an economy expands, for example, consumption increases, new factories are built, and employment rises. But this yang phase cannot last forever—yin within yang is always present, ready to contract what has expanded. Eventually the economy becomes overheated, inflation and interest rates rise, and recession looms.

Yin and yang analysis offers insight into the dynamic evolution of things. Yet the general nature of the qualities of yin and yang and their interaction, while allowing a high degree of flexibility in application, opens the way for a refinement and a description of more specific archetypal patterns of change. By representing yin with a broken line and yang with a solid line, the two lines are combined in groups of three to produce eight "trigrams." The trigrams, representing subtle sets of yin-yang interaction that appear on both cosmic and human scale, are given names and further combined in pairs to form sixty-four hexagrams. Each hexagram describes a configuration in time, and the study of these hexagrams offers insight into life circumstances.

The *I Ching* or *Book of Changes*, one of the five Confucian Classics, is a presentation of and commentary on the hexagrams. While continual change and transformation is a universal characteristic and starting point for the *I Ching*, it describes patterns and regularity within change that can be grasped. Implicit in the system of sixty-four hexagrams is the idea that the simple movement from yin to yang and from yang to yin—represented in the *I Ching* by a broken line (yin) becoming solid (yang) or solid line becoming broken—underlies the more elaborate trigrams which in turn combine to produce the hexagrams. The hexagrams are thus symbols for the subtle evolution of the universe with the dual forces of yin and yang as their root.

The Five Phases

Yin and yang and the complex, symbolic representation of the patterns of change found in the *I Ching* are not the only ways of understanding change in Chinese cosmology. The system of five phases—earth, metal, water, wood, and fire—also figure prominently in Chinese thought. Jesuit missionaries traveled to China in the seventeenth century, incorrectly interpreting these symbols as the five elements. They assumed that the Chinese were implying that earth, metal, water, wood, and fire comprised the fundamental stuff of the universe. The Jesuits' mistranslation highlights the underlying difference in Eastern and Western cosmology: the Western interest in material stuff and the Chinese emphasis on process.

The five phases (a more accurate rendering of the Chinese concept *wu xing* than "five elements") are not fundamental material substances, but five processes or activities with an interwoven set of relationships. Wood represents incipient growth, a stage of expanding activity, while fire is a symbol of an activity at its peak. Wood and fire are considered yang phases. Metal and water are yin complements, metal connoting a decline in activity and water a fully realized period of quiescence. Earth sits as the neutral balancing point between extremes.

The phases show cycles of positive and negative feedback, known as the engendering and restraining cycles. In the engendering cycle (the cycle of creation), metal is able to "create" water, water in turn engenders wood, wood gives rise to fire, fire fosters earth, and, in completion of the cycle, earth engenders metal. A pattern of change through the cycle of creation is found in the seasonal correspondences of metal with autumn, water with winter, wood with spring, fire with summer, and finally earth with late or Indian summer.

In the restraining cycle in contrast, metal controls wood, wood tempers earth, earth checks water, water restrains fire, and fire in turn moderates metal. The relationships between these symbolic processes do make literal sense: wood, for example, can give rise to fire and it is not hard to imagine water restraining fire. Since each phase has both yin and yang aspects, the five-phase system with its engendering and restraining cycles sets out a sophisticated set of systemic relations focused on self-regulation and organization. Such a system offers a framework for understanding the dynamic interplay between health and disease in terms of the self-regulatory organization of the complex human organism.[4]

Natural Medicine

Chinese medicine is set in the cosmological milieu of yin and yang, and so it is imbued with a mystical disposition. Yet, while the Chinese had one eye to the heavens they also had two feet planted firmly on the ground. As Joseph Needham emphasized, the Chinese had an intensely practical side with an inclination to distrust theories and directly engage nature through observation and experimentation.[5] Chinese medicine combines Eastern mystical tradition with this penchant for observation and practicality.

In the realm of medicine, the Chinese discovered techniques for working with natural systems and considered health as a state of dynamic balance—a configuration of mind-body, behavior and attitude attuned to the Tao. Health in Chinese medicine is something that can be qualitatively assessed, something that requires constant vigilance to nurture, and something that can be restored when lost. Healing techniques such as acupuncture are not oriented so much toward the elimination of disease as on restoring the natural dynamic balance inherent in the human mind-body system. As balance reestablishes itself, healing will take place from within the organism. This notion of health contrasts with the traditional tendency in Western medicine to concentrate on the negative aspects of health by focusing on disease states and defining health as the absence of disease.

Agriculture offers a parallel to this difference between looking at health in a positive and negative sense. Conventional agriculture, like Western medicine, is disease-centered, studying the various enemies of crops—insects, fungi, weeds, etc.—and developing the (usually chemical) means to eradicate them. Organic agriculture, like Chinese medicine, is founded on a different conceptual premise, one that seeks to support the health of agricultural systems in a broader sense by working with nature. Sick plants do not mean an enemy exists to be conquered with dangerous chemicals, but that the natural balance and harmony has been lost and needs to be restored.

Modern organic vegetable farmer Chester van Huisen expressed this idea clearly in an interview one summer day in his greenhouse as rain from a sudden cloud-burst pelted down on the glass covering: "Nature is a very delicate thing. It can be very harsh as well of course, but it is very delicate and you can ruin the delicate balance very easily. My desire is to learn as much as possible about this ecosystem that we have and work with it as much as possible, at times helping it along in a good way, not in a disastrous or destructive way."[6]

This sentiment echoes that of renowned market gardener Camel-Back Kuo, who lived in eighth century China. The essayist Liu Tsung-yuan, a contemporary of Camel-Back's, wrote about his success with fruit trees: "Old Camel-Back cannot make trees live or thrive. He can only let them follow their natural tendencies. In planting trees, be careful to set the root straight, to smooth the earth around them, to use good quality planting soil and pack it down well. Then, don't touch them, don't think about them....but leave them alone to take care of themselves and nature will do the rest."[7]

In the East the goal and quest of the sage was to comprehend the Tao fully. Sages did not seek this understanding for personal gain or power over nature, but to be able to attune their actions with the Way. Central to this quest to live in accordance with the basic patterns of nature is the principle of *wu-wei* or "non-action." *Wu-wei* does not literally mean non-action as a cursory study of the characters may suggest, but rather implies a spontaneous action with the current of nature.

Wu-wei—going with the grain of things, rather than against it—is an important idea for both sage and healer. *Wei* is forcing things without accounting for their inner nature. *Wu-wei* is allowing things to follow their fate according to their inner nature. "To be able to practice *wu-wei* implied learning from nature by observations essentially scientific," claims Needham.[8]

The Chinese sages felt that good health was achieved by studying and working with nature's ways. Success in following the Tao came in the form of a long and vital life. According to the *Yellow Emperor's Classic of Internal Medicine*: "Those who follow Tao achieve the formula of perpetual youth and maintain a youthful body. Although they are old in years they are still able to produce offspring."[9]

Following the Tao means attending to balance in all things or, in Chinese terms, harmonizing yin and yang. This road to good health was described by Huang-fu Mi, a third century Taoist scholar: "It is necessary to follow the disposition of the seasons and adapt to cold and heat, to balance joy and anger and be contented with what one is, to harmonize yin and yang and adjust the unyielding and tender. Thus, no evils can arise."[10]

Imbalance between yin and yang is at the root of disease; restoration of balance is at the root of healing. Yin and yang, while metaphysical concepts, have concrete and important application to medicine. Yin and yang are not absolute categories, but a means of describing relationships in a subtle, qualitative way. The outside of the body is yang relative to the inside. The liver is yin in contrast to the gallbladder which is yang, yet the liver itself has both yin and yang aspects that are important in clinical practice. If yin has waned it can be supplemented with yin herbs, while yin symptoms such as cold limbs and low energy would call for the balancing effect of yang herbs which warm and invigorate.

The Three Treasures: Jing, Qi, and Shen

Many of the basic concepts of Chinese medicine have direct Western counterparts. After all, a liver should be a liver no matter how you look at it. Strangely, however, the idea of a liver *does* depend on how you look at it. In Western medicine the liver is understood anatomically, as a particular thing in a particular place. Instead of using anatomical description as the foundation of physiology, Chinese reality is constructed from a study of patterns, processes, and relationships within the whole. The Chinese character *gan*, or liver, describes a set of corresponding physiological functions and mental/emotion phenomena. As American teacher, scholar, and practitioner of Chinese medicine, Ted Kaptchuk, claims: "The two paradigms embrace the body differently; there is no simple correspondence."[11,12]

While the Eastern and Western framing of seemingly similar medical concepts needs to be carefully differentiated, there are a number of Eastern ideas without clear Western counterparts. One such concept is qi, a particularly mysterious idea central to Chinese medicine and used pervasively throughout Eastern culture. Qi is variously translated as "energy," sometimes as "influence," but best remains untranslated and allowed to enter the English language on its own terms as with yin and yang.

Qi represents the active organization of matter into its various forms and patterns. It is the influence that precipitates change and the quality of organization that resists it.[13] In the medical sphere qi is life itself. As a seventeenth-century text claims: "When qi gathers, so the physical body is formed; when it disperses, so the body dies."[14]

There are five major functions and over 30 specific kinds of qi distinguished in human physiology. Qi is the activity behind growth, development, and physiological processes; it acts in a defensive capacity, offering protection against pathogenic qi; it provides the foundation for metabolic warmth; it is the catalytic factor in all transformative processes; and it is responsible for keeping the blood in the vessels.

Air qi—qi absorbed from breathing—combines with qi extracted from food and essential qi stored in the kidneys to produce original qi, the basis of physiological activity. The original qi associated with the various organs is called organ qi, while channel qi flows through a network of internal and external conduits (the acupuncture channels). *Wei* qi, or defensive qi, is a form of qi that nourishes the skin, controls the opening and closing of the pores, and resists invasion by pathogens.

Jing is another basic concept without a clear correspondence in Western science. According to Ted Kaptchuk, *jing* can be translated as "essence," and is "the substance that underlies all organic life."[15] Prenatal *jing* is inherited from one's parents: it provides the blueprint for growth and development and acts as a fundamental catalyst for digestion, thus providing a foundation for the creation of blood and acquired (or post-natal) *jing*.

In relation to each other, qi is yang, *jing* is yin, qi being active and energetic, *jing* being substantial. *Jing* helps to create qi and qi in turn plays a role in the formation of post-natal *jing*. In relation to blood—a fundamental substance, not completely equivalent to the Western conception, that circulates throughout the body providing nourishment—*jing* is yang, blood being a constant factor in regular nourishment and repair, *jing* being a guiding pattern over the scale of one's life.[16]

While qi is energetic, and *jing* substantive, *shen* or "spirit" is ethereal. *Shen* is awareness, consciousness, the foundation of self. Again Kaptchuk: "If *jing* is the source of life, and qi the ability to activate and move, then *shen* is the vitality behind *jing* and qi in the human body. While animate and inanimate movement are indicative of qi, and instinctual organic processes reflect *jing*, human consciousness indicates the presence of *shen*."[17]

While *shen* is linked more closely to mind than to body, it is important to appreciate that the Chinese do not isolate the mind from the body, as does the West. Mind and body, *jing*, qi, and *shen*, are linked in an inseparable web of matter, energy, and spirit that etches out an evolving pattern of self in space and time.

A Landscape of Pattern and Process

A first step in organizing the landscape of human physiology is the differentiation of yin and yang organs. The yin organs, or *zang*, are interior relative to the yang organs, or *fu*, and are considered "solid" or full compared to the yang organs which are "hollow." According to the *Su Wen*, or *Essential Questions*, one of the major sections of the millennia-old *Yellow Emperor's Classic of Internal Medicine*: "The five yin organs store essential qi and do not discharge waste. They are full, but cannot be filled. The six yang organs process and convey matter, and do not store. They are filled, yet are not full."[18] The yin organs are defined by the processes they carry out in relation to fluids, blood, *jing*, qi, and *shen*, including storage, formation, and transformation. The yang organs are receptacles that process food, playing a role in the extraction of the "pure" and the elimination of the "impure."

There are five yin organs, six yang organs, and a number of "curious" organs that fall outside of the yin-yang differentiation. The five yin organs—heart, lung, spleen, kidney, and liver—are of central importance for clinical evaluation and treatment. The six yang organs are the small intestine, large intestine, stomach, urinary bladder, gallbladder, and the triple burner, an "organ" without a clear correspondence in Western biology and medicine. The curious organs are the brain, bone and bone marrow, blood vessels, uterus, and the gallbladder, which is considered "curious" since it plays a role in the processing of food like other yang organs, but produces a substance (bile) that is not a waste material.

The heart has two main functions: first, as governor of the blood vessels, and second as the abode of the spirit. Being in charge of the blood vessels emphasizes the heart's role in maintaining circulation and securing the provision of nourishment to the whole body. The heart's role in housing the spirit, or *shen*, is an example of how different aspects of mind are ascribed to various organs in Chinese medicine. (In Western thinking, mind, while classically separate from the body, is associated with the brain.) If the heart is healthy the person will have clarity in his/her thinking, but if the heart is dysfunctional the *shen* may be disturbed, resulting in insomnia and agitation or in extreme cases delirium. Heart yin and yang, heart blood and qi, are all important in the clinical practice of Chinese medicine.

The spleen is the central yin organ of digestion, governing the transformation and transportation of food and derived nutrients. The spleen is the catalyst of digestion, extracting nutrients and helping to distribute them throughout the body. It also extracts qi from food, which it sends upward to combine with air qi extracted by the lungs. As a result of its primary role in the creation of blood and qi, the spleen is referred to as the foundation of post-natal life. The spleen governs the muscles through its primary role in blood and qi production, and also "manages" the blood, by helping to create it and helping to keep the blood in the vessels.

According to the Classics, the lung governs qi, referring to its role as the organ of respiration in which fresh qi is absorbed into the body and stale qi expelled. This fresh "air qi" is a primary component, along with the grain qi extracted by the spleen and the essential qi contributed by the kidney, of the true qi that circulates throughout the body. The lung has an important down-bearing function, sending absorbed qi downward to the kidneys and helping to move fluids down to the bladder. The lung plays a role in fluid metabolism, not only in the downward movement of fluids, but also in the distribution of fluids throughout the body, particularly to the skin. There is, in fact, a close relationship between the lung and the surface of the body, including the skin. *Wei*, or protective, qi, controlled by the lung, flows on the surface of the body, helping to resist invading pathogens, and healthy lung function is manifest in healthy skin and body hair.

The kidney governs water and is the storage depot for essential qi. As the governor of water it plays an important role in water metabolism, separating the pure from the turbid, discharging the impure, and regulating the distribution of fluids. The essential qi stored in the kidneys sets the pattern for growth and development and is closely linked to reproduction. At the same time, the kidney governs the bones and produces marrow. According to the Chinese medical classics, solid and strong bones result from health of the kidney. The brain, known as the "sea of marrow," is intimately related to kidney and weak kidney qi may show itself as a lack of concentration, dizziness, or poor memory.

The liver is considered the great regulator, for it governs flowing and spreading. This function is seen in its role in maintaining the smooth and even flow of qi, indicated by smoothly coordinated physiological function. The regular and healthy expression of emotion is also related to the free-flow of qi and the liver. Excessive emotional stimulation (too much fear or too much anger, for example) can impair the free movement of qi, or, conversely, a disruption in the liver's maintenance of free-flow can give rise to a emotional disturbance, like depression. The liver is also responsible for storing the blood.

Interconnections

Oriental medicine emphasizes fundamental interconnections between the processes described in terms of the yin and yang organs. The lung, for example, has a close relationship with the heart: the lung rules qi and the heart rules blood, so that their functions are intertwined. Blood passes through the lung, where it is invigorated by lung qi. The vigor of the lung qi contributes to a smooth and vital flow of blood.

The kidney is the foundation of qi and has a close relationship with the lung, the ruler of qi. While the lung plays a pivotal role in the movement of qi throughout the body, essential qi stored in the kidney is necessary for healthy qi. The kidney plays a role in helping the lung absorb qi. The kidney is also closely linked to the liver. While the kidney stores *jing*, the liver stores blood; *jing* and blood are intimately linked. The liver's regulatory function and the kidney's storage role are interdependent and counterbalancing.

The kidney is the root of the yin and yang of the whole body. Kidney yin serves as a structural foundation for the nourishment of the other organs' yin. The kidney yang is like a pilot light for metabolism, supporting the warmth of the body and stimulating the yang aspect of the spleen, thereby engendering a robust and healthy digestion. There is also an important connection between the kidney and the heart, a link between the lower and upper parts of the body.

Each yin organ has a paired yang organ with which it forms an exterior-interior relationship, in the sense that yang organs are considered more "external" and yin organs more "internal." These yin-yang pairs—heart and small intestine, lung and large intestine, spleen and stomach, liver and gallbladder, kidney and urinary bladder—are closely connected. Spleen and stomach, for example, are the primary organs of digestion. The stomach receives and ripens the food, preparing it for the spleen's function of transformation and transportation. The action of the spleen moves the qi extracted from food upwards, while the stomach moves the "ripened" food downward.

Some of these connections are less obvious. The lung is paired with the large intestine, for example, without the same obvious linkage seen between the stomach and spleen. Yet in Chinese medicine the lung and large intestine are linked functionally through their roles in water metabolism. The role of the lung in transporting and transforming water in the body is described in the classics as the lung being the upper source of water. The lung helps to disperse fluids and helps water descend to the kidney. The large intestine has a complementary relationship in its role in absorbing water in the final stages of digestion. More importantly though, the essence of the connection between the lung and large intestine, as with the other yin-yang pairs, lies in their energetic coupling through the meridians or channels.

The Web of Life

One of the most curious and perhaps startling facets of Chinese medicine—and one of great importance to the system—is its elaboration of a system of channels or pathways (called the *jing-luo*) for the travel of qi. There are both internal and external channels, and along the external channels are a series of points (called the *xue*). At these sites the qi can be accessed and manipulated for therapeutic effect using pressure, heat, or fine thread-like needles.

The channels provide an "energetic" linkage within the body, bringing otherwise disparate parts together into a harmonious whole. According to a modern Traditional Chinese Medicine textbook, "The organs, portals, surface skin and body hair, sinews and flesh, bones, and other tissues all rely on communication through the channels, forming an integrated, unified organism."[19] According to the two-thousand-year-old *Ling Shu*, "The twelve meridians are the place where life and death are determined, disease is generated, treated, and cared for; they are the place where beginners start and acupuncture masters end."[20]

The channels have many relationships important for the practice of acupuncture. The yin and yang organs have corresponding channels with which they connect. Also, yin-yang organ pairs are coupled by their channels. The lung channel, for example, has its origins in the middle of the body from where it travels downward to connect with the large intestine. From there it travels up to link with the lung, then courses up through the respiratory tract and throat to emerge on the surface of the body where it tracks along the edge of the arm to reach the thumb.

Fourteen channels have the greatest clinical and therapeutic value. Two of these run along the midline of the body dividing it into halves—the *ren mai* or conception vessel along the front and the *du mai* or governor vessel along the back. Twelve channels corresponding to the yin and yang organs have bilateral symmetry (they are the same on the right and left sides of the body) and are organized according to a six-fold division of yin and yang. (Yang is divided into yang ming, tai yang, and shao yang—yang brightness, greater yang, and lesser yang—and yin into tai yin, shao yin, and jue yin—greater yin, lesser yin, and terminal yin.) There are six channels, three yin and three yang, on each arm and six on each leg.

Tai yin channels move along the forward inner margin of the limb, shao yin along the back of the inner surface of the limb, and jue yin channels course the middle of the limb's inner surface. Yang ming channels move along the front outer edge of the limbs, tai yang channels along the back outer edge, and shao yang channels travel the middle of the outer surface. Hand tai yin, for example, is the lung channel, while foot tai yin is spleen. Hand yang ming is large intestine, while foot yang ming is stomach. Note that a sixth yin organ, pericardium, closely associated with the heart, pairs with the san jiao to complete the channel-organ system of correspondence.

Hand and foot channels in the same yin-yang category (tai yin, for example) are said to "communicate" with each other. Hand tai yin, lung, for example, communicates with foot tai yin, spleen, a linkage suggesting a close physiological relationship. Lung and spleen play complementary roles in the creation of qi and blood.

There are 365 classical points along the fourteen major meridians, and numerous other "extra" points. The acupoints were classically

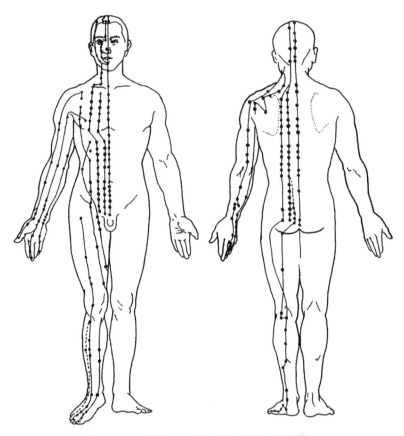

Acupuncture Points and Fourteen Major Meridians

described as "the joining places and confluences, 365 in all....the places where the vital qi enters in and leaves, traveling to and fro."[21] The Chinese character for acupoint, *xue*, symbolizes a cave, hole, or den and each point has an associated set of therapeutic functions.

In English, the points are assigned rather boring names, like stomach 36, the thirty-sixth point on the stomach channel. Points names in Chinese are much more poetic, rich with metaphor and multiple meaning hinting at a point's location and/or function. Stomach 36, for example, is "foot three li" (*zu san li*), which attests to the point's ability to relieve fatigue from travel by foot, so much so that one is able to manage another three *li* (a *li* is a Chinese "mile") after stimulating it. Points and their functions were often learned through poems and songs.

There are many groups of special points. Each of the twelve yin-yang organ meridians has five "ancient" points with five phase correspondences (see below). There are eight "influential" points that have a direct influence on qi, blood, and particular organs. Back *shu* and front *mu* points are filled with the qi of particular organs and are very useful in diagnosis and treatment. Of the over 1000 points known today, any given practitioner makes regular use of 150 or so.

The System of Correspondence

In Chinese cosmology the link between macrocosm and microcosm is expressed through a system of correspondence based on the five phases. This has practical significance for medicine. Each organ corresponds to one of the five phases, heart to fire, spleen to earth, lung to metal, kidney to water, and liver to wood. This correspondence sets out a series of relationships via the creation and control cycles of the five phases. Kidney, for example, being water, nourishes the liver, which is wood, in what is called a mother-son relationship of the creation cycle (water creating wood). In another example, the kidney exerts a restraining influence on the heart (water restraining fire) and is itself restrained by the spleen (earth restraining water).

Other correspondences link mind and body, person and environment, and are important in diagnosis. Emotional patterns correspond directly to the Chinese organs. For example, anger is associated with the liver and wood phase, grief with the lung or metal phase. An imbalance in the liver could predispose a person to anger, while at the same time a repeated pattern of anger arising from life circumstances could precipitate a disharmony in the liver. Environmental factors show five phase correspondences and linkages to the organs. Cold, for example, corresponds to water, dampness to earth, and so the kidney is susceptible to influence by cold, the spleen can be affected by dampness.

Tastes and colors, too, are found in this system of correspondence. Sweet has an earth and salty a water correspondence, while red is a fire color and white corresponds to metal. The correspondences suggest important consequences for health, as described in the second century *Nan Jing*, or *Classic of Difficulties*: "Being upset, gloomy, sad, or thinking too much upsets and injures the heart; drinking cold fluids or being cold injures the lungs; getting angry injures the liver; overeating and drinking or tiredness from overwork injures the spleen; sitting in a damp place for a long time or bathing in cold water after working hard injures the kidneys."[22]

Zi-wu Liu-zhu

One fascinating application of the correspondence system is the theory of *zi-wu liu-zhu*. *Zi-wu* refers to the organization of space and time, with *zi* and *wu* serving as reference points of extremes. For example, *zi* can refer to midnight and *wu* to noon. The couplet *liu-zhu* symbolizes the evolution and change inherent in all things. *Zi-wu liu-zhu*, then, is a system of calculating the effect of macroscopic patterns of change on the microcosm—in this case, on the human mind-body system.

The rhythm of the human mind-body system resonates with the regular patterns of the cosmos: humans are subject to the yearly rhythm of the earth's movement around the sun, the monthly lunar cycle, the daily rotation of the earth on its axis, the regular flux of yin and yang, and the evolution of the five phases describing these cosmological cycles. This resonance can be observed as the ebb and flow of qi in various acupuncture points.

In *zi-wu liu-zhu*, calculations can determine where any particular instant of time lies in relation to the cycle of heavenly stems and earthly branches—the Chinese emblems for positions in the cosmic cycle. Five phase correspondences with the heavenly stems and earthly branches then relate to specific acupuncture channels and points through their own five phase correspondences (the "ancient" points described above).[23]

Zi-wu liu-zhu directly relates the biorhythmic movement of qi in the human mind-body system to underlying cosmological patterns. We dance to a universal beat, one that the Chinese discovered and use for practical, therapeutic purposes. Since specific acupuncture points are in resonance or "open" at specific times and the method of *zi-wu liu-zhu* allows these times to be calculated, treatments using acupuncture and other methods that influence the flow of qi in the acupuncture channels can be optimized. Patients can receive treatment during the time of peak activity of points determined to be valuable for their particular problem.

A Different Way of Thinking

The Chinese system of correspondence is the result of a distinctive thought process, a "coordinative" or "associative" type of thinking. While Western scientific thought relies on an analytical process that breaks things down into component parts, Chinese medicine's underlying thought process centers on understanding the relationship between part and whole. While the West looks for specific causes and effects, the Chinese see patterns that emerge from underlying interconnections. Joseph Needham offers a particularly clear and insightful description of the Chinese way of thinking: "The keyword in Chinese thought is *Order* and above all *Pattern*....The symbolic correlations or correspondence all formed part of one colossal pattern. Things behaved in particular ways not necessarily because of prior actions or impulsions of other things, but because their position in the ever-moving cyclical universe was such that they were endowed with intrinsic natures which made that behavior inevitable for them. If they did not behave in those particular ways they would lose their relational positions in the whole (which made them what they were), and turn into something other than themselves. They were thus parts in existential dependence upon the whole world-organism."[24]

Chinese medicine is founded on this different way of thinking. Instead of searching for the cause of disease, practitioners strive to identify an underlying pattern of imbalance, a configuration of the mind-body system in which illness is set. Dampness, whether internal or external or both, is not a cause of disease, but simultaneously part of a pattern's description and a potentially aggravating factor.

In the same way, emotions and mental states are not causes of disease, but important parts of the pattern identification process of Chinese medicine. Excessive and inappropriate emotional states can aggravate organ disharmony, while at the same time arising from it. As Kiiko Matsumoto and Stephen Birch, contemporary Chinese medicine practitioners and scholars put it: "There is only one energetic pattern and it manifests both internal organ problems and emotional states."[25]

The system of Chinese medicine emerges from a self-consistent and holistic conceptual framework in which the human mind-body system is viewed in relation to the cosmological whole. We are part of a great Unity, a Universal Pattern, the Tao. Our health is dependent on maintaining harmony and balance in the midst of inexorable change. By understanding the Way, the true nature of this change, the Tao manifest in each moment, our path to health becomes spontaneous and natural.

Each person is intimately linked to his or her social and physical environment. Mind and body are flip sides of the same coin and each part of the body is linked to the whole through a web of functional and energetic relationships. It is via the energetic connections forged by the meridians that a point on the ear, for example, can be used to influence the condition of the kidney.

At times we lose balance and disharmony can become disease. The clinical gaze of Chinese medicine looks for a pattern of disharmony, a configuration that describes the state of the mind-body system. It is here, in the recognition of disharmony at the system level, that resolution, the Tao of healing, lies.

2 | Creating Balance with Needles and Herbs: The Healing Art of Chinese Medicine

Words alone cannot describe a pattern—it must be approached by determining the herbs and acupuncture points in the exact proportion, quantity, and quality that will match the exact movement of Yin and Yang in each individual patient.

—Ted Kaptchuk, *The Web That Has No Weaver*[1]

Introduction: An Ancient Healing Art for the Modern World

The great physician Fu Qing-zhu, born in 1607 to a scholarly family with a tradition of medicine, was caught in the politics of the era. The early seventeenth century found China in the last years of Ming rule, a dynasty that was several centuries old and had already reached a peak of cultural achievement. Chinese silk, porcelain, and printing were at that time unmatched anywhere in the world, and the Son of Heaven, the Chinese emperor, ruled more subjects than all European countries combined from a palace with a scope and grandeur having few equals.

But true to the cycle of yin and yang, expansion and accomplishment led inevitably to collapse and decline. Problems with taxes and unpaid armies, famine and pestilence, and economic destabilization from an influx of Western silver coalesced in such a dramatic fashion that the last Ming emperor committed suicide. The year was 1644 and Fu was in his thirties. The northern tribesmen, the Manchus, filled the void with their military and diplomatic skill, creating the Qing dynasty that was to last until 1912 when the last emperor, Puyi, abdicated the throne.

China, for millennia, had a unique political system known as bureaucratic feudalism. The emperor ruled a vast territory with the help of a bureaucratic elite of Confucian scholars or Mandarins. Unlike the European system of hereditary aristocracy where "blue blood" was the ticket to success, it was through a rigorous system of exams that one could advance and build a career in the ruling elite. From an early age, helped by a photographic memory, Fu Qing-zhu excelled in literature, painting, scripture, and history. He succeeded in passing the county-level exams at the age of fourteen, setting the stage for advancement in the bureaucracy. By the age of twenty Fu had achieved a position for which others spent a lifetime struggling.

But the life of a ruling bureaucrat was not Fu's cup of tea. Disgusted by the political machinations and corruption he saw, he dedicated himself instead to the study and practice of medicine. His skills as a physician became legendary, and his clinic was crowded with patients from sunrise to sunset. Even the most difficult and longstanding illnesses yielded to his penetrating insight. A master of the classics, Fu was always quick to point to the failings of past theories and push the practice of medicine to new levels. The "Divine Doctor," as he became known, set up a school—still in existence today in Taiyuan, Shanxi Province—and many of the most famous physicians of the Qing dynasty were his students.

Fu was a Han Chinese and ethnically different from the Manchus who set up the Qing dynasty. Fu refused to accepted Manchu rule and fled to the mountains, living as a mountain hermit. He changed his name, using characters with the same sound but a different meaning, as a symbol of his resistance. Instead of *Qing-zhu*, meaning green (*qing*) bamboo (*zhu*), he became *Qing-zhu*, conqueror of the *Qing*, the name of the new dynasty.[2] Fu's defiant actions landed him in the Imperial prison, and it was only through his friends in high places and a Manchu policy of appeasement to Ming loyalists that Fu was released.

Fu Qing-zhu's lifetime of insights on the practice of medicine are recorded in two books, aptly titled *Fu Qing-zhu's Men's Diseases* and

Women's Diseases According to Fu Qing-zhu.[3] Chinese medicine has always been aware of women's susceptibility to subtle shifts in functional balance and the consequent disharmony in the menstrual cycle. Fu was never content to treat menstrual problems using traditional approaches and was always breaking new ground. He argued, for example, in a chapter titled *Balancing the Menses*, that while a condition of irregular menstruation is often attributed to a deficiency of qi and blood, the practitioner should carefully consider whether the liver was involved. The liver is the great regulator, and any disruption in the smooth flow of liver qi could affect bodily function, including menstruation. Further, claimed Fu, in such cases it is important to appreciate the close link between liver and kidney, and the fact that the menstrual flow has its root in the kidney.

Fu developed a special formula, comprised of eight herbs, to treat cases of irregular menstruation with a pattern of liver qi stagnation and kidney deficiency. The formula, called *Ding Jing Tang* or *Fix the Menses Decoction*, uses herbs that relax, nourish, and open the liver, while supplementing the kidney. It includes herbs like the famous "women's herb" *dang gui* (Radix Angelicae Sinensis), which strengthens and invigorates the blood and harmonizes menstruation, and *bai shao* or white peony (Radix Paeoniae Lactiflorae), which simultaneously nourishes blood and "softens and comforts" the liver. *Chai hu* (Radix Bupleuri) is added for its ability to move stuck liver qi and regulate menstruation.[4]

Some of Fu's several-hundred-year-old formulas are still popular today, in China and throughout the world. North Americans exploring Chinese medicine may encounter herbal formulas with origins that can be traced back several thousands of years. When Nancy visited a Chinese medicine specialist—part of her health maintenance "team"—she was diagnosed with a pattern of kidney yin deficiency. She had sensed something was not quite right. She often felt flushed, sometimes she woke at night in a sweat and experienced a lack of regularity in her menstrual cycle. This, together with other symptoms including a sore back and increased thirst, led her to visit her family doctor for a thorough check-up. While everything seemed to be in order according to routine tests, her physician suggested that she may be encountering some first symptoms of menopause and that they continue to evaluate the situation over the next months.[5]

Her Chinese medicine specialist found that her pulse was very thin with a "thready" and rapid quality, and her tongue was redder than normal with a rather dry appearance. This pulse and tongue assessment, together with the symptoms Nancy was experiencing, pointed to a pattern of a weak kidney, particularly its yin aspect. Since Nancy had just celebrated her fiftieth birthday, it was likely that she was experiencing an age-related decline in kidney energy. With age the yin withers and the *jing* stored in the kidney wanes, a fact that accounts for the enduring popularity of special tonic mixtures designed to counteract this natural decline with kidney-supplementing herbs.

Nancy was prescribed a variation of the formula known as Six Ingredient Pill with Rehmannia (Liu Wei Di Huang Wan in Chinese and often called Rehmannia Six). This formula first appeared in a twelfth-century text and was itself a variation of a formula recorded two thousand years ago in *Essentials from the Golden Cabinet*. The formula Rehmannia Six is an elegant combination of herbs designed to enrich the kidney yin. In Chinese herbal medicine, combinations of herbs are used to harmonize and restore balance in the mind-body system, carefully chosen to achieve specific therapeutic goals without side effects. Nancy's prescription contained, in addition to the six herbs of Rehmannia Six, Fructus Schisandrae Chinensis (*wu wei zi* or five-flavored seed), a red wine-colored berry the size of a pea, and Radix Astragalus (*huang qi*), a woody, yellow root shaped much like a tongue depressor. This variation was developed by the great master Fu Qing-zhu. Nancy's herbal therapy was complemented with acupuncture at points that strengthened her kidney and supplemented her waning yin, like kidney 3 (*tai xi* or great ravine) and bladder 23 (*shen shu* or kidney shu), and over a period of several months the soreness in her back vanished, her sweating gradually declined, and a sense of well-being returned.[6]

Making Sense of Sickness: The Art of Diagnosis

The Four Examinations

In Chinese medicine, illness is synonymous with imbalance in the mind-body system. The overriding therapeutic goal is the restoration of balance. Over several millennia, fundamental patterns of imbalance have been catalogued and serve as the template for diagnosis, a process of bringing order to the chaos of signs and symptoms found in a particular patient. Through this pattern-identification process specific diseases are set in the broader milieu of the mind-body and parts are viewed in relation to the whole. These basic patterns serve as a guide to assessing the pattern of imbalance of an individual at a particular time, a unique pattern that is reflected ultimately in the herbs and acupuncture points used to restore harmony and balance.

The diagnostic process of pattern identification is carried out through what are classically described as the four examinations: looking, listening-smelling, asking, and feeling. Each is a group of methods for gathering information about the state of the mind-body system. This process is logical and rational, yet not analytical, for the Chinese physician does not strive to pinpoint a specific disease location nor a precise causal agent, but works to weave the constellation of information obtained from the four examinations into a recognizable pattern.

Looking is a means of obtaining information about a patient's appearance, and can include everything from general body characteristics and facial complexion to the condition of the tongue. An obese and sluggish person with a pale, white complexion would trigger a practitioner to consider different sets of possible patterns than would a flushed, red-faced person with a nervous disposition.

Tongue observation falls into the looking category and is one of the two pillars of diagnosis. Tongues come in all shapes and sizes, colors and characteristics. There are fat, swollen tongues, red, dry tongues, furry, yellow tongues, and cracked, pale ones. These prominent differences help with pattern discrimination and (to the skilled practitioner) other subtle features help pinpoint the herbs and acupuncture points to be used for a particular case. In sticking out her tongue, the patient is presenting a mirror of the basic condition of the mind-body with characteristics matching those of the organs. Tongue diagnosis was already an important part of Chinese medicine by the time the *Yellow Emperor's Classic* was written, and was further developed during each successive era.

Tongue assessment centers on several essential features, including the color, shape, and coating, and a judgment of the deviation from the normal, healthy tongue. A healthy tongue is not too red or too pale, it is not too thin or too swollen, and it has a healthy coating or "moss" that is not too thick or moist and not too dry. Tongue signs, as with other information gleaned from the four examinations, do not have an absolute significance but must be set in the context of other signs and symptoms. A swollen tongue, for example, must be combined with tongue color, among other things, to offer meaning. A swollen, pale tongue, for example, may signify that the spleen and possibly kidneys have become deficient to the point where the movement of fluids is affected, causing the tongue to swell.

Skilled tongue observation can be compared to a walk through a vegetable field with a talented farmer who senses the close relationship between microclimate and plant health. In some areas of the field the soil might be too dry and parched, in others it may be soggy and moist, all indications of sub-optimal plant health. A broccoli crop, located in an area of full sun with exposure to the wind, might do better in a cooler, slightly moist site. The corn might be growing in depleted soil, while the rich, moist soil of the carrot bed may lack sufficient drainage. Like the farmer, the physician has an intuitive feel for the qualities that foster a healthy inner environment.

Included in the listening-smelling examination are voice quality, cough characteristics, and odors. Odors, particularly unusual ones, are a useful clue to the nature of imbalance.

From the asking examination much vital information is obtained about the history of a patient's health, details of his or her problem, and general characteristics that hint at the underlying pattern of disharmony. According to the *Essential Questions,* a major division of the *Yellow Emperor's Classic of Internal Medicine,* asking is an integral part of diagnosis: "If, in conducting the examination, the physician neither inquires as to how and when the condition arose, nor asks about the nature of the patient's complaint, about dietary irregularities, excesses of sleeping and waking, and poisoning, but instead proceeds straightaway to take the pulse, he will not succeed in identifying the disease."[7] Questions about hot and cold, perspiration, diet, sleep, and medical history are part of every exam.

The last of the four examinations, feeling, offers the opportunity for direct physical contact between patient and practitioner. There are special acupuncture points, called the back-shu and front-mu points, where the qi of the zangfu (the yin and yang organs) is "infused" and "converged," allowing the condition of the organs to be evaluated. The back-shu point of the heart, for example, is Xin Shu, the 15th point of the bladder channel beside the spine in the space between the shoulder blades. The heart's front-mu point is Ju Que, or conception vessel 14, along the midline of the abdomen below the sternum. Problems with the heart may be reflected in soreness or sensitivity at these points.

The second pillar of diagnosis, pulse taking, also falls under the category of feeling examination. While it is still an important part of the diagnostic process today, the art of the pulse was inflated to mystical heights in earlier times. The pulse is felt on the radial artery at the wrist. There are three positions at each wrist and three levels for each position, along with some thirty different qualities that can be felt, making pulse reading a complex and subtle art.[8] Each of the three positions on each wrist corresponds to particular organs and the pulse at each site reflects the health of corresponding organs.

It was Li Shi-zhen who long ago warned of overinflating the usefulness of the pulse. Li was a renowned physician of the sixteenth century and today is hailed as China's greatest naturalist. "The pulse ranks last among the four examinations," wrote Li, "and must be placed against the background of all the information gathered. All four examinations must be carried out."[9] Li wrote *The Pulse Studies of Bin Hu*, in which he set out the foundations of pulse assessment, discussing pulse states and their relationship to different diseases. According to Li, a rapid pulse is simply one that "beats six times per respiration," while the more elusive slippery pulse is one that "feels round and smooth and flows evenly. It is like a greasy round ball, which slides under the fingers. It always remains even, like a smooth stream of water."[10]

Like Fu Qing-zhu, Li was a brilliant youngster, passing the first level of bureaucratic exams at the age of fourteen. And like Fu, Li turned his attention away from the bureaucracy to the study of medicine. Obsessed with his medical studies, Li did not leave home for a decade and read every book he could acquire. His enthusiasm and interest in every aspect of the plants, animals, and minerals used in medicine—the materia medica—was like the compulsion some feel toward sweets. Li divided his time between the practice of medicine—again like Fu, he had patients coming from far and wide because of his great skill—and the study of the materia medica. For thirty years he traveled across China collecting specimens and examining plants and animals in their natural environment, eventually combining this firsthand knowledge with the study of 800 books to produce an encyclopedic work on the natural history of medical substances. Li's *Ben-cao Gang-mu* (*The Great Materia Medica*), first published in 1596, was much more than a book on medical substances, it was a comprehensive discussion of every aspect of the plants, animals, and minerals known at that time along with his own observations, reflections, and findings.

The purpose of Li's great work was clear from the introduction by Wu Thai-chung: before making use of a medicine, one should know everything about it. "One has to know the ways of the starry heavens," wrote Wu, "the profitable kindly fruits of the earth, the principles of natural things, and all that the mountains and valleys

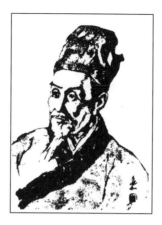

Li Shi-zhen

produce in the form of herbs, trees, metals, and minerals from gold to iron; likewise one must penetrate to the deepest essentials of their manifold changes and transformations, following their likenesses and differences whether on the minutest or the grandest scale—then alone may one venture to employ a single drug."[11]

It was this quest for knowledge that led to Li's experiments on such things as the synergistic or combined effect of different herbs and the origins of various animals. At that time, there was a pervasive belief in spontaneous generation—the idea that life could mysteriously appear from non-living material. Li was skeptical and argued that tiny insects emerged from eggs. Li described how hormone disorders were treated with steroid hormones prepared from urine, a technique that had been employed for several hundred years. Li pointed out the connection between sweet foods and tooth decay, provided one of the first clear descriptions of job-related illnesses (like lead poisoning), and offered insight into the nature of diseases caused by parasites. As Li Shi-zhen himself claimed, this was more than simply a book about medicine, it was a text dealing with the fundamental patterns of the natural world.

The Origin of Disease

Health is a state of balance, balance between person and environment and among the physiological and psychological components of the body-mind system—qi, blood, yin and yang, the organs and the meridians, *shen*, and emotions. Such a state of balance ensures a natural resistance against disease. Disharmony—a loss of balance—is the origin of disease. As the Yellow Emperor claimed: "If blood and qi fall into disharmony, a hundred diseases may arise."[12] When the pleasing symphony of life strikes a dissonant chord, we become susceptible to disease.

There are three general types of factors that play a role in patterns of imbalance: factors related to the external environment, factors of the internal environment, and other "independent" factors, many connected to lifestyle. These factors are much more than causes of disease: they are so intimately bound up with patterns of disharmony that they can simultaneously be considered causes and effects. In the practical art of medicine, they are part of the descriptive landscape of a pattern, offering a clue to its true nature and the means of resolution through acupuncture or herbal therapy.

Life in modern society has largely isolated us from our environment. With our dependence on central heating and cooling we are buffered from the extremes of heat and cold. Humidifiers and dehumidifiers keep our homes from becoming too dry or too damp. It is perhaps difficult, then, to appreciate the emphasis Chinese medicine places on the meteorological factors of the external environment. Until modern times people have been under the powerful influence of wind, cold, summer-heat, dampness, dryness, and heat—the six environmental "excesses"—all of which can affect our health and, because of their constant change, to which we must continually adapt.

It is this constant need for adaptation that makes the six environmental excesses a direct factor in the development of disease. Even modern folk tradition highlights the relationship between weather and health. Exposure to a cold draft might precipitate a cold or flu, what is termed "catching a chill." A damp environment may aggravate an arthritic condition, while a sudden change in the weather might bring on a migraine headache. Other connections are obvious, like the heatstroke caused by excessive sun.

In Chinese medicine, these factors are not only catalysts for illness but the characteristics and qualities of these environmental factors are mirrored in the illnesses they generate. Wind is swift and changeable, causing movement; signs and symptoms of wind may include sudden onset, tremors, and pain that shifts location. Cold is slow, congealing, and associated with diminished activity; its signs and symptoms include lack of warmth, aversion to cold, and low energy. Heat is warm, often red and drying; it can manifest as a red face or eyes, thirst, and agitation. Dampness is wet, heavy, and lingering; its presence may be indicated by a heavy feeling in the limbs, aching joints, and lack of thirst. Similarly, dryness is indicated by signs and symptoms such as dry mouth and dry skin.[13]

These qualities and characteristics—signs and symptoms of illness in Chinese medicine—may appear without a connection to meteorological phenomena. Dampness can be generated internally by a weak spleen failing to transform and transport fluids. Weakness in the spleen and kidney yang may create a condition of cold. If the body's yin becomes deficient, the yang will no longer be held in check and heat will be generated. In this way, environmental qualities are used as descriptions of internally generated disharmonies.

These internal and external qualities—the microcosm and the macrocosm—may both play a role in a pattern of disharmony. Someone with a tendency toward an internally damp condition may be predisposed to the deleterious effects of living in a damp environment, creating a circular chain that dissolves the distinction between cause and effect. As the damp environment affects the body, the internal condition of dampness worsens, making it more susceptible to the damp environment. Damp is a description of one aspect of a pattern, a pathological process with signs and symptoms characteristic of the environmental condition that can affect it.

According to the system of correspondence, these climatic influences are linked to particular organs and to the seasons. Wind corresponds to the wood phase, the liver, and spring; heat to the fire phase, heart, and summer; damp to earth, spleen, and late summer; dryness to metal, lung, and fall; and cold to water, kidney, and winter. Various organs are thus noted as being susceptible to particular environmental excesses. The yin organ spleen, for example, has a vulnerability to damp, while its paired organ, stomach, can be affected by dryness. Environmental excesses can also combine to create a pattern of disharmony. Damp can combine with heat, for example, as part of a pattern of disharmony affecting the liver.

Emotions, the internal environmental factors, can become part of a pattern of disharmony. Joy, anger, anxiety, pensiveness, sadness, fear, and fright are healthy and natural responses to personal circumstances. Yet they can become unhealthy when extreme or recurrent. Emotions have five-phase correspondences and can be related to patterns of disharmony in particular organs. Anger, for example, may be part of a liver disharmony, while pensiveness or brooding may be a reflection of a spleen pattern. These internal factors, like the external ones, are both causes and effects. A liver disharmony may predispose a person to anger, yet the repeated expression of anger reinforces and exacerbates the liver disharmony.

The Chinese system also discusses a number of independent factors—the majority of them related to lifestyle—that play a role in patterns of disharmony. Good eating habits and proper nutrition are a foundation of qi and poor diet can create disharmony. Too much fatty food, too much sweet food, or too many raw foods can disrupt the digestive functions of the spleen and stomach, and may become part of a pattern of dampness. Too much alcohol or hot, spicy food can create or exacerbate a hot, damp condition.

Like emotions, sex is a normal, healthy part of life, but too much can weaken the body, particularly the kidney *jing*. Similarly, any kind of excessive strain can create problems. According to the *Yellow Emperor's Classic*: "Prolonged vision damages the blood; prolonged recumbency damages qi; prolonged sitting damages the flesh; prolonged standing damages the bones; and prolonged walking damages the sinews."[14,15] From this perspective, there is always a healthy balance between extremes. Too little exercise—or sex—is not good for you, but it is also possible to get too much.

Eight Principal Patterns

In Chinese medicine, there is a structured framework with which to organize the array of signs and symptoms gathered from the four examinations into a recognizable pattern of disharmony. This framework is known as the eight principal patterns. The eight principal patterns are four pairs of complementary distinctions that assist the pattern-identification process: yin and yang, interior and exterior, deficiency and excess, cold and heat.

Exterior patterns arise when the body's exterior is assailed by external environmental pathogenic factors, especially cold and heat guided by the penetrating action of wind. As the body struggles to resist the invasion of the offending pathogen, symptoms are generated—like aversion to cold or wind, fever, and a "floating pulse." The floating pulse is a strong indicator that the pathogen is at the exterior of the body. Such exterior patterns can, if the pathogen is strong, the person's defenses weak, or the disharmony unsuccessfully treated, penetrate to the interior. Disharmony affecting the interior—an interior pattern—emerges from a variety of causes, including the inward movement of an exterior pathogen.[16]

Cold patterns are characterized by signs and symptoms reflecting cold, including a white complexion, cold limbs, desire for warm fluids, and aversion to cold. The pulse will be slow, suggesting the inhibiting influence of cold on physiological function. Heat patterns, in contrast, are indicated by signs of heat, ranging from a red complexion, thirst, and restlessness to a rapid pulse indicative of the effect of heat on physiological function.

Deficiency implies weakness; excess is associated with a vigorous pathogen. Deficiency signs such as a pale face, pale tongue body, lack of energy, and a weak pulse suggest a deficit in function or substance. Any of qi, blood, yin or yang may be undersupplied, a distinction that must be made clear as the pattern recognition process proceeds. Excess is indicated by pain that is intensified by pressure, a strong pulse, and a thick tongue fur. There are several possibilities here: blocked qi and blood will form accumulations; an overenthusiastic appetite can result in digestive organ stagnation; or various environmental factors can become pathogenic.

Yin and yang, the last of the four pairs, are general qualities that shape the pattern-recognition process and can be applied to the other three pairs of complementary distinctions. Cold, deficiency, and internal are yin, while heat, excess, and external are yang. Yin and yang can also refer to specific aspects of the body-mind system, yin to the nutritious and thicker fluids of the body, and yang to the yang qi, the functional force animating physiological function and stoking the metabolic fire.

Pattern Possibilities

Starting with the information collected from the four examinations and further organized with the eight principal patterns, the practitioner must progress to a more specific pattern of disharmony. It is only possible to sketch a few of the myriad possibilities here as examples, but patterns based on combinations of the eight principal patterns can center on qi, blood, the organs, and the environmental pathogenic factors. Since patterns can be quite complex, the more years of experience the practitioner has, the easier it is to interpret them. Cold and heat can exist simultaneously, as can excess and deficiency. Disharmony can involve multiple organs and combinations of pathogenic factors.

Nancy, whose case was discussed earlier in this chapter, had a constellation of symptoms—flushed face, waking up at night with sweating, sore back, and thirst along with a thin, rapid pulse and red, dry tongue—interpreted as kidney yin deficiency. Yin and yang had lost their usual balance, in this case a result of a decline, or deficiency, of yin. Because the yang was no longer held in check by yin, heat was produced. The flushed face, sweating, thirst, and rapid pulse are all signs of this "deficiency heat"—a condition of heat arising not from an over-exuberant yang, but from deficient yin. The dry tongue and thin pulse, on the other hand, pointed to the deficiency of yin.[17] Yin deficiency can affect various organs, including the kidney. In Nancy's case, a sore back and pulse that was weak in the kidney position signified the involvement of the kidney.

Dave, a third-year university student, was concerned about falling grades. For the past year he had been sleeping more than usual and was struggling to concentrate on his studies. As a budding biologist, he was required to memorize a large number of facts, something he was usually good at but now found made him tired and "foggy." Dave complained that he lacked appetite and felt full and "bloated" after eating. His pulse was weak and slippery, his tongue somewhat pale and quite "furry," and his stools were often watery.

This constellation of signs and symptoms fit a pattern of spleen qi deficiency with a complication of dampness. Dave's poor appetite, low energy, pale tongue, and weak pulse pointed to deficient spleen qi. The spleen controls transportation and transformation, and as the spleen weakens the digestive function wanes, causing poor appetite and a feeling of fullness after meals. Over time fluids may build up, since the transportation and transformation function of the spleen is deficient, and generate a pattern of dampness, further impairing spleen function and creating a combination of deficiency (the spleen qi) and excess (the damp pathogen). Dave's thick tongue fur, his "foggy" feeling, and poor concentration were clues to the presence of dampness. The stress of school and shift from Mom's nutritious home-cooking to institutional food were likely factors in the emergence of Dave's disharmony.

Alex always felt as if she were on an emotional roller coaster. On a good day she was frustrated; on bad days she was angry at everything. This made her depressed. Her coworkers had learned to avoid her on "PMS days," during which she often complained of sore breasts and slight nausea, and soreness just below her ribs. Her pulse, particularly in the liver position, was wiry, a feeling like a hard and taught wire under the fingers without the natural, rolling undulation of a normal pulse. Her tongue was normal except for a slight redness along the sides.

Alex presented a pattern of stagnant liver qi. The liver, the great regulator, controls "flowing and spreading," and Alex's emotional instability and repeated experience of anger and frustration pointed to a disharmony in the free flow of liver qi. The wiry pulse is a classic sign of liver involvement, and menstrual disharmony is also commonly part of a stagnant liver qi pattern. Stuck liver qi can generate heat and this is evident from the redness along the side of her tongue, the area corresponding to the liver and gallbladder.[18] Her slight nausea associated with PMS suggested a subpattern of "liver invading stomach," which occurs when stuck liver qi "counterflows" and disrupts digestive function.

Restoring Health with Herbs and Needles

From this diagnostic model the principles of therapy become apparent: heat is balanced with cold and coldness warmed; deficiencies require supplementation while excesses are cleared; yin and yang must be harmonized. To paraphrase Ted Kaptchuk, exaggerated activity must be calmed, too little activity must be tonified, a build-up of substances must be cleared, heat must be treated with cold, cold must be buffered with heat, and movement must follow its proper direction. In short, balance must be restored to the system.[19]

Over the millennia, an array of methods have been developed to accomplish these goals. Herbs can be used to cool or warm, clear or supplement, and harmonize. Through acupuncture, the qi can be manipulated to supplement deficiencies or eliminate excesses. Diet, exercise, massage, and qi gong can also help with the transition from disharmony to harmony. It is here, grounded in the perennial challenge of healing, that theory merges with practice, coming to life as the art of medicine.

Herbs: From Folklore to High Medicine

One day while picking herbs in the mountains Master Shan noticed two young men chasing a vigorous and lithe teenager. He was told by the empty-handed and fatigued men that the girl had escaped from a foster home. Wanting to learn the girl's secret of health, the herbalist's curiosity got the best of him. Carefully placing a bowl of rice and spiced bean curd in a nearby cave, he hid in a bush by the entrance. After some hours had passed the girl appeared and began eating. Shan ran to the entrance and asked about the abundance of energy, perfect complexion, and robust health she possessed. Without hesitation the girl attributed her ability to survive the rigors of mountain life to the regular consumption of a local plant's fleshy roots. After finding the plant, Shan named the root yellow essence (*huang jing*).

Herbs are an important part of Chinese culture. Many herbs like *huang jing* are famous not for their ability to heal the sick but because they are able to build intrinsic health and prevent illness. For millennia the farmers and craftsmen of China have used herbs to strengthen and improve health. Taoists discovered and made use of herbs in their search for the elixir of immortality, while martial artists found herbs gave them strength and durability. The wealthy praised the ability of herbs to maintain youthfulness and beautify the complexion. Today, Chinese herb shops—timeless apothecaries where both abacus and calculator are used to tabulate customer accounts—throughout the world attest to the continuity of this tradition.

The use of herbs—including plants, animals, and minerals—is a key therapy in Chinese medicine. Over several thousand years Chinese herbal medicine has evolved, blending folk tradition with the learned medicine of the scholar-physicians and empirical discovery with the theory of systematic correspondence. The first book dedicated to describing the substances used in medicine was *The Divine Husbandman's Classic of the Materia Medica*, attributed to Shen Nong, the legendary Divine Husbandman, who is credited with introducing agriculture to China and honored as the patron saint of herbal medicine. From the 364 herbs recorded in *The Divine Husbandman's Classic* in 200 A.D., the materia medica grew to include 1000 herbs by the year 1000 and close to 2000 herbs by 1600, thanks in part to the work of Li Shi-zhen. In 1977, the Jiangsu College of New Medicine completed a massive twenty-five year project cataloguing 5,767 medical substances.[20]

Chinese herbs are classified according to function. There are tonifying herbs to supplement blood, qi, yin and yang, herbs to expel dampness, herbs to clear heat and expel cold, and herbs to move or "regulate" stuck qi, among others.[21] All herbs have a taste—a combination of sweet, spicy, salty, bitter, sour, and bland—and temperature—a ranking on the cold to hot scale—which guide their application. Herbs are also discussed in terms of the meridians they enter, their major functions, important combinations, correct dosage, and cautions, including toxicity.

The materia medica includes many substances of plant origin, a spectrum of colorful and exotic-looking roots, berries, twigs, flowers, and fungi. Some of these, such as ginseng root and walnut, are well known in the West, while others, such as broomrape (Herba Cistanches)—a fleshy parasitic plant—are unfamiliar in the west. Minerals like gypsum and animal substances like deer antler are also widely used. In some cases, herbs are used fresh, but often they are processed to neutralize toxicity or enhance a particular function. Many herbs, particularly those in the tonic category, are used for their nutritional, rather than medicinal, value.

Dang gui (Radix Angelica Sinensis) and *shu di huang* (Radix Rehmannia Preparatae), for example, are two of the most important blood tonic herbs. *Dang gui* is a white, hard-as-rock root that releases a unique fragrance as it is cooked. It helps invigorate and harmonize the blood and its ability to regulate menstruation makes it an important women's herb. *Dang gui* is classified as sweet, pungent, and bitter; it enters the heart, liver, and spleen meridians, and was first recorded as far back as *The Divine Husbandman's Classic*. The sticky-black root *shu di huang* is prepared by steaming it with wine, a process that changes its temperature from cool to warm. It is a sweet herb that enters the kidney, liver, and heart meridians, and is used to tonify blood and nourish yin.

The earthy-colored root *dang shen* (Radix Codonopsis Pilosulae) is a sweet-flavored qi tonic with a neutral temperature. *Dang shen* strengthens qi, tonifies the lung and spleen, and nourishes fluids. *Dang shen* is similar in function to ginseng root (*ren shen* or Radix Panax Ginseng), although not as strong. North American ginseng root (Radix Panax Quinquifolium), unlike its Asian cousin, is classified as a yin tonic and has a cool temperature. It has been exported to the Orient for over 250 years, since it was first spotted by Jesuit missionaries who were familiar with ginseng through their travels to China. In addition to major areas of production in states such as Wisconsin, Canadian farmers produce close to one million pounds a year; most of this crop is exported to Asia. *Xi yang shen*, or "root from the Western seas," as it is called in Chinese, enters the lung, stomach, and kidney meridians, strengthens the qi, and supplements yin.

Wu wei zi or "five-flavored seed," a deep-red pea-sized berry of the magnolia vine, is predominantly sour, but contains hints of the other four flavors: sweet, spicy, salty, and bitter. Fructus Schisandra Chinensis (*wu wei zi*) is placed in the astringent category, enters both lung and kidney meridians, and has several functions related to its sour taste and astringent property. It can check excessive sweating, help stop cough in cases of lung deficiency, and is used for diarrhea with a pattern of spleen and kidney yang deficiency. *Wu wei zi* has the secondary function of calming the *shen* and is valuable for insomnia and poor memory. Modern research indicates that *wu wei zi* has an "adaptogenic" effect, normalizing various physiological functions and helping to buffer the impact of stress.

Creating Combinations

Despite the large number of substances used in herbal medicine, the goal is not to match single herbs with particular diseases, but to create a combination of herbs that can address an individual pattern of disharmony. The first step toward this goal is recognizing effects that appear when herbs are used in combination, so that unwanted synergistic effects are avoided and the best use is made of beneficial ones. White peony root (Radix Paeonia Lactiflora), for example, can relieve pain and spasm when combined with licorice root (Radix Glycyrrhiza Uralensis), and has a special function related to the resolution of lingering wind cold patterns when combined with cinnamon twig (Ramulus Cinnamomi Cassia).[22]

Combinations of herbs are constructed according to a fourfold hierarchy of king, minister, assistant, and messenger. King refers to those herbs whose function reflects the fundamental goal of the formula, while minister herbs either support this goal or are directed toward a secondary purpose. The assistants offer support for the king and minister or buffer their potential side effects. The messengers harmonize the actions of their superiors. The result is a combination that is more than the sum of its parts, a therapeutic agent that can address even a complex pattern of disharmony. A modern text on formulas states: "The formulas in Chinese medicine are not mere collections of medicinal substances in which the actions of one herb are simply added to those of another in a cumulative fashion. They are complex recipes of interrelated substances, each of which affects the actions of the others....It is this complex interaction which makes the formulas so effective...."[23]

This means that the practitioner not only has to study individual herbs and their synergistic actions, but also must be familiar with many of the hundreds of formulas that have been developed over the past two thousand years. These formulas are classified functionally in a manner similar to that of the herbs themselves. There are formulas that tonify, combinations that calm the spirit, and others that treat dryness. Such formulas serve as the starting point for developing a combination matching a patient's particular pattern of disharmony.

Rehmannia Six, used as a basis for Sue's prescription, is a skillfully crafted formula designed to tonify the kidney yin. At the core of this formula is *shu di huang*, the tarry-looking prepared root used to supplement kidney yin. *Shu di*, as it is called by pharmacists, is used in the highest dosage in the formula and its actions are supported by the astringent herb Fructus Corni (*shan zhu yu*), the purple-red fruit of the Japanese cornelian cherry, and Radix Dioscorea (*shan yao*), the tuber of a species of Chinese yam. Cornelian cherry strengthens and stabilizes the kidney, while yam is a tonic to the kidney and spleen. Support for the spleen helps to strengthen the kidney indirectly, since the spleen is the foundation of postnatal *jing* stored in the kidney.

These tonic actions are not without potential side effects, chief among them congestion from the sticky, hard-to-digest *shu di*. The heat that is part of a pattern of kidney yin deficiency must also be addressed. The underground stem of the water plantain (*ze xie* or Rhizoma Alismatis Orientalis) has the specific action of clearing heat, as does the "blood cooling" herb *mu dan pi* (Cortex Moutan Radicis). Together with the sixth herb completing Rehmannia Six, the subterranean mushroom *fu ling* (Sclerotium Poria Cocos), water plantain also acts to support fluid metabolism, buffering the potential congesting effect of the tonics. Together with the yam, *fu ling* bolsters spleen function, ensuring that the digestive function is not impaired by the richness of *shu di*. *Mu dan pi*, a cool herb, counterbalances the warmth of the cornelian cherry. These supporting and counterbalancing interactions make Rehmannia Six an effective way to address a pattern of kidney yin deficiency, strengthening and restoring physiological functions with a minimum of side effects.

In contrast to Sue, Dave presented a pattern of spleen qi deficiency with a complication of dampness. Dave's prescription was constructed by adding several herbs to a classic formula known as the Four Gentlemen. The king of the Four Gentlemen is *dang shen*, the spleen-supplementing herb discussed above, while its minister is *bai zhu* (Rhizoma Attractylodis Macrocephalae), a woody-looking and pungent spleen tonic with a significant drying quality. The assistant is *fu ling*, the white, chalky subterranean fungus that appeared in Rehmannia Six. *Fu ling* supports the spleen through its ability to activate the spleen's ability to transform and transport moisture, a

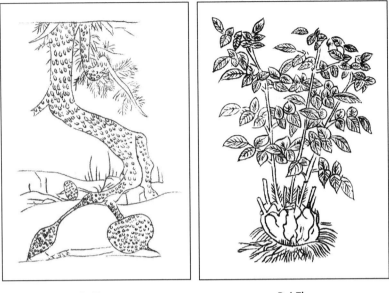

Fu Ling   Bai Zhu

function that is ideally suited for Dave's pattern. The messenger herb
is *gan cao*, or Chinese licorice root, which supports the spleen qi and
harmonizes the action of the other herbs. Although his underlying
pattern was one of spleen qi deficiency, Dave's problem with dampness required the addition of other herbs, including dried orange peel
(Pericarpium Citri Reticulatae) and *sha ren* (Frutus Amomi).
Addressing a pattern of disharmony is a dynamic process set in a
constantly changing landscape. During the course of his herbal
treatment, Dave will change in response to the formula, and the formula will be changed to reflect his new condition.

Acupuncture: The Art of the Needle

Acupuncture and herbal medicine are the foundations of Chinese
medical therapy. Many aspects of acupuncture are comparable to
treatment with herbs, and its therapeutic goals, derived from the
patterns of disharmony identified through the diagnostic process, are
the same. Like herbs, needles can counteract excesses—relieving
stagnation by circulating stuck qi, for example—or can strengthen

specific meridians to overcome deficiencies. Hot conditions can be cooled; cold conditions warmed. With her fine needles the acupuncturist, like the herbalist (who are often one and the same), works to harmonize yin and yang.[24]

For the patient, acupuncture is a relatively painless procedure. It is very important that the practitioner "gets the qi"—which means obtaining a needling sensation—and when this occurs there may be a sense of pressure or fullness at the point. In the thirteenth century, Dou Han-qing noted that "a hollow, smooth, and loose sensation around the needle suggests the absence of qi, which lets you feel as if you are walking on a wild and empty ground, but a heavy, uneven, and tense feeling suggests [the practitioner has obtained the qi], which is felt as a fish biting at the hook and pulling the line downward."[25] Over the centuries, many authors have stressed the value of "getting the qi," including Yang Ji-zhou, who wrote in the *Great Compendium of Acupuncture and Moxibustion*, published in 1601, that "[getting the qi] alone is the measure of the treatment. If the qi does not arrive, there is no treatment."[25] During treatment it is common that a patient will experience "propagated sensation along the channel," a tingling or warmth that extends along the channel being needled.

Points, like herbs, are rarely used alone and point "prescriptions" typically include from six to twelve needles. Prescriptions of points are chosen from a variety of strategies, including the king, minister, assistant, and messenger hierarchy. Needling technique is also an important part of a point prescription since various needling techniques have different effects. The two most important techniques are reinforcing and reducing; reinforcing is used to balance deficiency, reducing to balance excess. As *The Yellow Emperor's Classic* warns: "The disease will be aggravated by treatment with the wrong reinforcing or reducing method of manipulation, that is, reinforcing in excess syndromes and reducing in deficiency syndromes."[26]

In addition to using points based on the therapeutic principles required for a particular pattern of disharmony, points can be chosen based on the location of the disease, since points can affect their surrounding area. For example, large intestine 20, a point beside the lower edge of the nose, can be used to treat nose problems. Since the effect of needling is transmitted along the channel, points far from the problem can also be chosen. Large intestine 4, a point on the edge of the hand close to the vertex of the V formed by the thumb and index finger, can be used for toothache, since the large intestine channel extends from the hand along the arm, traversing the gums to end at large intestine 20 by the edge of the nose. There are also a host of points with special functions—including the front-mu and back-shu points which bear a special relation to the qi of the organs, the eight influential points which directly affect the qi, blood, and six other areas of the body, and the crossing points where two or more channels meet.

June and Heidi had both suffered for months with sleep problems, and both found that acupuncture, along with cutting out coffee and exercising regularly, virtually eliminated the problem. As they discussed their experiences over a cup of herbal tea at the office, they were surprised to learn that the treatments they received for such similar problems were different. Both recalled receiving needles at a point in the crease of the wrist, but the other needle sites appeared to be different. When they asked their acupuncturist about this strange difference, she explained that heart 7, the point on the crease of the wrist, is an important point for nourishing the heart and calming the *shen*, and this was used in both treatments. However, June, who was diagnosed with a pattern of deficiency affecting the blood, heart, and spleen, also had needles placed at spleen 6, a major point for spleen and blood tonification, bladder 15, the back-shu point of the heart, and bladder 20, the back-shu point of the spleen. Heidi, in contrast, presented a pattern of hyperactive liver and needles were placed at bladder 18, the liver back-shu point, and liver 3, a point that can settle the liver by nourishing the yin aspect of the liver. Perhaps, suggested the acupuncturist, it was their opposite traits that made them good friends—Heidi, a bundle of energy, always excited about something but often edgy and tense, and June, the calm in the center of the storm, relaxed but often unmotivated and sometimes fatigued.

The subtle power of Chinese medicine lies first in its perception of the whole and systematic organization of signs and symptoms into a pattern of disharmony. This "pattern thinking" places the clinical gaze on the milieu in which illness is set, defining the relationship between part and whole. This focus on patterns of disharmony is like a farmer who perceives a connection between the fungus on her strawberry crop and the field's poor drainage, recognizing that excessive dampness allowed the fungus to thrive. Adding sand to the soil and installing drainage pipes does not kill the fungus, but fosters the kind of environment that strawberry plants love and fungus loathes.

Intimately intertwined with Chinese medicine's "pattern thinking" is the development of therapies directed toward the restoration of balance. Patterns of disharmony are addressed using means that are subtle but persevering, flexible while precise, gentle yet effective, dynamic although directed. A contemporary practitioner can draw on an empirical body of knowledge going back thousands of years. The result is a process of healing—a realignment over space and time, rather than an event or singular solution—from which health can grow.

3 | A Story of Clocks and Genes: Uncloaking the Old Biology

It is impossible to understand the present without knowing the past.
—Johann von Goethe

A well-known cardiologist asked Dean Ornish why he was interested in such a "radical intervention." (Ornish, the maverick young doctor from Texas, was searching for funding to do a study on the treatment of heart disease with dietary and lifestyle change.) He replied by asking the eminent physician what avenues of research would be, in his opinion, less radical. The senior physician suggested several possibly fruitful avenues of exploration: the weekly filtering of patient's blood to remove cholesterol; the surgical bypassing of the intestine; or perhaps even the aggressive use of drugs to lower cholesterol level.

Still too early in his career to "know" that reversing heart disease was impossible, let alone with a low-tech program of dietary and lifestyle change, Ornish felt the whole approach to cardiology was upside down. What appeared to him to be common sense was often considered as radical heresy, while routine medical practice seemed to be overly invasive. Ornish, undaunted by the lack of enthusiasm for such a study among his peers, went on to discover that a comprehensive program of change in eating and living habits could not only reverse heart disease, but it could do so with a staggering success rate. (Ornish's work is explored in more detail in Chapters 4 and 8).[1]

This exchange between Ornish and his fellow physician illustrates the conceptual gap that often must be bridged before a new discovery can be made. It also shows how the practice of medicine is dependent on a predefined conceptual framework, a coherent collection of ideas that defines the conventional and acceptable and differentiates it from the radical and undesired. Ornish's colleague reflects a conceptual framework—one that now dominates the practice of medicine—with an emphasis on technological intervention and molecular understanding (in this case, surgery and drugs and a focus on the cholesterol molecule).

Medicine is intimately linked to science, and so its conceptual framework is rooted in the Scientific Revolution that took place in the sixteenth and seventeenth centuries. The conceptual framework that current medicine employs can be called the "old biology" to emphasize its long history and to distinguish it from a "new biology," which is starting to take root. (The new biology is described in Chapter 4.)

Early Origins

The old biology is a way of thinking about living systems that emerged from the mechanical ideas of René Descartes and Isaac Newton. It is founded on a model of the human body as complex machine, a machine that can be understood by taking it apart. Biology, under the direction of this taking-things-apart approach, moved from a study of anatomy to the cell and the discovery of microscopic disease-causing bacteria—and ultimately to the molecules of life. Medicine simultaneously evolved to develop ever more refined surgical techniques, powerful drugs to kill bacteria, and a molecular understanding of disease. The result of this several-hundred-year-old chain of practical and conceptual development is a powerful system of medicine that, while Western in origin, is now used throughout the world.

Understanding the roots of the old biology requires an exploration of European history, particularly that remarkable constellation of events clustered about the seventeenth century. Science in its modern form was based on the work of men like the Italian Galileo, Frenchman René Descartes, and Englishman Isaac Newton—and along with science came the shift from agrarian to industrial culture. Arising from within this new science, biology and medicine charted a course that would eventually produce the technologically advanced, molecular-based medicine we know today. These momentous and remarkable developments were stimulated, in part, by a seemingly simple invention: the mechanical clock.

The Clock: Metaphor and Instrument of Transformation

The invention of the mechanical clock was one of the most important turning points in the history of science and technology, indeed of all human art and culture.

—Joseph Needham, *The Grand Titration*[2]

In trying to make sense of their world, people throughout the ages have used models and analogies. For those thinkers and doers of the sixteenth and seventeenth centuries, a time of unparalleled transition, the clock was a source of inspiration and metaphor. The mechanical clock is a link among the Scientific Revolution, the Industrial Revolution, and the democratic ideal—and a starting point for understanding the old biology.

Time is the rhythm of astronomical change—like day and night arising from the Earth's rotation—and clocks are a means of marking this change. The earliest clocks were sundials which simply charted the movement of the sun in the sky by the movement of its shadow on a dial. The water clock, or clepsydra, and the sandglass were also used to track the movement of time.

It was not until the 1300s that the mechanical clock appeared in Europe, first used—somewhat ironically as we shall see—by monks. The word clock itself originated from the Dutch word for bell, because the earliest timepieces rang bells to assemble the monastic order for prayer. These early clocks were powered by the force of hanging weights, and later, spring-power was harnessed to create a more portable "watch." The technological breakthrough that made the mechanical clock possible was the "escapement," a device that governed the regular transfer of energy into the movement of the clock's cogs and wheels.

The gap between the simple sundial and the complex mechanical clock was filled by the Chinese, who used escapement devices at least 600 years earlier than Europeans. The Chinese developed water-powered escapement-regulated timepieces that were much more elaborate than what is usually thought of as a clock. The greatest of these was the magnificent clock-tower constructed at the Imperial Palace by Su Sung in the latter part of the eleventh century. This five-story astronomical clock had an upper platform containing a rotating celestial globe and lower platforms with bell-ringing manikins who marched on the quarter-hour to announce the time. The heart of this grandiose contraption was a three-story water-driven clockwork! Originally built at Kai Feng, in Henan Province, the clock was disassembled and moved to Beijing as dynasties shifted. Unfortunately, the same political events that precipitated its move soon led to its demise, and the Chinese forgot about their clock-making achievements, greeting imported European clocks with amazement hundreds of years later.

While clock-making ingenuity had little or no impact on Chinese society, the same thing cannot be said about the clock in Europe. Every European town and city soon had their own public clock—a prominent feature of the growing urban form—and eventually the desire for clock ownership spread among the citizenry. The rhythm of human life was always intimately connected to the heavens, something the sundial and even the clepsydra did not change. But the mechanical timepiece paved the way for a new type of culture, one that pulsed to the tick-tock of the clock. With the clock, the cyclical, flowing time of agricultural society was forever transformed into the linear, discrete time of industrial civilization.

The mechanical clock fostered the development of industrial culture in other ways. The craftspeople and artisans needed to manufacture and maintain clocks, the technical skills they acquired and their tools were the seed of technological capability. Science itself arose from the fusion of natural philosophy, a "high" tradition of metaphysics, with the empirical and pragmatic, the "low" technology exemplified by the clockmakers. This tight blend of theory and experiment is a key to the power and success of science.

With science came the idea that the Earth and planets moved around the sun, replacing the earlier notion of the Earth as the center of the universe. Italian scientist Galileo Galilei's house arrest for supporting this view foreshadowed the collapse of church authority. As the church slowly lost its iron grip on European society, the clockmakers and their mechanically skilled brethren, together with merchants, lawyers, and other members of the new middle class, helped to shape a radical, rediscovered form of social organization—democracy.[3]

The clock had another profound effect. It became a metaphor and model for understanding the universe, a model whose ripples are with us today. The French Bishop Nicholas Oresmus in the four-teenth century described the universe as a great mechanical clock, constructed and set in motion by God. This powerful image was adopted with zeal during the Scientific Revolution of the sixteenth and seventeenth centuries. As the German astronomer Johannes Kepler, an enthusiastic supporter of Polish astronomer Nicolaus Copernicus's heliocentric revelation, said in 1605, "My aim is to show that the celestial machine is to be likened not to a divine organism but rather to a clockwork."[4]

Here we return to the irony of the monks who first used clocks to regulate their daily prayers, for the clock set in motion the idea of the universe as a grand mechanical clockwork. God was still necessary as the Great Clockmaker, but over time the idea of God became superfluous to the understanding of the world machine.

If the universe was a machine, so were living organisms, albeit elaborate ones. The French wandering philosopher-scientist René Descartes (1596–1650), for example, enthusiastically described living things as machines. Descartes argued forcefully that just as men can make various automatic machines with performing figures—these were popular upper-class toys of that era and Descartes himself had built several—nature produces its own automata: "For I do not recognize any difference between the machines made by craftsmen and the various bodies that nature alone composes."[5] He also used the clock in his imagery and metaphor: "My thought … compares a sick man and an ill-made clock with my idea of a healthy man and a well-made clock."[6] Yet Descartes held back from a complete theory of mechanism, feeling that human intelligence, in contrast to the body, would never succumb to mechanical description. This led to his famous "Cartesian dualism," the separation of the mind from the body.

The machine model of living systems was powerful, and it had a strong impact on biology and medicine. French physician Julien Offray de la Mettrie (1709–1751), following in Descartes' footsteps, argued that while Descartes was the first to prove animals were pure machines, he was wrong in separating mind from body. La Mettrie wrote in his controversial book *Man a Machine* that "The human body is a machine which winds its own springs" and "The body is but a watch..."[7] He also argued that mental phenomena were simply derived from the substance of the body. *Man a Machine*, published in 1748, was controversial not for its mechanical approach to biology and psychology, but for its questioning of the existence of God.

In the twentieth century, even Joseph Needham, the great China scholar, argued in favor of the machine model of understanding life, the universe, and everything. His 1927 book, *Man a Machine*, was a vigorous defense of La Mettrie's materialism. Needham claimed that from a scientific perspective, humans are machines. Needham, of course, went on to have a dramatic change of heart, becoming an ardent supporter of the organismic or systems view of the world and a brilliant chronicler of Chinese science and civilization, which he saw as embodying this view.

Exploring the Mechanical Body

The new science that emerged in the seventeenth century was a remarkable achievement. The Italian genius Galileo helped to put the final nail in the coffin of Earth-centered astronomy by using the newly invented telescope to make careful observations of celestial phenomena. Galileo emphasized measurement over metaphysical speculation and used mathematics to describe his data. René Descartes added a method of rational, deductive analysis through which complicated problems could be broken into smaller, more bite-sized pieces.

If men like Galileo and Descartes poured the foundation of a grand palace of human achievement, Isaac Newton, the great English philosopher-scientist (1642–1727), set the bricks and mortar of the upper floors. Newton combined experiment with theory and mathematically described the motion of astronomical bodies with a general theory of gravity. Among a constellation of achievements, his celestial mechanics was able to predict the path of comets, astronomical objects previously surrounded by considerable fear and superstition. Halley's Comet, for example, was visible in 1682 and Newton predicted its return in about 76 years. When it returned in 1758, the hero Newton was elevated to superhero.[8]

Newton's mechanics soon spread widely, at academic institutions and even through wandering lecturers who traveled the cities and towns speaking to enthusiastic audiences who wanted to learn about the new science. Mechanics was a key to industrial development and the ticket to financial and social advancement. The success of Newtonian mechanics only enhanced the mechanical view of living systems and the Newtonian method had a strong influence on biology.

One of the great physicians of that era, the Dutch medical professor Hermann Boerhaave (1668–1738), became a Newtonian convert, using gravitational principles to describe the body and bringing Newton's emphasis on real observation into medical practice. Boerhaave was known for actually traveling to study disease in its natural setting: in the residences of the sick and poor.[9] His biological theories centered on the mechanical pressures and forces involved in the movement of fluids throughout the body. Going beyond the simple clock-like models of other mechanically inspired physicians, Boerhaave felt disease arose from an obstruction of the smooth and harmonious movement of fluids.[10]

These new, albeit largely unfruitful theories, were indicative of a new attitude of openness and exploration permeating European culture. Medicine was then completely dominated by the ideas of Galen and Hippocrates, Greeks whose ideas had been rediscovered during the Renaissance that took Europe out of the Dark Ages. While the authority of these ancient physicians rivaled that of the church, cracks were beginning to appear in their views of anatomy and physiology. This was a time when excitement about the possibility of new discovery was tempered by the danger of questioning established views. Italian philosopher Giordano Bruno, for example, was burned at the stake in 1600 for his radical views and Galileo was placed under house arrest.

Anatomy was always of great interest—the ancient Greeks themselves had dabbled in dissection—but prohibitions on desecrating the dead had always limited opportunity. With the Renaissance, barriers to dissection and even vivisection—cutting and experimenting on live animals—began to break down, and interest in anatomy grew. (The supply of corpses, often executed criminals, never could fill demand, creating a new profession of grave robbery and adding to the shady reputation of the anatomists. Vivisection was particularly appalling to many people unable to accept its practitioners' claims that animals do not feel pain.)

Anatomy appealed to academics and even artists. Theatres of anatomy—centers of university-based medical education—became popular places. The famous theater in the Dutch city of Leiden was decorated with skeletons holding flags appropriately displaying the adage "Know Thyself." Artists at that time were struggling for greater accuracy in their work and many turned to anatomy. The famous artist and inventor Leonardo da Vinci (1452–1519), for example, dissected everything from insects and oxen to pigs and people.

The physician and anatomist Andreas Vesalius (1514–1564), who taught at the famed Italian University of Padua, went to great lengths to fulfill his fondness for anatomy. The University of Padua professor slipped the bones of an executed criminal—fleshless but still chained to the gallows until "liberated" by Vesalius—into the city under his coat and fought off wild dogs to gather bones in the local cemetery. In his book, *Fabrica,* Vesalius demonstrated the deficiency of Galen's anatomical ideas, setting the stage for further anatomical investigation.

Spanish philosopher-anatomist Michael Servetus (1511–1553) did not share the fortune of his Italian contemporary Vesalius. While Vesalius spent his latter years as physician to the kings of Europe, Servetus was burned at the stake twice for his religious ideas: once in the flesh by Protestant Calvinists in Geneva and once in effigy by the Catholic Inquisition. Galen taught that blood traveled through pores to get from the right to the left side of the heart, a generally accepted "fact." Servetus, however, found that blood actually traveled from the right chamber of the heart to the lungs, where it was mixed with air and returned to the left chamber. Unfortunately, most of his heretical books describing this discovery were used as fuel for the inquisition's flame.

William Harvey (1578–1657) traveled to Padua to complete his medical education, returning to England to practice medicine and carry out research. Despite being steeped in Galenic medical theory and of a generally conservative disposition, he worked hard to overcome the inaccurate theories of his time. Through careful observation, including vivisection on a variety of animals, Harvey rediscovered that blood traveled from one side of the heart to the other through the lungs and demonstrated that the heart acted as a pump, pushing blood through the arteries to the veins and back to the heart in a continuous circulation. He was able to calculate that every hour the heart pumped an equivalent of blood greater than the weight of the body. Harvey was afraid of making an enemy of "mankind at large," preferring to discuss his discoveries in the safe environment of lectures to his peers. Many years passed before he published his physiologically heretical results.

Harvey's mechanical explanation of the circulatory system was greeted with enthusiasm by the mechanical physicians who liberally applied mechanical metaphor to other parts of the body. Jaws were pincers, the stomach was seen as a mill, muscles and bones were cords and pulleys, the lungs were bellows, and the kidneys were filters and sieves. While crude and with few lasting implications for medical therapy, this frenzy of theoretical speculation hinted at the many new and often fruitful ideas that were to come in biology and medicine.[11]

Alchemy and the Chemist-Physicians

Alchemy arose in both ancient Egyptian and early Chinese civilization. Practiced by Arabs and popular in the Middle Ages, it may still be practiced today in secrecy and seclusion. From a historical distance, alchemy's essence is elusive. It involved magic and mysticism and could be deeply spiritual, but it was also an extremely practical and empirical art, a precursor of science, particularly chemical science.[12]

Alchemists were concerned with longevity and esoteric doctrines. They wanted to turn common metals into gold, the most ideal of substances, perfecting themselves in the process and perhaps even the world. In their attempts at transformation and manipulation of metals and other substances, the alchemists—who among other things worked with mercury, antimony, sulfur, and learned to distill ethyl alcohol from fermented beverages—helped give birth to the science of chemistry.

While the Scientific Revolution is usually credited with throwing off the yoke of mysticism and magic, it is curious that the superhero of the Revolution, Newton, was himself an avid alchemist.[13] Newton was greatly disturbed by the atheism of a purely mechanical universe, a world of dead atoms and uniform forces. Such a world could never have produced richness and diversity: a divine, vital spark was needed to animate the universe and produce its spectacular living variety. This vital spark, the agent that would reconcile science with theology, was what Newton sought in alchemy.

Newton agreed that the universe had a mechanical part that was shaped by gravity and "ordinary" chemistry. But he felt it also had a "vegetable" part imbued with the divine breath. The "vegetable" part included animals, plants, and even metals. For Newton, alchemy—or "vegetable" chemistry—was something quite different from "ordinary" chemistry, providing a means of studying the vital agent. Metals were much less complex than plants and animals, but still contained the same vital activity, making them ideal subjects for study.

Philippus Aureolus Theophrastus Bombastus von Hohenheim—luckily known simply as Paracelsus (1493–1541)—was an alchemist and physician who died about a hundred years before Newton was born. Paracelsus was a vigorous opponent of Galenic medicine and a man who knew how to attract attention to his ideas. While a professor of medicine and city physician of Basel, Switzerland, he performed a public burning of Galen's books—much to the chagrin of his conservative colleagues.

Paracelsus and his followers introduced many radical ideas into biology and medicine. While Galen talked about humors and animal spirits, the Paracelcians saw life as a chemical process. The body and its diseases could be described in terms of chemistry, and specific remedies, chemicals, could be used to cure specific chemically described diseases. The Paracelcians also felt that the complex mixtures of herbs and other substances used therapeutically by Galenic physicians were unnecessary. Through alchemy, the active agent could be purified and administered by itself. Diagnosis could also proceed by chemical analysis: instead of visually inspecting urine for indications of pathological change as did his contemporaries, Paracelsus recommended breaking it down and studying its various components.

Paracelcian medicine sounds remarkably like contemporary Western medicine with diseases described in terms of chemical changes, purified chemical drugs used as therapy, and diagnosis by chemical analysis. However, it would still take hundreds of years for medicine to evolve to its present form. Despite the resonance between Paracelcian notions and contemporary medicine, Paracelsus was not necessarily a leap forward from Galen. Alchemically refined mercury, antimony, lead, copper, and sulfur were popular Paracelcian remedies, as was "laudanum," a mixture of opium and wine. Such "medicines" were certainly not a breakthrough in the treatment of disease. Analyzing urine chemically sounds impressive for the sixteenth century, but the crude distillation used was hardly an improvement over the visual inspection used by Galenic physicians.

Yet, Paracelcian ideas did set the stage for the transformation of biology and medicine into their present form. Over time, chemical physicians who believed that chemistry was the means to advancing physiology, pathology, and therapy took their place alongside their more mechanically inspired brethren. Together, these physical and chemical approaches generated the concept, central to modern biology and medicine, of the body as a complex physical and chemical mechanism.

The Rise of Scientific Medicine

The simplistic mechanical models of living organisms were abandoned, but the essence of the Cartesian idea survived. Animals were still machines, although they were much more complicated than mechanical clockworks, involving chemical and electrical phenomena.
—Fritjof Capra, *The Turning Point*[14]

The Chemistry of Limes

The crystallization of the science of chemistry in the eighteenth century was essential to the development of biology and medicine. With the understanding of and techniques to work with the chemical substances of living systems, new light was shed on the mysteries of life. The understanding of respiration and the discovery of a cure for scurvy are two interesting examples of the impact of chemistry on biology and medicine.

Bleeding gums and weakness are the first signs of scurvy, a disease once commonly found in European soldiers and sailors. Scurvy was a miserable disease and the overwhelming cause of death among sailors who ate salt pork and biscuit and lived in fifth-class accommodations on long sea voyages. Scurvy is caused by a nutritional deficiency that many of the world's peoples had learned to avoid. An Australian plum, the Asian bean sprout, and even the uncooked fish and partially digested stomach contents of the caribou used by Far Northern peoples provided protection against scurvy. Indigenous North Americans used tree needle and bark tea to prevent and treat scurvy, a technique they taught to Jacques Cartier and his crew in the winter of 1536 while in the midst of a scurvy outbreak on an exploratory voyage from Europe. Perhaps European arrogance prevented their learning from the experience, for it took another 200 years before Europeans "discovered" a cure for scurvy.[15]

The naval physician James Lind (1716–1794) was not ready to accept the view held by many of his colleagues that scurvy was a disease of sin and heavenly retribution. Most curious was the fact that officers were rarely afflicted. Diet, it seemed, held the key to scurvy. Indeed, earlier writers had pointed to the lemon as a cure and common lore held to the value of fresh fruits and vegetables. Lind's contribution was clinical experimentation.

Dividing stricken sailors into groups, Lind tried out a number of possible cures ranging from vinegar, sea water, oranges and lemons, diluted sulfuric acid with alcohol, and a mixture of garlic, mustard, myrrh, and barley water. It took less than a week for the winning cure to emerge: the sailors taking oranges and lemons were soon up and about. Lind had finally solved the puzzle of scurvy.

Even though scurvy-preventing citrus fruits were eventually included in the daily rations of sailors (this simple step took years to be implemented by conservative officials with contemptuous attitudes towards the "inferior" classes), outbreaks continued, and many theories of scurvy's origin were bandied about. Animal and even human experiments helped to confirm scurvy was a nutritional deficiency disease as Lind hypothesized. Physician William Stark acted as a human guinea pig in the eighteenth century, deliberately limiting his diet until symptoms of scurvy appeared. Stark helped prove the cause of scurvy, but unfortunately died of his self-induced deficiency before he could help to confirm the cure. Over a hundred years later Theodor Frölich and Axel Holst showed that scurvy could be induced and cured by diet in real guinea pigs.

It finally took the application of chemistry to biology and medicine and twentieth century technology to definitively prove Lind right. It was renowned Hungarian-born American biochemist Albert Szent-Györgyi von Nagyrapolt (1893–1986) who accidentally discovered the scurvy-preventing nutritional factor in Lind's limes. Szent-Györgyi was intrigued by the fact the flesh of an apple would turn brown when exposed to air and, further, that citrus fruits contained an anti-browning agent. He chemically isolated this agent, which turned out to be vitamin C, the scurvy-preventing factor in citrus fruit. Vitamin C is also called "ascorbic" acid in honor of its anti-scurvy ability.

Another longstanding physiological mystery, respiration, was also solved with the help of chemistry, this time the chemistry of gases. Joseph Priestley (1733–1804), an Englishman known as much for his radical politics as his experimental chemistry, was an avid explorer of gases and is credited with discovering ammonia, carbon monoxide, and hydrogen sulfide, among others. Priestley also discovered oxygen, a gas which he found exaggerated the flame of a burning candle. He noted that air could be "spoiled" by both animal respiration and burning candles, but restored by plants. Priestley was burdened conceptually by the theory of phlogiston and never succeeded in deciphering the mystery of respiration. (Phlogiston was a fictitious substance used to explain why things could burn. All combustible materials were thought to contain phlogiston, a mysterious vital agent whose nature was elusive and alchemical.)[16]

It was not phlogiston theory that cut short Antoine-Laurent Lavoisier's (1743–1794) contribution to science, but the blade of the French Revolution. Lavoisier, considered the father of modern chemistry, worked for the French King as a tax collector (an occupation thoroughly despised by the people) and sadly met his fate at the guillotine, the new invention of a French physician who gave his name to the device. Lavoisier built on Priestley's study of respiration and combustion. He coined the word oxygen to describe the gas discovered by Priestley and helped to purge chemistry of phlogiston theory by burning the books of the theory's creator Georg Stahl.

Instead of using a phlogiston-based explanation, Lavoisier described respiration as a process that used up oxygen and created carbon dioxide. He linked respiration to combustion by measuring the heat produced in a respiring animal. As the nineteenth century dawned, chemistry had established itself as a pillar of progress in the understanding of physiological processes.

The Miraculous Microscope

While the clock was a catalyst for the Scientific Revolution, the microscope was an agent of transformation for biology and medicine. The microscope emerged in the seventeenth century from a long line of practical work with lenses and spectacles. While early versions offered a magnification of no better than ten times, the first glimpses of a hitherto invisible world proved irresistible and a flurry of investigation was soon underway. Of course, not everyone was thrilled with these new visions: critics warned that the new devices showing strange creatures tricked the mind or, worse, were instruments of sorcery.

Anton van Leeuwenhoek (1632–1723) was one of the greatest microscopists of all time. The Dutchman's accomplishments remained a legacy long after his death and despite the fact he did not begin to dabble in science until almost forty, his tremendous productivity was supported by an energetic constitution and a long life. He outlived two wives and five of his six children. Perhaps it was an advantage that Leeuwenhoek approached science as an amateur without formal training, for he was not burdened by preconceived notions that might have hindered his seeing things for what they really were.

Leeuwenhoek developed high-quality microscopes—up to two hundred times magnification—and special techniques that helped in his discoveries. In fact, it took until the nineteenth century for microscope technology to surpass that acquired by early pioneers like Leeuwenhoek. Without a defined research agenda, his studies cut a broad swath across the field of biology. Microorganisms were a special fascination, and his excitement can easily be imagined by anyone looking at a drop of pond water under the microscope for the first time. He was a keen observer of sperm and believed that these vigorous, microscopic creatures were the source of life. Leeuwenhoek even discovered the microscopic capillaries that connect the arteries with the veins, solving one of the remaining puzzles left in Harvey's description of the circulatory system.

Leeuwenhoek's contemporary Robert Hooke (1635–1703) found that plants were made of honeycomb-like structures, which he called cells. Physical science was founded on the notion of a universe of empty space filled with miniature, indivisible units called atoms. For biological science, the cell was the atom of life, the fundamental structural unit of plants and animals. Despite the complexity of plants and animals, there was an underlying unity in their construction.

Matthias Schleiden (1804–1881) first described plants as a collection of cells, pointing out that cells were independent entities on one hand while being parts of the plant on the other. He also felt that the physiological functions of the plant resulted from cellular activity. Theodor Schwann (1810–1882) extended this notion to include animals, since, as Schwann demonstrated, even complex animal tissue developed from cells. For Schwann, the scientific understanding of complex living systems lay in understanding the inner workings of the cell, something that could be described in terms of physical and chemical mechanisms. Schwann used the word "metabolic" to describe the chemical activity occurring inside the cell.[17]

The Microscope Applied to Medicine

From Sickness to Disease

While some physicians looked to mechanics for biological understanding, some to chemistry, and some to both, still others turned to anatomy. These anatomically inspired physicians felt it was necessary to go beyond the clinical observation of signs and symptoms to a true understanding of disease, something they felt could be found in the specific pathologies observed in dissection. Medicine, in their view, should adopt the analytical approach used in physics and other sciences, breaking complex things down into their parts. By focusing on "localized lesions," diseases could be described more accurately and therapies improved. This was a very powerful idea in medicine, one that would separate illness (something the patient experiences) from disease (a breakdown in a specific part, the "localized lesion").

Curiously, many of the early anatomically focused physicians had an aversion to the microscope, keeping them from entering the world of microanatomy. Marie François Bichat (1771–1802), for example, argued that the microscope was an unreliable tool for anatomical study because there was so much variation in what different people claimed to see. But by the nineteenth century, the microscope had improved and biologists and physicians were using it with enthusiasm to investigate disease at its finest level. This was a turning point for medicine, marking a shift of attention away from the sickness experienced by the whole person toward his or her disease, something he or she "had" rather than "was."

The Struggle Against Pestilence

The microscope helped illuminate the nature of disease, and also shed a powerful light on the problem of infectious disease. European history is largely a study of war and pestilence. For centuries, waves of plague, smallpox, cholera, and other deadly infectious diseases ravaged defenseless citizens. There were many theories about the origin of these frightening diseases. Sin and filth were popular explanations but more thoughtful speculations centered on "miasma" and "contagion," an often vague combination of foul air and mysterious infective agents.

Europeans learned to cope with the dreaded smallpox during the eighteenth century. Many of the world's peoples—including Africans, Arabs, and the Chinese—had realized it was possible to induce a mild case of smallpox during favorable circumstances, a process that offered immunity to the disease during subsequent virulent epidemics.[18] While entailing some risk, smallpox inoculation was safe enough when done properly that it became popular in England after being introduced by Lady Mary Wortley Montagu (who learned of inoculation while in Turkey accompanying her ambassador husband). Robert and Daniel Sutton began mass inoculation in England and claimed to have performed the technique on some 400,000 people with few deaths. The technique also found its way to the United States, promoted by the Reverend Cotton Mather, who learned of it from an African slave.

The next breakthrough came when British physician Edward Jenner (1749–1823) investigated a local folk tradition holding that people who got cowpox, a bovine disease often acquired by milkmaids, rarely got smallpox. Jenner's experiments using cowpox to provide immunity against smallpox were very successful and this procedure of "vaccination"—coined from *vacca*, the Latin word for cow—proved to be safer than inoculation.[19] The technique was soon carried around the world, including to China, where, as Jenner himself noted, it was eagerly adopted by the people.[20]

Such progress in the prevention of smallpox came with little gain in understanding about the disease itself. Again, it was the microscope that made new discoveries possible, and it wasn't long before German Robert Koch (1843–1910) and Frenchman Louis Pasteur (1822–1895) offered conclusive proof of the role played by microorganisms in infectious epidemics.[21] While the idea that disease could be spread by "germs"—invisible agents of contagion—was not so strange by the time Koch and Pasteur turned their microscopes to the problem, they faced opposition on many fronts. Yet because of its remarkable practical success, the "germ theory" of disease quickly became a fundamental medical concept.

Koch graduated from the University of Göttingen medical school and settled down to a country practice well suited for his reserved temperament. A meticulous, patient worker, Koch was a skilled microscopist who conducted research in a modest laboratory adjacent to his clinic. Working with an oil immersion microscope outfitted with the latest illumination technology, he carried out painstaking experimental work using special dyes and staining techniques that enabled him to reliably "see" what others could not. (Koch's disposition shifted with fame. At fifty years of age the now pompous and opinionated physician added zest to a dull personal life with marriage to Hedwig Freiberg, a twenty-year-old artist's model. His affair with Hedwig attracted more attention than the scientific research at an 1892 conference.)

Koch's first success came in the study of anthrax, a devastating disease afflicting domesticated animals and causing a variety of symptoms in humans. Koch isolated the bacteria responsible for the disease, demonstrated that laboratory cultures of the organism could be used to infect animals, and described in detail its natural history. (It was Koch's arch rival Pasteur—war and hostility between France and Germany provided a fertile ground for animosity between the two great bacteriologists—who developed a vaccine against anthrax.)

While it was well known that microorganisms were associated with wound infection, scientists debated whether these organisms *caused* infection or were simply its *result*. Using techniques perfected in his work with anthrax, Koch used animals to show that microorganisms were responsible for the deadly infections often associated with surgery and traumatic injury. He also opposed a prevailing theory that bacteria did not exist as distinct species, but rather led a plastic existence of shifting forms. The shifting form theory, said Koch, was simply the result of poor experimental technique failing to eliminate contamination. Koch proposed instead that specific microbes were responsible for specific diseases.

Koch won the 1905 Nobel prize in medicine for his study of tuberculosis, a disease with chronic and often debilitating symptoms. Using special microscopic methods and with plenty of patience and determination, Koch was able to finally see the elusive tuberculosis bacteria. "Koch's postulates"—his rigorous rules for proving a particular microbe is the cause of a particular disease—were also codified during work with tuberculosis. According to the postulates, a microbe must be isolated, grown in the laboratory, and be shown to cause the disease in an appropriate animal before it can be confidently considered a cause. (Despite years of trying, Koch failed to find a cure for tuberculosis. While now rare in industrialized nations, it is still a serious problem worldwide and drug-resistant forms are making treatment a challenge.)

Like Koch, Pasteur's list of accomplishments is spectacular. While Koch struggled against the shifting form theory, Pasteur was a vigorous opponent of spontaneous generation—the theory that living things could spontaneously arise from non-living matter. He demonstrated that fermentation was caused by microorganisms. Others had argued microorganisms were the result of, not the cause of, fermentation, and some used fermentation as an example of spontaneous generation. In the course of these investigations, Pasteur developed techniques of sterilization and "pasteurization" important not only to the beer and wine industries, but to biology and medicine.

Pasteur discovered the microorganisms associated with various silkworm diseases that were then a serious problem for the French silk industry. This success led him to study human diseases. He developed a vaccine against rabies that made him instantly famous and found the microscopic organism associated with childbed fever, a devastating illness that struck women after childbirth. Pasteur felt this microorganism was transmitted largely by doctors and other hospital staff.

"Germ pioneers" Pasteur and Koch were opposed on many fronts. Some in the medical profession did not appreciate Pasteur's theory that medical staff carried the fever from sick to healthy women. One went as far as to challenge Pasteur to a duel to protect the honor of the medical profession. Others were afraid Pasteur's work would lead to widespread prevention of disease, diminishing the need for physicians.

Max von Pettenkofer (1818–1901) was a powerful opponent of the germ theory and an outspoken advocate of the theory and practice of hygiene. He believed filth was the cause and hygiene the cure of epidemic disease, and founded the world's first Institute of Hygiene. The feisty German was seventy-four in 1892 when he challenged Koch by drinking a glass containing a culture of cholera vibrio, the microorganism Koch felt was responsible for cholera. (Pettenkofer claimed to have suffered only minor intestinal discomfort.) Members of the French hygiene movement were more open to germ theory, hoping that their compatriot Pasteur's work would lend support to their own efforts.

Because of his extensive work with germs and acute awareness of their ubiquitous presence, Pasteur became paranoid about the malevolent microbes lurking on every surface. He was known to carefully wipe the dust from plates and glasses. Curiously, while Pasteur's paranoia is widely found today among Americans, his fellow French maintain a more ambivalent attitude toward environmental germs. According to medical journalist Lynn Payer, there are vastly different attitudes about microbes in France compared to America. Americans are obsessed with cleanliness and are prodigious users of cleaning chemicals and disinfectants. American doctors freely prescribe antibiotics and if an illness has no clear cause it is often attributed to a virus. The French, in contrast, do not share the American "cleanliness is next to godliness" approach to life. They consider too much washing bad for the skin and hair, and feel that at least some exposure to germs provides a natural form of vaccination.[22]

The Good, the Bad, and the Sometimes Dangerous: The Evolution of Medical Therapy

Despite the exponential increase in biological and medical knowledge, the ability of physicians to effectively treat disease was much slower in coming. There were notable exceptions—such as Jenner's vaccination and the use of quinine for malaria—but the public's less than exalted attitude about physicians was indicative of the failure, and even danger, of many common therapies. Medical historian Lois Magner describes the medical man—they were almost without exception male—of the sixteenth and seventeenth centuries: "The average physician resembled Molière's caricature of the pompous snob whose prescription for any illness was always 'clyster, bleed, purge,' or 'purge, bleed, clyster.'" ("Clyster" is an old word for enema.)[23]

George Washington died in 1799 after two days of purging and bleeding under the care of three top doctors—his problem: a sore throat. In the 1840s, the renowned Vienna General Hospital recorded a mortality rate of about 10 percent—sometimes as high as 50 percent—in its maternity ward. Interestingly, a section of the ward attended by midwives rather than physicians recorded a mortality rate in the range of 2 to 3 percent, a difference explained as a fatal fear of male doctors.[24]

Two of the longest lasting and most widely used therapies were mercury and bloodletting. Mercury was considered a treatment for syphilis, a venereal disease thought to have been brought to Europe by Columbus and his crew. The enthusiasm for mercury therapy, which lingered until the 1940s, has been described as the biggest fraud in medical history. Mercury is highly toxic—with even the still widespread use of mercury by dentists being phased out in many countries—but was often applied as a salve in such high concentrations that mouth sores and salivation occurred in patients. While a few physicians saw these as signs of toxicity, others saw them as signs of an effective treatment.[25]

While mercury was used for centuries as a treatment for syphilis, bloodletting was popular for millennia. Therapeutic bleeding was a mainstay of Greek medicine and its use continued until the early part of the twentieth century. Indeed, it underwent a revival around 1900. The therapy centered on the idea that a build-up of blood in the body was an underlying cause of disease, and Harvey's description of bodily circulation only seemed to generate more enthusiasm for it. Eminent physicians argued about the finest technical aspects, including the quantity, location, and technique. Leeches were so popular that the preferred species of leech was extinct in Europe by 1800.[26] The Lancet, today one of the world's top medical journals, was named for that all-purpose tool of bloodletting.

Although the medical use of leeches for wound healing and other purposes has undergone a revival in recent years, traditional bloodletting was an entirely different kettle of fish—with or without leeches. Even laypeople would bleed themselves several times a year just to stay healthy. Benjamin Rush, physician and American revolutionary, felt medical practice was held back by excessive faith in the healing power of nature and encouraged the liberal application of bleeding and purging. Convinced the average patient had at least 25 pints of blood, Rush advocated bleeding until at least four-fifths was removed.[27]

Surgeons developed many skills during centuries of dissection and vivisection, but without anesthetic or germ-free procedures, surgery was not a very successful or desirable enterprise. The danger of infection and lack of effective and consistent pain relief hampered public enthusiasm for the surgeon's blade. The first breakthrough was the introduction of anesthetics, made possible by developments in chemistry. Joseph Priestley, the Englishman who first isolated oxygen, also discovered nitrous oxide or laughing gas. During the 1840s, American dentists found it useful for their profession, and laughing gas, along with other anesthetics such as ether and chloroform, soon found wide use in dentistry and medicine. Morphine was extracted from opium in the early 1800s, and with the invention of the hollow-tipped needle in the 1850s, the drug could be effectively used for local pain relief.

Pasteur's work on fermentation and the germ theory inspired British surgeon Joseph Lister (1827–1912) to introduce antiseptic practices into medicine. Lister struggled to prevent infection in his patients and carried out experiments on animals to test his ideas. Pasteur had called attention to the presence of microbes in the air and on surfaces. Motivated by this vision of unseen lurking microbes, Lister searched for appropriate disinfectants, eventually turning to carbolic acid, which had been used with success to treat sewage. Carbolic acid was sprayed as a fine mist into the air of the operating room and used to treat wounds and instruments. While misting the air turned out to be unnecessary, and better sterilization techniques, such as the autoclave, which sterilized by pressure and heat, were soon introduced, Lister helped transform surgery from a game of Russian roulette into a lifesaving and essential part of medical practice.

While surgeons could now help to prevent infection, they still had little hope of treating it when it did occur. Paul Ehrlich (1854–1915) helped change that early in the twentieth century. The German scientist was interested in the relationship between pathogenic microbes and the immune system. He was particularly intrigued by the finding that the lethal effects of some bacteria were due to the toxins they produced and that the body manufactured "antitoxins" to protect itself. If the body could produce substances to counter bacteria and other toxic agents, thought Ehrlich, so, too, substances could be manufactured artificially to accomplish the same task. Ehrlich began the search for "magic bullets"—chemicals that could destroy pathogens without destroying the patient—pitting various chemical agents against pathogens in the test tube. He eventually discovered salvarsan, a successful treatment for syphilis.

Two decades later, fellow German Gerhard Domagk (1895–1964) discovered another magic bullet, the so called sulfa drugs, which proved effective against pneumonia and other infections. While the microbes quickly evolved resistance and the sulfa drugs lost their effectiveness by the 1940s, more and better "antibiotic" drugs were soon to come. In 1928, the Scottish scientist Alexander Fleming (1881–1955), for example, serendipitously found a bacteria-killing mold growing in his dirty lab, leading to the development of penicillin during the Second World War. With anesthetics and antiseptics, surgery and antibiotics, medicine was now powerful and effective, and the status of physicians rose to the highest rungs of the social pecking order. (Unfortunately, Domagk's warning of the need to account for resistance when using future drugs fell on deaf ears, and we are now facing an epidemic of drug resistant microbes.)

Modern Medicine

The Flexner Revolution

This historical rendering of Western medicine suggests a sense of progress, a continual and relentless accumulation of improved theory and technique. Yet it is not always so clear why biology and medicine took the course they did at various critical moments in their history. Culture, politics, and even serendipity must be accounted for, together with science, in order to understand the evolution of medical knowledge—a story that has not yet been adequately told.

Medicine in China was never a coherent and consistent body of theory and practice. The "medicine of systematic correspondence" represents but one thread of an often contradictory and competing collection of Eastern approaches to health and healing.[28] The same can be said of medicine in the West. Even by the early part of the twentieth century, such tremendous "progress" did not necessarily imply a universally effective system of medicine that automatically superseded other approaches to healing. "Conventional" physicians trained at the best medical colleges competed with doctors graduating from a profusion of small and sometimes inadequate schools as well as homeopaths, hydrotherapists, natural healing enthusiasts, and plenty of homestead and fairgrounds medicine.

Homeopathy, in particular, was a prominent feature of the North American and European health care landscape. There were homeopathic colleges, associations, and hospitals. A homeopathic doctor, Duncan Campbell, was the first to use anesthesia in Ontario and in its first year the Homeopathic Hospital of Montreal boasted the lowest death rate in the British Empire.[29]

For a number of reasons, Western "scientific" medicine grew during the 1900s to eventually monopolize health care and spread itself around the world as a universal system of healing. One reason was its spectacular success. Scientific-based medicine offered the possibility of improvement through the experimental method and the incorporation of sophisticated technology; the germ theory offered a profound insight in the understanding and control of infectious disease; and the magic bullet concept offered a glimpse of better things to come.

Technological, scientific medicine also resonated with the society of which it was a part. A world that was being transformed by machines of every size, shape, and color was open to what science could bring to the field of medicine. Lifesaving magic bullets and miraculous surgical skills were more than enough to turn any skeptic into a true believer. Medical historian Lois Magner reports that in the United States 95 percent of all births occurred in the hospital by 1955. This was before the hospital birth became generally safer than home birth—a hint of the complex social factors at work in the creation of the conventional medical system we know today.

The Flexner Report of 1910 was another catalyst for the change from medical diversity to a rigidly homogeneous medical system. Scientific medicine had coalesced into a fairly concrete and well-defined entity by the early 1900s. The biomedical model was based on the idea of the body as a physical and chemical mechanism, the germ theory of disease, and the use of human-created chemical substances as therapeutic magic bullets. Supported by the Carnegie Foundation, Abraham Flexner toured medical schools in the United States and Canada, evaluating their adherence to the biomedical model. He then wrote a damning report.

Flexner judged only 20 percent of schools as adequate, recommending stricter standards and certification procedures. His report prompted many changes in medical education, with many ramifications for the practice of medicine, both good and bad. On the good side, shoddy schools were closed and the public could now have more confidence in the professional abilities of their physicians. But on the bad side, the report effectively made all healing practices that did not conform to this narrow view of science illegal, restricting acceptable medical practice to a well-defined and state-enforced pigeonhole from which it would take more than another half century to be extricated.[30]

This purging of the unorthodox and "unscientific" from the practice of medicine initiated by Flexner was never as complete in Europe as in North America. Perhaps because they were more thoroughly interwoven into the European cultural fabric, traditions like the use of herbs and spa therapy remain popular there. German physicians prescribe herbs like St. John's wort and echinacea with enthusiasm. Spa therapy, sometimes part of the national health care system in Europe, is considered a vacation, not a valid medical treatment, from the American medical point of view, which maintains a Rush-like disdain for the healing power of nature. Finally, it is ironic that as medical science progresses, more pluralistic possibilities are now being explored with interest, some of the same possibilities that Flexner helped to banish almost a century ago.

Molecular Medicine for the Twenty-First Century

The success of medicine is embedded in its steady progression from the macroscopic to the microscopic. The clinical gaze gradually shifted from the complex of signs and symptoms involving the whole person to the specific microbe and the "localized lesion," diseases separate from the patient and with which the physician must do battle. Attention to the balance of "humors" and the constitution of the patient inherited from Greek medicine gave way to an anatomical and later a cellular model of medicine. As the twentieth century picked up steam, startling technological developments in physics and chemistry brought biology and medicine to their present frontier: the world of the molecule.

Paul Ehrlich won the Nobel Prize in 1908 for his research into the immune system. In his acceptance speech he outlined a vision for the future of biology and medicine that would shift attention to yet another level. Ehrlich described the cell as the "axis around which the whole of the modern science of life revolves." But, he claimed, it was now necessary to take the cell apart into its component structures and functions. Scientists must now turn to study the fundamental chemical processes that take place within the cell, adopting a chemical strategy that would offer a true insight into the nature of living systems and form the basis for a "truly rational use of medicinal substances."[31]

Ehrlich's speech proved to be a visionary description of the future emphasis on the molecular machinery of the body. The body was now a complex machine understandable in terms of physical and chemical mechanisms, mechanisms that could be studied with new and improved physical and chemical technologies. Using electron microscopy, X-ray diffraction, and nuclear magnetic resonance, together with sophisticated methods of chemical analysis, scientists began to probe the molecular level of living systems.

In 1944 Erwin Schrödinger (1887–1962), a physicist famous for his contribution to quantum theory, wrote an inspiring book that helped bring the molecular approach to new heights. In his *What Is Life?*, Schrödinger put forth intriguing questions and hypotheses about the gene, the still mysterious unit of heredity. While basic principles of inheritance were uncovered by the Austrian monk Gregor Mendel and scientists had observed the behavior of the subcellular structures called chromosomes, the physical basis of heredity remained a riddle. Schrödinger speculated that the gene was a real physical entity serving as a source of information, suggesting also that information might be coded in its physical structure.

The effort to "crack the genetic code" was a competitive one, won by American biologist James Watson and British biochemist Francis Crick with help from X-ray crystallographer Maurice Wilkins. They discovered that the large molecule called deoxyribonucleic acid, or DNA for short, found in the chromosomes in each cell, had a peculiar "double helix" structure containing a code of hereditary information. (Imagine the double helix structure as two interwoven spiral staircases. The information is encoded in a sequence of objects placed along the stairs.) Proteins—large and complex molecules composed of basic building blocks called amino acids—fill essential structural and functional roles in living systems. The gene is a segment of the DNA molecule containing the information for the amino acid sequence for a particular protein. (Every three consecutive objects along the DNA staircase act as a code for a particular amino acid. There are four possible objects that can be placed on each stair, so that the code has room for sixty-four amino acids.)

Molecular biologists are now involved in a massive research effort, called the Human Genome Project, designed to uncover the complete set of information in human DNA. In the summer of 2000 scientists announced that they had completed a "rough draft" of the entire sequence of genetic information. But this achievement is as much a beginning as an end. It is not yet clear how many genes are to be found in the over three billion bits of information or what the majority of the genes actually do. Researchers hope to uncover genes linked to various human diseases, and to develop genetic treatments. According to this "genetic cause" theory of disease, since genes contain the code for proteins, malfunctioning genes cause disease by creating faulty proteins. There are proteins in the liver, for example, that help control the level of cholesterol in the blood. If these proteins do not work properly—because of a faulty gene—the result may be high cholesterol and hardening of the arteries.

W. French Anderson, medical doctor and professor of pediatrics at the University of Southern California, believes gene therapy will "revolutionize medicine in the next century," and optimistically claims that gene therapy should be able to cure "the vast majority of disorders, including many that have so far resisted treatment," since most illnesses result from malfunctioning genes.[32]

Are we now at the end of our long search for a complete understanding of disease and the panacea for all human ills? Likely not. While molecular research and gene therapy offer great hope for the reduction of human suffering, it is always wise to temper one's reaction to talk of a panacea.

A century ago physicists had reached a pinnacle of success using so-called classic approaches, methods initiated by the great Isaac Newton. Many physicists proclaimed that the end of physics was near: they were close to knowing all there was to know about the physical universe. Yet within several decades, physicists like Niels Bohr, Erwin Schrödinger, and Albert Einstein had turned the world upside down and inside out, and the quantum theory was born. The classical model, it turned out, is powerful and useful, but is a limited view that cannot explain all phenomena. The quantum universe is a complex and strange one that physicists are still trying to understand.

Biology and medicine are at a similar junction. Some biologists perceive the complete understanding of the molecular machinery of living systems to be just around the corner and feel that the end of biology is near. Yet just like physicists a century earlier, who traveled to the end of one railway line suddenly to realize there were other tracks to take, biologists are approaching a station along a single track where a tangled web of routes awaits the next journey.

4 | Embracing Complexity: An Exploration of the New Biology and Medicine

The list of accomplishments of Western medicine is impressive—organs transplants, a panoply of magic-bullet antibiotics, and the discovery of insulin to name a few. It is little wonder that the mystique surrounding it is so great. There is an ever-present air of enthusiasm for the new discoveries that seem to be just around every corner. Faith and expectation are pervasive.

Western medicine also has its weaknesses and problems. While powerful drugs and lifesaving technologies have improved the quantity and quality of life, these benefits have not come without costs.

To overcome the limitations of conventional biological science, some scientists and medical doctors are now thinking about fundamental problems in new and fresh ways. These "frontier" researchers have opened the way to new approaches in biology and medicine. The emerging ideas of the new biology, with its more "ecological" world view, offer exciting implications for medicine.

The Limits of Traditional Biology and Medicine

Western scientific medicine has had tremendous success in many areas. But its success in other areas has been more limited. For example, Western medicine has not dealt as successfully with chronic, degenerative disease as it has with illnesses of an acute, infectious nature. Its technological emphasis and molecular model of disease have separated medicine from the person behind the problem and severed the link to the timeless art of healing, an art that honors the innate capacity for self-healing and the value of caring and connection.

Another problem is the financial burden of technological medicine. The rising costs of medical care do not correlate with a rise in the health of the population: countries that spend more on high-tech medicine are not necessarily healthier. For example, despite its high per capita health care expenditure, the United States ranks eighteenth in infant mortality, well behind countries like Sweden, Finland, Japan, and the United Kingdom,[1] and access to medical care for those in the lower rungs of the socioeconomic ladder is a major problem.

These issues, however, can be viewed in other ways than as fundamental problems with medicine. Access to medical care is a political issue, cost limitations are economic in nature, and the dilemmas of reproductive technologies like cloning fall in the realm of ethics. Yet deeper questions arise about the basic approach of the biomedical model. The success of biology and medicine has come by moving from anatomy to the world of the microscope and ultimately to the level of the molecule. Is the molecular cause-molecular cure model of Western medicine a handicap in the study of chronic, degenerative disease? Indeed, the history of science shows that breakthroughs come from the ability to think about problems in a new way. Harvey did not simply "discover" the circulation of blood, but thought about the problem in a way that overcame the limitations of past approaches.

While disease can be described in terms of the molecules involved—such as heart disease and the cholesterol molecule—there is always the question of context. The human mind-body system is complex, interacting with an equally complex social and physical environment. Set in this intricate web of interaction the molecular changes underlying disease processes are descriptions and not necessarily causes. Chemical drugs can powerfully and positively alter an illness, but the frequency of negative effects—so-called side-effects—shows the degree to which complexity remains a problem. Each patient is unique, making side effects difficult to predict, and the multitude of complex physiological interactions virtually ensures that powerful chemical agents will have more than their intended beneficial effect.

The Problem of Complexity

"Reductionism" in science means reducing things down to their smallest elements in an attempt to understand them. In a way, that's like trying to understand the Pacific Ocean by studying the sex organs of a shrimp. You can only go so far with it.

—Jim Unger, in *The Complete Herman*, 1992

The tremendous success of science has come from a concept called "reductionism." This is an approach to science derived from the rational method of analysis developed in a flash of intuitive insight by Descartes, an approach whereby complex problems can be solved by breaking (or reducing) them down into simpler pieces. Wholes can be understood by breaking them into their parts and the parts can be understood by breaking them down into their parts, and so on. In biology, reductionism is combined with the notion that living organisms can be considered machines. Thus, "mechanistic reductionism," the dominant approach in biology, is an attempt to understand the physical and chemical mechanisms that comprise living organisms.

Over one hundred years ago the great British biologist Thomas Huxley (1825–1895) described the basic model of animal biology, which "regards animal bodies as machines impelled by various forces and performing a certain amount of work which can be expressed in terms of the ordinary forces of nature."[2] In its more modern form, the model is directed toward a complete understanding of the intricate chemical and physical mechanisms of living systems. Tremendous progress in describing the fundamental molecular machinery of life has been made, and many molecular biologists feel that the cause and cure of many chronic, degenerative diseases lies "in the genes."

Yet, despite such success, exclusive attention to molecular detail has left behind many interesting questions related to the complexity of living systems. In real life, narrowly considered solutions sometimes mask a quagmire of complication. In agriculture, for example, it would seem obvious that replacing a water buffalo with a tractor would be of great benefit. Yet in Sri Lanka this agricultural "improvement" unleashed a surprising chain of consequences. Buffalo create shallow pools (wallows) that serve as a home for fish during the dry season. The fish provide food for people and are voracious eaters of malaria-carrying mosquito larvae. Thick plant growth next to the wallows provides a home for rat-eating snakes and crab-eating lizards—rats and crabs are pests to the rice crop—and a source of roofing material for people. As natural rat, crab, and mosquito control is replaced with the use of chemical agents, another chain of ecological events is unleashed.[3]

This agricultural example serves as an interesting metaphor for medical intervention. The human body, like an agricultural ecosystem, is a tightly coupled system. With all the parts so closely linked, it is limiting to think about parts without considering their interactions. Even a small change in one seemingly insignificant part can have a large impact on the system as a whole, an impact that cannot be predicted by studying parts in isolation.

Returning to a medical example, antibiotic therapy can unleash a surprising chain of events and lead to consequences hard to connect to their source. Antibiotics, which are bacteria-killing agents, can disrupt the natural microfloral ecology (the human body is a living garden of micro-critters, especially in the intestinal tract). If too many bacteria are killed, yeast can proliferate and the loss of beneficial bacteria can deprive the host of nutrients.[4] If antibiotics are over-used, resistant strains of disease-causing bacteria develop.

Doris, a middle-aged mother with a serious case of the autoimmune disease lupus, illustrates the complexity of medicine. Her physician, writing in the popular science magazine *Discover,* described the relentlessness and devastation of lupus as "an empty and demoralizing vision of how far we have yet to go in treating and curing chronic disease." Hospitalized for complications of her illness, Doris was suddenly unable to lift her hands. Specialists were consulted and as her physician lamented, "No two seemed to agree about what was wrong." The rheumatologists felt that the inflammation associated with lupus was now affecting her nerves and blood vessels and recommended a higher dose of steroids, drugs that were already causing her skin to become "exceptionally fragile," and making her more susceptible to infection. The neurologists, in contrast, felt that the steroids themselves were causing the problem, advising that Doris be taken off steroids and subjected to further tests. The infectious disease experts thought some kind of bacteria or virus might be at work, suggesting appropriate tests and a prescription of antibiotics. Her physician persevered through this confusion of consultation, eventually locating the root of the problem: a side effect of one of the twenty-five drugs she was taking.[5]

The Challenge of Infectious Disease

When the tide is receding from the beach it is easy to have the illusion that one can empty the ocean by removing water with a pail.
—René Dubos, *Mirage of Health*[6]

Ever since the dawn of civilization—when humans began to gather into villages, towns, and cities—plague, smallpox, cholera, and other deadly infectious, communicable diseases swept through nations. Miraculously, during the nineteenth century the force of pestilence began to recede and by the later part of the twentieth century optimists proclaimed that the problem of infectious disease had been solved once and for all. This decline in sickness and death from infectious disease is commonly believed to be the crowning achievement of scientific medicine, the result of Pasteur and Koch's germ theory and the development of vaccination, immunization, and antibiotics for prevention and treatment.

However, the curious thing is that medicine had only a small role to play in this defeat. Medical historians and others who have studied the decline in death from germ-based disease have discovered what has been called "a most fundamental heresy of our time." The decline in death from measles, typhoid, pneumonia, diphtheria, and a host of other dreaded diseases was already well underway by the time specific preventative or therapeutic interventions were developed. The most important factors in the decline were better living conditions, especially better nutrition, and specific sanitary measures introduced in the later part of the nineteenth century.[7]

Research suggests that in the United States only 3.5 percent of the decline in mortality since 1900 can be attributed to specific medical measures for major infectious diseases and about 92 percent the decline in mortality since 1900 had already occurred by 1950, the point when medical spending began to dramatically increase.[8] This is not to strip medicine completely of its claim to fame—indeed, many lives were saved by medical intervention—but to acknowledge the ecological complexity of infectious disease and the crucial role played by factors like public health and good nutrition. The germ theory has come to dominate popular and medical thinking and this, coupled with an almost irrational confidence in antibiotic drugs, has meant the neglect of many important mysteries of germs: the environmental, social, and host factors related to their spread. As Dubos pointed out, "The more important reason for the stubborn persistence of infection lies in our lack of understanding of the inter-relationships between man and his biological environment."[9]

The great Pasteur himself began his exploration of infection with the study of silkworm disease and he was painfully aware of the intricate web linking germ, silkworm, and environment. In reflection he wrote: "If I were to undertake new studies on the silkworm diseases, I would direct my effort to the environmental conditions that increase their vigor and resistance."[10] Pasteur was keenly aware of the importance of the *terrain*, a concept encompassing those factors that pertain to the natural resistance of the host and a concept still important in French medicine. (While an American doctor might battle the germ, the French doctor might attempt to shore up the terrain with "terrain building" prescriptions or spa therapy.) Pasteur felt that improvement in a patient's resistance should be an underlying

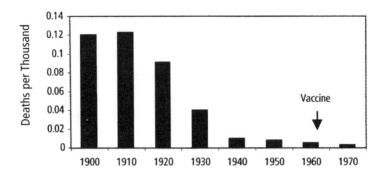

Measles Rates in the United States [11]

focus of therapy and even went as far as to suggest psychological factors played a role in the interplay between man and microbe.[12]

From an ecological perspective, poverty and filth can be as important in generating disease as the microbes themselves. The sanitation movement of the nineteenth century made a major contribution to the decline of infectious disease before the advent of the germ theory and even after the germ theory was developed some proponents of sanitation refused to accept its premises. The great German hygienist Max von Pettonkofer publicly drank a glass of water containing the cholera-causing bacteria in an attempt to disprove the germ theory. Pettonkofer was interested in what he saw as the disease-generating potential of foul air, peculiar soil conditions, and climate, a theory that led him to improve water and sewer systems. It is an irony of history that Pettonkofer and those in the sanitation movement who were opposed to the germ theory did so much to reduce mortality. (Of course, many in the sanitation movement did accept the germ theory and in doing so were all the more effective in enacting successful public health measures.)

Today in Canada, tuberculosis—to pick a dreaded disease from the past that still lingers in the population—occurs most commonly among native people who live in a First World country in Third World conditions with poor housing and poor nutritional status. The life expectancy of Canada's native people was 42.4 years in 1977.[13]

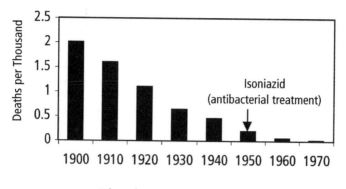

Tuberculosis Rates in the United States [14]

Contrast this with the parish of Hartland in the southwestern English county of Devonshire where people had a life expectancy of fifty-five years or more from the entire period from 1558 to 1837. The parish population had abundant food and good nutrition, infectious disease was rare because of the area's isolation, and the infant mortality rate was low for the time because of extensive breastfeeding.[15]

Sadly, the slow realization of the complexity of infectious disease has come at the expense of the lifesaving antibiotics that were to spell its end. Bacteria have a remarkable capacity to evolve, and have over decades of enthusiastic antibiotic (over)use learned to resist the best and brightest drugs. And their adaptive abilities are stunning.

Antibiotics act as magic bullets by affecting parts of bacteria that are different than anything found in human cells. (That way the drug can kill the bug without damaging the person.) Penicillin, for example, works through the action of a special enzyme which destabilizes the bacterial cell wall when the bacteria tries to divide—its way of reproducing. The "bugs" have evolved numerous strategies to counter this threat to reproductive success. They are able to generate a counter-enzyme, for example, or narrow their cell wall cavity to stop the penicillin enzyme from entering. Worst still is the fact that the bacteria can trade resistance genes—even exchanging genes with completely different kinds of bacteria! In this way, a dangerous germ can pick up resistance from a harmless microbe that has become insensitive to antibiotics.

It was arrogant to declare the end of infectious disease. Since as one expert put it, "No magic bullet stays magic for long," the prospect for the future is not so clear.[16] Some authors—such as Laurie Garrett in *The Coming Plague*—offer discomforting predictions and physicians are now struggling with resistant forms of many pathogens. But perhaps with a more ecological perspective accounting for host, bug, and environment, the magic bullets that still have some firing power can be used more wisely and their lifesaving potential will be with us for some time to come.

The Unsolved Problems of Biology and Medicine

> *By reducing biological functions to molecular mechanisms and active principles in this way, biomedical researchers necessarily limit themselves to partial aspects of the phenomena they study. As a consequence they can achieve only a narrow view of the disorders they investigate and the remedies they develop.*
> —Fritjof Capra, *The Turning Point*[17]

The history of biological and medical science is a steady progression from whole to parts, from parts to subparts, eventually ending at the level of the molecules. Because of the success of this program of reduction, all biological and medical problems are often thought to begin and end in the molecules themselves. Behavioral patterns, intelligence, and chronic diseases are all thought to be "in the genes." Taken to its extreme, organisms do not really exist—there are only "selfish" genes.

While the study of the molecules of living systems can offer essential insight, many unanswered problems of biology remain, problems surrounding the exquisite organization of living systems. In physics, all systems move from order to disorder. But biology moves in the opposite direction—from disorder to order. How do all these molecules work together to form an organism? What are the regulatory and organizational principles of living systems? How do ecosystems—complex webs of interaction between living and non-living things—function, and what part does humankind play in the global ecosystem? What is mind and what is its connection to the physical basis of life? What are the relationships between chronic disease and social and environmental factors like climate, diet, activity level, and stress? These tough questions have been, for the most part, swept under the rug, although not entirely out of sight and out of mind.

Organizational understanding is needed to better describe the evolution of living systems. The conventional model of evolution envisions random changes in genes causing favorable or unfavorable traits in organisms, traits which are then "selected" according to their contribution to the organism's survival and reproduction. In this theory of "natural selection" a creature without wings could in principle evolve a pair through a series of small gradual changes; bits and pieces would emerge and eventually add up to a functional wing. It is easy to see the survival advantage of a wing, but the problem lies in the fact that many changes would be needed over a long period of time before a useful wing evolved. It is hard to imagine the selective advantage of a still useless half-wing, and so, while the theory of natural selection can explain changes in simple traits like the wing color of a moth, it lacks the ability to explain major organizational shifts and the emergence of complex parts like wings. (Such problems with the theory of natural selection do not, of course, represent support for "creationism," but rather point to the need to evolve the understanding of evolution.)

Evolution, the big picture of life, is framed around the little picture of life—the molecular stuff from which organisms are made, and both suffer from a lack of organizational understanding. Genes, molecular sources of biological information, contain the blueprint for the proteins found in living systems and despite the popularity of genetic determinism—the idea that practically everything is "in the genes"—genes are only part of the story. Biologists distinguish

between the genotype—an organism's genes—and the phenotype—
the actual organism that results from those particular genes. While
an organism's potential is restricted by its genotype, what it actually
turns out to be—its phenotype—is shaped and molded by its environment. Some critics of determinism, such as the Harvard biologist
Richard Lewontin, deny that human behavior is "in the genes," and
argue that the role of genes in complex biological processes is not as
straightforward as claimed by enthusiastic molecular biologists.
(Lewontin is one of the authors of the 1984 book *Not in Our Genes*.)

Cystic fibrosis is a genetic disease that affects the lungs and pancreas
and causes a potentially life-threatening build-up of mucus in the
lungs. By the 1930s it became clear that the disease was inherited.
Armed with the powerful tools of molecular biology, scientists hoped
to find the gene that was the "cause" of the disease—the first step
toward a cure. In 1985, the chromosome harboring the cystic fibrosis
gene was located and in 1989 the actual gene was found and copied.
Cystic fibrosis patients can have mutations in at least several hundred
sites in the gene, some of which cause a severe form and others a more
benign form of the disease. Still other mutations can result, not in
cystic fibrosis, but in lung diseases like asthma and chronic bronchitis
or even infertility resulting from a congenital malformation of the
reproductive organs in males. Stranger still is the fact that some mutations do not result in any apparent symptoms, while other mutations
may cause cystic fibrosis in some people but not in others.[18]

With the June, 2000 announcement that a rough draft of the
human genome had been completed ahead of schedule, the public
was left with a sense that cures for many diseases are now just
around the corner. But scientists still only have a vague idea of how
many genes exist in the more than 3 billion letters of the genome, or
of what purpose the vast majority of this code serves. Few diseases
appear to be the simple consequence of a single, malfunctioning
gene. Rather, it appears that most diseases result from multiple genes,
interacting together in complex non-linear ways and with the environment. Clearly, just as infectious disease will continue to plague

humans for some time to come, chronic disease is not likely to yield to simple ideas. Genes, like germs, are a complex story that will occupy the human intellect for a long time to come.

The Search for a New Biology

Our vision of nature is undergoing a radical change toward the multiple, the temporal, and the complex.
—Ilya Prigogine and Isabelle Stengers, *Order Out of Chaos*[19]

The evolutionary biologist Stephen J. Gould once remarked that: "We debase the richness of both nature and our own minds if we view the great pageant of our intellectual history as a compendium of new information leading from primal superstition to final exactitude."[20] As Gould suggests, the quest for knowledge is much more complex than a steady accrual of facts moving us relentlessly from ignorance to certainty. Old ideas are not automatically wrong or "superstitious" if they cannot easily be explained "scientifically." Science itself is a process of creating models to be used as tools for exploration and understanding. New models replace old ones not only because they might work better, but also for their aesthetic appeal and their resonance with the spirit of the times.

Thomas Kuhn, philosopher and historian of science, explained the progression of science in terms of ordinary and extraordinary phases. In a period of ordinary science, scientists in a particular discipline work from within the framework of a particular model—a broadly accepted collection of facts, assumptions, and methods that Kuhn called a "paradigm." The model delineates what is true from what is untrue, the acceptable from the unacceptable, and contains a large number of "puzzles" that keep the scientists busy. This, said Kuhn, is what most of the scientists do most of the time.

At some point the model fails. Too many unexplainable or contradictory facts accumulate, precipitating a practical, intellectual, and even emotional crisis. This is extraordinary science, a period when old models dissolve and new ones are forged. Often it is the young scientists and those from other disciplines that rise to the challenge of creating a new model because they are less indoctrinated in the old way of doing things and more open to new ways of thinking. Some older scientists remain intransigent, refusing to work with a new model even long after it becomes widely accepted.[21]

Physics, usually seen as the exemplary science for its precision and mathematically predictive theories, underwent a major shift in its underlying model as the twentieth century dawned. The Newtonian approach, with its material bodies acted upon by the force of gravity, proved inadequate to describe the physical universe at the level of the atom and quantum physics—with its legendary figures such as Albert Einstein, Erwin Schrödinger, Neils Bohr, and Werner Heisenberg—was born. The usefulness of the quantum model, a strange one of probability waves, uncertainty and non-local connections, is unquestioned; its implications remain a fascination and challenge.

Conventional mechanistic biology is based on the idea that living systems can be understood completely in terms of the laws of physics and chemistry. Since, as the argument goes, quantum physics is only needed when exploring unimaginably small things like electrons and protons, biology—which deals only with big things—remains firmly in the framework of centuries-old Newtonian physics.

At the dawn of the twenty-first century, biology is poised for a shift in framework equal in magnitude to that of physics a century earlier. Facing a collection of thorny problems, intractable and largely ignored in the old biology, frontier scientists have begun to initiate a period of extraordinary science. A model centered on the reduction of living systems to their basic structures using old physical ideas is giving way to a new biology, one focused on the complexity and organizational features of life. In this new biology the quantum theory is being applied to the understanding of biological organization, and a new theory of complex, dynamical systems is offering completely new perspectives on embryology, evolution, and the centuries-old mind-body dilemma. The new biology is based on a much more appealing conceptual framework, a framework attuned to the ecological spirit of the times. And there are now hints of what this new biology will mean for medicine.

From a Dead to a Living Universe: The Philosophy of Organicism

Life is an offensive, directed against the repetitious mechanism of the Universe.

—Alfred North Whitehead, *Adventures of Ideas*

Mechanistic biology, based on Newtonian physics, always suffered from a serious problem. The physical world of Newtonian physics was dead, uniform, and predicable. Living systems, in contrast, were alive, diverse, and unpredictable. Ironically, Newton himself was loath to accept that the ideas he pioneered to describe a dead physical world could completely describe living systems. While Descartes described animals as machines, Newton recoiled at the thought. The richness of the world could not have arisen from the mechanical interaction of uniform matter: it required a vital agent, an agent that for Newton connected the world to the divine. This divine vital agent was what Newton sought in his alchemical research, research that was to occupy much of his time and energy.[22]

Although Newton helped forge science in to its modern form—with a dead, material world replacing a timeless, organic vision—his work also helped to split biology into two camps. The intellectual battle between mechanists and vitalists became a dominant theme of biology, and even into the early part of the twentieth century the spark of vitalism burned brightly. Champions of vitalism, like biologist Hans Driesch (1867–1941) and philosopher Henri Bergson (1859–1941), did not deny the material basis of life, but added to it a vital organizing agent. For Driesch this was "entelechy," for Bergson the "élan vital."[23]

Despite the vitalists' penetrating critiques of mechanistic biology, vitalism could not offer a concrete and useful alternative to mechanism. Vague talk about mystical-sounding "vital agents" responsible for the organization of matter in living systems could not compete with the spectacular insights of the mechanistic molecular biologists. The mechanists soon claimed victory and declared their hated enemy, vitalism, dead and buried. For modern students of biology vitalism is but a historical curiosity, a heresy of earlier times.

Yet the victory party was premature. Despite the success of molecular biology, the problem of understanding biological organization remained and a third conceptual thread, a bold new perspective beyond the perennial mechanism-vitalism debate, emerged to challenge the primacy of mechanistic dogma. This third way, the philosophy of organicism, has spawned a concrete and viable approach to the study of living systems. And its champions have included eminent thinkers like Joseph Needham, a converted mechanist and the great chronicler of Chinese science and civilization.

Alfred North Whitehead (1861–1947) played a central role in describing the basic ideas of organicism. The remarkable British mathematician and philosopher, who spent his later professional years teaching at Harvard University, rebelled against the materialism of science and shifted the focus from matter to process. The essence of the universe was not matter, immutable and eternal, but structures of activity which he termed organisms. Mechanists saw the universe as dead, and were comfortable thinking of living things as machines, while vitalists accepted the idea of a dead universe, simply adding that a mysterious vital agent was needed to account for life. For Whitehead, the whole universe was alive. His "organisms" were not only animals, plants, and cells but also minerals and molecules. As he put it: "Biology is the study of the larger organisms, whereas physics is the study of the smaller organisms."[24]

In the philosophy of organicism, each organism has properties that arise from the relationships and interactions of its parts, parts which are themselves organisms at another level, and which, in turn, are composed of further parts, organisms at yet another level. Thus, there is a hierarchy of levels, each with organisms possessing unique properties that emerge as a result of the relationships among its components. Animals are composed of cells, which are composed of molecules, which are composed of atoms, which are composed of subatomic particles and so on.

Ant colonies, for example, have properties that emerge from the relationships between individual ants. In an ant colony, as in its human counterpart, there is a spectrum of work effort: some individuals are lazy, others are ambitious. This is more a property of the colony arising from the social dynamics of the group than a property that can be reduced to a feature of individual ants. If the hard-working ants are separated from their lazy brothers, two colonies are produced with the same spectrum of working characteristics as in the original colony. For a complete understanding of its properties a system must be studied in its entirety. Ant colonies cannot be fully understood by the study of individual ants. Plants and animals cannot be understood by the study of cells in isolation, nor solely in terms of their individual molecular constituents.

Organisms as Complex Systems

From the perspective of organicism, organisms are wholes with properties that emerge from the relationships of their parts. An organism is thus appropriately described as a "system," a word with Greek origins suggesting "a composite whole" and "to bring together." The new biology is thus a "systems biology" that uses "systems thinking" and the effort of those working in the new biology has been to understand the properties and organization of complex systems.[25]

Two pioneers of systems theory were the Austrian biologist Ludwig von Bertalanffy and Alexander Bogdanov, a Russian whose interests roamed from medicine to philosophy and economics. Bogdanov developed a theory of the organizational principles of both living and nonliving systems, which he called "tektology" and described as a step toward a "universal science of organization." Many of his ideas were precursors of important features of systems thinking that only became more widely incorporated into the new biology many years later. A German edition of Bogdanov's *Tektology* was published in 1928, over a decade after the Russian original. Von Bertalanffy described decades of systems research in his 1968 book *General System Theory*.

Systems theory is distinctly different from mechanistic biology. Instead of dissecting wholes into parts as a means of understanding, parts are examined in the context of the whole. This sense of context suggests a network or web of relationships that characterize a system at each level, a web of relationships that combine to produce a unique pattern of organization. Fritjof Capra, who presented an overview of the emerging new biology in his 1996 book *The Web of Life: A New Scientific Understanding of Living Systems*, notes that the pattern of organization of a system is distinct from its structure. The pattern of organization is "the configuration of relationships among the system's components that determines the system's essential characteristics," while the structure refers to the actual components themselves.[26]

Cybernetics, the study of regulation and control in living and non-living systems, is an important facet of the new systems biology. Organization is achieved with the help of regulatory networks of positive and negative feedback. If A affects B and B affects C, feedback exists when C affects A. This means that something A does is transmitted in a circular fashion back to itself. Positive feedback can be harmful, like an ultimately self-destructive device that increases the volume of a speaker when it records an increase in sound. Negative feedback, on the other hand, is important for achieving balance, like a thermostat which turns a furnace off when the temperature exceeds a set value and turns it on when the temperature goes below that value.

One of the interesting and important things about networked systems with multiple loops of communication and feedback is the blurring of cause and effect. Analyzing things in terms of cause and effect is a hallmark of traditional science. Yet in complex systems the causes and effects can become blurred into a chicken and egg scenario: it is hard to distinguish which came first. Multiple factors can be involved in the breakdown or disruption of a complex system. Breakdowns can be described in terms of the factors involved and the system's altered pattern of organization.

Networks of interacting components with multiple feedback loops are a challenging mathematical problem, one that has required many years and the help of powerful modern computers for solutions to emerge. For most of its history, science has concentrated on simple cases and ignored the more complex problems. These simple cases are described as "linear" and have basic mathematical relationships, often existing only as the exception rather than the rule in the "real world." Complex systems, in contrast, exhibit non-linear relationships and, although the non-linear mathematics describing these systems is hard to solve, they are much more relevant to biological problems.

While linear systems exhibit simple and predictable behavior, non-linear systems are complex and unpredictable. In the linear case, a small input will generate a small change in the system and a large input, a large change. In the non-linear case, small inputs can give rise to large changes, while stability of the system can sometimes be maintained in the face of a large input. Non-linear systems can also experience catastrophe, a sudden and often unpredictable change after a period of stability.

The complex systems that are relevant for biology are also characterized as "open" and "non-equilibrium." Open means that the system is in constant connection with its environment, taking in and giving off or "dissipating" matter and energy. Non-equilibrium means that the system is not in balance with its environment. The human body, for example, is maintained at a constant temperature despite the changing and varied temperature of the surroundings, a feat that is accomplished by various heating and cooling mechanisms. After a plant is pulled out of the ground, it will quickly wilt and die. Cut off from a supply of water through its roots, the plant is unable to maintain the "turgor pressure" that generates its stiffness and structure. The plant is in effect maintaining itself in a non-equilibrium state.

The Russian-born scientist Ilya Prigogine is famous for his studies of open, non-equilibrium systems. Prigogine, who, as *Scientific American* put it, "oscillates between the international Solvay Institute in Belgium and the University of Texas at Austin," has explored how in such systems order can arise from chaos.[27] The order and complex pattern of organization that can arise in random, disordered systems offers a hint of the exquisite organization seen in living systems. The Bénard cell, for example, is an ordered, dynamic structure that arises in an open, non-equilibrium system. If a thin layer of fluid is heated, heat will flow by conduction from the bottom to the colder top. In conduction, the fluid does not move, but heat is carried by the bumper car effect of adjacent molecules. As more heat is applied, conduction alone cannot transmit sufficient heat and convection begins, with heat-carrying currents of fluid moving in a random, disordered way. Strangely, as more heat is applied, the random convection currents form a beautifully ordered hexagonal pattern that allows cold fluid to descend and hot fluid to rise.

Prigogine, who called these dynamic patterns of organization "dissipative structures" because their existence is related to the dissipation of matter and energy, won a Nobel Prize for his work in 1977. Prigogine emphasizes the importance of fluctuations and feedback in these complex systems. While the system can maintain stability in this non-equilibrium state, internal fluctuations are amplified through feedback and the system can reach a "bifurcation" point, a point of instability from which it evolves to one of several possible new patterns of organization.

Dissipative structures are an example of self-organization, a spontaneous ordering that occurs in the face of a transfer of energy and matter and that offers a glimpse of a fundamental characteristic of living systems. Living systems share other characteristics with such complex, self-organizing systems, including the need for a constant input of matter and energy, internal feedback and fluctuation, and system evolution. The basic units of biological systems which interact to produce organisms with these characteristics are processes, not structures, for biological structures emerge from the web of inter-acting processes of each organism. The structures that comprise the human body, for example, are constantly being broken down and built up. Yet, despite this constant recycling and replacing there is an evolving pattern of organization with enough constancy to create at least the illusion of a fixed sense of self.

Organism and Environment, Mind and Body: The Relationship Between the Part and the Whole in the New Biology

> We know today that both the biosphere as a whole as well as its com-ponents, living or dead, exist in far-from-equilibrium conditions. In this context life, far from being outside the natural order, appears as the supreme expression of the self-organizing processes that occur.
> —Ilya Prigogine and Isabelle Stengers, *Order Out of Chaos*[28]

An organism is a dynamic pattern of organization with a tension between its individuality and its role as part of whole. A cell, for example, is a distinct entity, yet its activity is constrained and shaped by its role as part of a multicellular organism. A liver cell can be studied in terms of its components and functions, but these only make sense in the context of the liver's physiological role in an animal body. At another level, an animal's behavioral pattern only makes sense in the context of the animal's relationship to its envi-ronment.

The conventional reductionist approach to biology draws a sharp line between the organism and its environment. The various characteristics of an organism are thought to be shaped by distinct innate and external factors and the problem is thought to be one of determining what percentage of a particular characteristic is biologically determined ("in the genes") and what percentage is the result of the influence of the environment. Yet from a systems per-spective the line between the organism and its environment is not so clear. The organism and its "environment" interact in a dynamic way—the organism affects the environment and the environment affects the organism. They co-determine each other as part of a broader evolving process, making it difficult to think about one or the other in isolation.

The complex and intimate relationship between organism and environment is demonstrated by the behavior of bacteria, who actively choose their environment by moving toward a sugar-rich region. The bacteria will "eat" the sugar and excrete waste products, eventually altering the environment to the point where it becomes hostile. Finding themselves in a poisoned environment of their own making, the bacteria leave to find more hospitable territory. The "environment" is not a fixed external reality in which an organism must struggle to survive, but an evolving set of conditions with which organisms interact, shaped in part by the activity of the organisms themselves.[29]

This intimate intermingling of organism and environment reaches to the level of the entire planet. Indeed, one of the most profound revelations of twentieth century science has been the realization that the planet is a complex, self-organizing system—an organism. James Lovelock, a British scientist and inventor, first noticed that the atmosphere of the Earth was not in equilibrium. Searching to explain this startling fact, he concluded that the Earth's special atmosphere was connected with the existence of life on the planet. As he put it: "Could it be that life on Earth not only made the atmosphere, but also regulated it—keeping it at a constant composition, and at a level favorable for organisms?"[30]

Working with American biologist Lynn Margulis, Lovelock traced a variety of complex cycles, complete with feedback loops, that link the planet's living and non-living systems so that conditions favorable for life are maintained. The startling conclusion is that living things play a central role in producing the very conditions upon which their existence depends. Lovelock called this self-organizing planetary system Gaia after the Greek goddess of the Earth. The Gaia theory shows that the miracle of life is literally and not just figuratively a planetary phenomenon, and changes the view of evolution from one where only the fittest organisms survive against the hostility of their environment to a complex, co-evolutionary process involving organism and environment as parts in a larger whole. It also offers an ecological vision of human place in the biosphere that contrasts sharply with the values of growth-oriented technological society.[31]

Systems theory not only sheds light on the relationship between organism and environment, but also it offers a fresh perspective on the age-old problem of mind and body. Since the birth of modern science and Descartes' pronouncement "I think, therefore I am," Western civilization has felt uncomfortable about its conception of mind and the relationship between mind and body. Descartes took a "dualist" position, arguing that while mind could influence body through the pineal gland, they were separate and distinct. Today, confusion reigns. Descartes' dualism lingers alongside a strictly materialistic perspective that simply denies the existence of mind by reducing mental and emotional phenomena to brain events. An understanding of mind is equated with an understanding of the brain: emotions like anger, for example, are reduced to brain chemistry.

From a systems perspective, mind is not synonymous with brain. Mind is not a thing at a specific location, but an intimate and interwoven feature of complex, self-organized systems. As Fritjof Capra explains in *The Web of Life*:

According to the theory of living systems, mind is not a thing but a process—the very process of life. In other words, the organizing activity of living systems, at all levels of life, is mental activity. The interactions of a living organism—plant, animal, or human—with its environment are cognitive, or mental interactions. Thus life and cognition become inseparably connected. Mind—or, more accurately, mental process—is immanent in matter at all levels of life.[32]

Seen in this way mind is fundamentally inseparable from the physical basis of life. Mental activity is reflected in the physical embodiment of a living system, while the physical reality of the system shapes and constrains its mental reality. This is far more than simply suggesting that mind affects body and body affects mind. Mental responses to the environment are also physical responses; physical responses to the environment *are* also mental responses. Such a new understanding of mind and its relationship to the body has profound implications for health and healing and is congruent with a plethora of new research showing the fundamental connections between the nervous system—with its organ the brain—and the hormonal and immune systems.

Fields of Organization

A "field" is a special concept widely used in physical science to describe the distribution of a physical property in time and space. Think of a flowing stream. At each position in the stream the water is moving with a particular speed in a particular direction. The speed and direction of flow at each position also changes in time. A "flow field" describes the pattern of movement of the stream by specifying the velocity of the water at each point in space and how it changes in time. This flow or velocity field is a useful way of describing the organized pattern of moving water.

Biological systems also display a pattern of organization across space and time. The human form, for example, begins with the meeting of sperm and egg, moves through a startling sequence of forms during the development of the embryo, and continues with a series of changes in form through childhood to adulthood and old age. Regeneration—the ability of creatures like starfish and salamanders to regrow parts—also shows the remarkable ability of organisms to organize themselves in space and time.

The maintenance and evolution of an organism's form over the course of its life has always been a mystery to biologists. Every cell in the human body, for example, contains the same genetic information. Yet some genes are switched on and others off to form particular cells, like liver cells or skin cells, and all these different cells are organized to form a whole person. Vitalists used the idea of a mysterious vital force to "explain" the exquisite organization that characterizes life. Instead of a vital force, conventional mechanistic biology talks about an equally mysterious genetic "program" as the source of biological organization. Searching for a more concrete understanding, organismic biologists have applied the field concept to the understanding of form and pattern in living systems. These organizing fields are called morphogenetic fields because they shape an organism's form and pattern of development over the cycle of its life.

University of Toronto biophysicist Lynn Trainor and his colleagues have successfully applied the morphogenetic field concept to a simple, single-celled organism called tetrahymena. Their morphogenetic field model describes the dynamic changes associated with the growth and replication of the organism. Tetrahymena is a strange critter. Two of these miniature, single-celled creatures can fuse together into one, and in the course of doing so they change from a form with two complete "mouth parts" to a form with only a single mouth part. That by itself is not so strange, but during this conversion process a configuration with three mouth parts occasionally appears. Trainor's mathematical model of the morphogenetic field explains "why 3 is between 2 and 1," making detailed predictions about the location and orientation of the mouth parts. Trainor has also used biological fields to gain insight into regeneration in the salamander, a creature with a spectacular ability to regrow its legs and tail. This research shows that fields can describe and even predict biological patterns, making them an exciting part of the new biology.[33]

One of the most prominent advocates of the morphogenetic field concept has been the maverick British biologist Rupert Sheldrake. His popular book *A New Science of Life* generated a lively debate when it was published in 1981. An editorial in the British science journal *Nature* was titled "A Book for Burning?," illustrating the radical character of his ideas. He has even discussed his ideas before a United States Congressional Clearinghouse on the Future. *A New Science of Life* and his subsequent book *The Presence of the Past* present an elaborate vision of the morphogenetic field concept. Sheldrake's organizing fields shape living and non-living forms ranging from protein structure to the shape of individual organisms as well as behavioral patterns, instinct, and learning. They also evolve and influence each other through a kind of resonance, a fundamental connection across space and time.

This "morphic" resonance, as Sheldrake calls it, is an important feature of his morphogenetic field model. An organism's field is connected across space and time to those fields that bear the most similarity and the more often a pattern occurs in nature, the more likely it will occur in the future. Because of morphic resonance between similar patterns of behavior and learning, as rats in one location learn to negotiate a maze, rats in another locality will then find it easier to negotiate the same maze.[34]

Biological field research is still in its early stages, and Sheldrake's effort is more speculation than science. Yet the idea of organizing fields associated with living systems has interesting implications for health and healing. Can one person help heal another with prayer because of the morphic resonance between their fields? Can healing take place, even without actual physical contact, through the interaction of the human bio-field?

Electricity and Magnetism in the New Biology

Now there is evidence that it is the informational aspect of biological systems that characterizes the essential view of life. And this is less reflected by biochemical findings but rather by a level beyond the domain of chemical reactivity, namely that of electromagnetic fields. Within the framework of electromagnetic bioinformation a basic explanation of biological processes, e.g., communication, health, aging, cancer, biological rhythms, regulation, and biochemical control may be found and not just their description.

—K. H. Li, *Electromagnetic Bioinformation*[35]

Since the discovery of electricity and magnetism, scientists have wondered what role, if any, they play in the organization of living systems. Italian physiologist Luigi Galvani (1737–1798), for example, spent many years studying "animal electricity," an electrical phenomena associated with the injury of tissue. Galvani was convinced that the biological electricity he observed was the long sought after vital force. But as the enthusiasm for vitalism waned, the idea that electricity might be relevant to biology fell out of favor. Even the electrical characteristics of the nerve signal were shown to result from the movement of charged ions (like sodium and potassium) across the nerve membrane.

In more modern times, the spectacular successes of chemical-based biology led to a pervasive view that any electromagnetic phenomena associated with living things were secondary to chemical events. Yet some scientists remained convinced of an important relationship between electromagnetism and biology. The Belgian scientist Georges Lakhovsky, for example, wrote *The Secret of Life* in the 1920s, in which he claimed that living things emit and receive electromagnetic radiation and that health was related to the oscillatory equilibrium of living cells.

Electromagnetic technologies improved as the twentieth century progressed and more scientists, especially in the former Soviet Union, became interested in bioelectromagnetic research. The Russian scientist A. S. Presman discussed the results of hundreds of experiments in his 1968 book *Electromagnetic Fields and Life*. Presman concluded that electromagnetic fields were important biologically. Organisms, he argued, could use fields for gaining information about their environment, for integration and regulation, or for communication with other organisms. Since the publication of Presman's book, more has been learned about all three of these bioelectromagnetic phenomena.

Organisms ranging from bacteria and bees to salmon, pigeons, and dolphins use the earth's magnetic field for navigation, a feat which they seem to accomplish with the help of a built-in magnetic "compass." Joseph Kirschvink, a scientist at the California Institute of Technology, explains the interaction between magnetic fields and organisms in terms of a special cellular structure containing magnetic material of biological origin. Kirschvink's group even announced in 1992 the discovery of magnetic particles in the human brain.

W. Ross Adey, another California-based scientist, has studied the role played by electromagnetic fields in cellular communication, describing cellular electromagnetic signals as the "whispering" of cells. Adey describes bioelectromagnetics as one of the most significant new scientific frontiers of this century and is quick to criticize other scientists for dismissing the biological importance of electromagnetic fields. He stresses that progress in understanding bioelectromagnetic regulation and communication will come from work on the highly cooperative nature of living systems using nonlinear, non-equilibrium concepts.

The German scientist F. A. Popp has explored the electromagnetic waves given off by living organisms—called biophotons by Popp. The conventional view holds that these electromagnetic waves are by-products of chemical reactions and of no biological importance. Popp, in contrast, feels that biophotons act as regulatory signals, controlling phenomena ranging from cell differentiation and growth to the activity of enzymes and the immune system.

Robert Becker, an American orthopedic surgeon interested in healing processes, picked up where Galvani (and others) had left off in their work on the relationship of electrical currents to injury. Beginning in the 1960s, Becker explored, in several decades of brilliant experimental work, the basic processes associated with healing and regeneration. He (re)discovered the electrical current generated in injured tissue and went on to describe a "second" nervous system, more primitive but more fundamental than the nerve impulse system. Becker found that very weak electrical currents could affect a cell's DNA, stimulating a phenomenon called dedifferentiation. (All the cells in the body have the same genetic information. Some genes are turned on and others off to produce particular kinds of cells—"specialized" cells like skin cells or liver cells. This is called differentiation. In dedifferentiation, specialized cells revert back to their more primitive, undifferentiated state. Interestingly, Becker's work on dedifferentiation foreshadowed the recent success in cloning, a controversial biotechnology which made use of dedifferentiation stimulated in part by electricity.)

Bioelectromagnetics, despite a long history, has only recently coalesced into an important field of study, one that will play a prominent role in the new biology. As suggested by the preliminary work of pioneering scientists like Becker, Popp, and Adey, electromagnetic phenomena are an important part of the regulatory and communication systems in organisms.[36]

The Medicine of Complexity

From the point of view of the new biology, each human is a unique and complex system with a network of internal and external interactions. Each organ system affects every other organ system. Mind and body are mutually interacting facets of a dynamic whole linked with the social and physical environments, themselves complex systems at another level. Disease—a disruption in the mind-body system—can at times be described and successfully treated in terms of narrowly defined causes and specific cures. This model has been particularly successful with infectious disease, allowing disease-causing microbes to be effectively treated with "magic bullet" antibiotics. This approach has proven less valuable for chronic diseases such as cancer and coronary heart disease, two of the plagues of modern industrial civilization.

Conventional medicine has searched for the cause of coronary heart disease by examining the biomolecular processes involved, and has centered much of its attention on the cholesterol molecule. A number of drugs have been developed to lower the cholesterol level in the blood, and these drugs, together with techniques like bypass surgery, have been used with limited success to treat the disease.

As a medical student in Houston, Texas, Dean Ornish became discouraged by what he saw as "the limitations of technological approaches that literally and figuratively *bypassed* the underlying causes of the problem." Instead, he looked for more fundamental causes of heart disease and found research suggesting many factors were involved. A high fat and high cholesterol diet could increase blood cholesterol, something that was widely implicated in the development of heart disease, and stress, smoking, and (lack of) exercise were other clearly important factors. It was surprising to Ornish that no one had studied whether a program combining potentially positive lifestyle changes could affect the processes underlying heart disease.[37]

Ornish developed a comprehensive program combining dietary change (see Chapter 8), stress management, exercise, smoking cessation, and group support. He borrowed many elements of his program from ancient Indian yoga, incorporating yoga-based techniques of relaxation, visualization, and meditation as used by modern researchers like Herbert Benson, Jon Kabat-Zinn, and Carl Simonton. Program participants stretched, meditated, and ate their way to health.

Ornish's results were very impressive. Over 80 percent of program participants showed an actual *reversal* of their coronary artery blockage and the more rigorously they followed the program the greater the improvement. Data suggested that all parts of the program are important, but according to Ornish each participant might benefit more from some parts than others. Stress management might be very important for someone with a high-stress life; dietary change might be crucial for someone else with a history of poor eating habits.

Ornish emphasizes the importance of taking a multi-factorial perspective. Cholesterol is an important part of the heart disease puzzle, but by itself it does not form the whole picture. The same thing can be said about blood pressure, smoking, and exercise. Ornish was surprised his research demonstrated little link between change in blood cholesterol level and improvement in arterial blockage, but explains that cholesterol is simply not *the* critical factor because other factors—such as stress, poor social support, and negative emotions—also play a significant part in the development of coronary heart disease. "The farther back in the causal chain of events we can address a problem," says Ornish, "the more powerful the healing can be."[38]

Ornish is not averse to conventional treatments and makes use of appropriate drugs and lifesaving measures when they are needed for the short term. Yet over the long term the goal is to activate the innate healing power by correcting the myriad factors that disrupt the system in the first place. Side effects from this approach are positive ones: participants lose weight, experience a decrease in blood pressure, and have more energy. Such success with a multi-factor model of cause and cure in dealing with an important chronic disease demonstrates that a "systems approach" can indeed be an effective means of medical therapy. In this interesting example of the new medicine, conventional treatments and the full power of science are combined with ancient insights into health and healing to create a comprehensive therapeutic regimen that is cost effective and empowering rather than invasive.

Like heart disease, cancer has also proven challenging. In the traditional model, cancer is an entity separate from the person with a specific cause and a specific cure. Despite the enormous amount of money spent to study cancer from this perspective, no specific cause has yet been found nor is there a magic bullet on the horizon. Like heart disease, many factors seem to be involved in the disease and the development of magic bullet cures is hampered by the difficulty of killing the cancer without harming the patient.

In a pessimistic 1997 study of cancer death rates, published in the *New England Journal of Medicine*, University of Chicago researcher John Bailar concluded that little progress has been made in the treatment of the disease. "In 1986, we concluded that some 35 years of intense effort focused largely on improving treatment must be judged a qualified failure," claimed Bailar, adding "Now, with 12 more years of data and experience, we see little reason to change that conclusion."[39]

One group of researchers is working to forge a completely new approach to the cancer problem based on systems thinking. The team, led by Harvey Schipper at the University of Manitoba, argues it is time to throw out the old cancer model—a model that has been used for over one hundred years and one that has clearly reached its limits—and begin looking at the problem in a new way. Cancer is not composed of cells with any great difference from normal cells and trying to kill the cancer cells can even make the problem worse since invasive therapies depress the immune system.

Cancer is really a problem of cellular regulation and communication involving the interactions of a complex system. Cancer cells are normal cells that are not doing what they should. The problem is not the cancer itself but the distorted channels of regulation and communication. Rather than trying to kill cancer cells, the solution is to restore the natural regulatory environment so that the pathological growth processes that characterize cancer are brought back under normal control. This means a wider focus on both the cancer and its surrounding environment—what the researchers describe as "a complex, multi-component non-linear system." Rather than using cancer-killing drugs and radiation, this new approach is based on the use of agents designed to "reregulate" in the effort to reverse or at least stabilize the pathological, unregulated processes that characterize the illness.

Critics of organicism have often argued that it is nothing more than a different way of talking about complex physical and chemical machines. Organicism might be philosophically appealing, but it does not lead to anything distinct from the mechanism model. Yet as Ornish's work on heart disease shows, thinking about the complex interactions of humans themselves, rather than just the molecules, can lead to success in the treatment of disease. And Shipper and his colleagues make it clear that the real breakthrough in cancer research might simply be thinking about the problem in a new way: "We now have data that suggest a subtler paradigm based on cellular and intercellular communication and biologic control. The upshot will be an approach to cancer that is distinctly different from that to microbial and viral diseases, in which we recognize an intruder and kill it. In the case of cancer, we may come to recognize aberrancy in our normal self and reassert control."[40]

Technological medicine is a mixture of miracle and muddle, promise and peril. Within this contradiction it is possible to celebrate the accomplishments of Western medicine while acknowledging limitations that both engender the evolution of its theories and therapies and leave room for complementary approaches. As a new biology and medicine eclipses the old, progress will come from looking at problems in fresh ways while building on the accomplishments of the past—accomplishments of both technological medicine and other ancient and evolving traditions.

5 | Exploring the Cosmic Tapestry: Chinese Medicine and the New Biology

There is a web of relationships throughout the universe, the nodes of which are things and events. Nobody wove it, but if you interfere with its texture you do so at your peril....[W]e shall be able to trace the later developments of this web woven by no weaver, this Universal Pattern, until we reach, with the Chinese, something approaching a developed philosophy of organism.

—Joseph Needham, *The Grand Titration*[1]

In their book *Between Heaven and Earth: A Guide to Chinese Medicine*, Harriet Beinfield and Efrem Korngold offer a metaphor to compare Eastern and Western medicine, describing the doctor of the West as a mechanic and the doctor of the East as a gardener. These TCM practitioners stress the vast chasm between Western and traditional Chinese medicine, and their complementary nature: "What works in the garden may be inappropriate in the factory. Compost doesn't nourish a machine, and oil and gasoline do not enhance the soil. Chinese medicine readjusts balance, enhancing self-healing and helping chronic, long-term problems. Western medicine affects the structural components, suppressing and eliminating pathologic phenomena, intervening in life-threatening crises."[2]

It is valuable to view Eastern and Western medicine as complementary systems, but there is another interesting perspective. While Chinese medicine has little in common with conventional Western medicine, its conceptual framework and therapeutic perspective share common ground with the new biology. As scientists work to push forward our understanding of living systems, they are offering insights that parallel more ancient insights from the East.

The organismic, systems thinking that permeates the new biology resonates deeply with the Chinese conception of the organism and its environment. Systems thinking is central to the theoretical framework of Chinese medicine, leading to concrete, practical medical intervention. In East and West, organism and environment as well as mind and body are seen as intimately interlinked facets of a complex, multilevel network. The search for health and healing takes place in the context of such interconnections, both the internal relationships that define an organism's organizational pattern and its external relationships with its environment. The Way or Tao of healing is a re-stitching of distorted threads in the universal pattern—the internal and external web of relationships that defines the human organism.

The parallels between Chinese medicine and the new biology range from the emphasis on process and pattern that is part of the new biology and a mainstay of Chinese medicine to the mind, which in the new biology as in Chinese medicine is an inseparable facet of the organizational processes of living systems.

Chinese Thought and the Not-So-New Physics

Contraria Sunt Complementa
(Opposites are complementary.)
—Inscription on Niels Bohr's coat-of-arms.

It was physics that gave birth to the mechanical world view so central to science. Physics was also the first to shift away from a mechanical to an organic universe, when, a century ago, Newton's physics began to fail. Scientists found that small things did not behave as they should. Electrons were waves at time, particles at others and measurements of atomic phenomena revealed discontinuous jumps—called quanta—rather than smoothly varying values.

While the new theories of quantum mechanics and relativity—crafted by some of the greatest thinkers of all time including Dane

Niels Bohr, German Werner Heisenberg, Austrian Erwin Schrödinger, and German-born American Albert Einstein—could successfully describe this strange world, it was a world turned upside down and inside out. Space and time did not constitute an absolute and universal reality, but were shaped by the observer. The material "stuff" of the world appeared not as substantive and immutable, but as nodes of coalescence in an indeterminate dance of potential and being.

This new conception of the world resonated in many ways with that of the Chinese. Niels Bohr, for example, was knighted in 1947 for his accomplishments. He chose for his coat-of-arms the Latin inscription "opposites are complementary" together with the Chinese symbol representing the dynamic relationship between yin and yang. Bohr had visited China a decade earlier and came to appreciate the Chinese dualism in relation to his own concept of complementarity.[3]

Complementarity helped Bohr reconcile contradictions in atomic behavior. Classical physics was familiar with particles and with waves, but electrons were both, sometimes displaying a wave nature and sometimes acting like a particle. Worse still was the fact that, as Werner Heisenberg demonstrated with his uncertainty principle, it was only possible to know about one or the other of these aspects with any certainty. Bohr felt that the electron's wave and particle natures were complementary facets of reality, each incomplete without the other, and that complementarity was a general principle that could be widely applied, even outside of physics.

Joseph Needham, too, often pointed to a fundamental congruence between the cosmologies of East and West. He compared the ideas of modern physics with those of the Neo-Confucian philosophers, who described the universe in terms of a pair of concepts, *tai ji* and *wu ji*, borrowed from Confucianism and Taoism. (Neo-Confucianism was a grand synthesis of Taoist, Confucian, and Buddhist ideas in the eleventh and twelfth centuries.) *Tai ji* was the fundamental pivot or great basis of the universe; *wu ji* described the fact that this organizational focus was without form or any relationship to space.

As Needham put it, these Neo-Confucian concepts described an "immanent power informing the wholeness of the universe, and present everywhere within it." There is a universal pattern or field which shapes the dynamics of matter-energy, a pattern inseparable from that which it shapes. "[O]ne cannot but admit," wrote Needham, "that the Sung [dynasty] philosophers were working with concepts not unlike some of those which modern science uses....Here again the Chinese shot an arrow close to the spot where Bohr and Rutherford were later to stand, without ever attaining to the position of Newton."[4] (Ernest Rutherford was a British physicist who played a key role in the early study of atomic phenomena.)

Physicist Fritjof Capra was the first to systematically explore parallels between Eastern thought and modern physics. In his book *The Tao of Physics*, Capra convincingly chronicled an underlying world view shared by the mystical East and the materialistic West under the influence of modern physics. Fundamental to this shared world view is a sense of the "basic oneness of the universe." In the East, all things are perceived as parts of a cosmic whole, distinct and differentiated in outward appearance yet reflections of a greater unifying reality. Similarly, in the quantum theory particles are not independent and distinct. According to Bohr: "Isolated material particles are abstractions, their properties being definable and observable only through their interaction with other systems."[5]

Another central feature of this common world view is the inherently dynamic nature of the Universal Pattern. All phenomena—the myriad things of the world—are in constant transformation, growing and decaying, manifesting and disappearing. The Chinese expressed this most profoundly in the *Book of Changes* or *I Ching*, the great Confucian Classic. While words cannot be found to describe the Tao, which is formless and boundless, it is through the dynamic relationship between yin and yang—the polar opposites that emerge from the undifferentiated Tao—that the various things of the world come into being.

In the *I Ching*, broken and solid lines are used to represent yin (broken) and yang (solid). These lines are combined in sets of three to create eight "trigrams" which are further paired to produce sixty-four "hexagrams." Each of the hexagrams, symbolic representations of archetypal patterns of change, is discussed in the *I Ching*, making it a guide for understanding. Change is not random and chaotic, but patterned. Just as yin and yang represent the dynamic relationship between polar opposites like day and night and hot and cold, the trigrams and hexagrams, complex arrangements of sets of yin and yang, offer insight into the greater richness and complexity of the world. By deeply understanding these patterns of change one can successfully follow the Tao.

Capra compares the *I Ching*, with its emphasis on patterns of change, to the S-matrix theory of modern physics. S-matrix theory, based on the S-matrix originally devised by Werner Heisenberg, combines quantum theory and relativity to describe subatomic particle behavior. The theory does not center on the particles themselves, but on their interaction. Particles are not things, but processes in four-dimensional space-time. As Heisenberg emphasized: "The world thus appears as a complicated tissue of events, in which connections of different kinds alternate or overlap or combine and thereby determine the texture of the whole."[6]

In *The Tao of Physics* Capra notes the similarity between East and West: "Because of its notion of dynamic patterns, generated by change and transformation, the *I Ching* is perhaps the closest analogy to S-matrix theory in Eastern thought. In both systems, the emphasis is on processes rather than objects. In S-matrix theory, these processes are the particle reactions that give rise to all the phenomena in the world of hadrons. (Hadrons are strongly interacting particles, including protons and neutrons.) In the *I Ching*, the basic processes are called 'the changes' and are seen as essential for an understanding of all natural phenomena...."[7]

The *Book of Changes* also reflects another Eastern idea that strikes a chord with modern physics. In conventional science, things behave the way they do because of distinct and discernable causes. By knowing the motion of all the bumper cars on the track, for example, it is possible to predict the path of any one car as it gets tossed and jolted by other cars. Yet for the Chinese philosopher and modern physicist a world of interconnection and interdependence is not governed by simple bumper car cause and effect.

For the Chinese, things behave the way they do because of their relationship to the whole. There is a "resonance" between seemingly separate parts of the universe, parts that nonetheless connect with each other through their roles as correlating parts of a greater pattern. (Resonance is a well-known phenomena in physics. By placing a tube that "likes" to vibrate at a particular frequency next to a tuning fork with the same frequency, for example, a loud sound will result from matching the vibratory nature of tuning fork and tube.)

A fifth-century text discussed the *Book of Changes*: "Mr. Yin, a native of Chinchow, once asked a Taoist monk, 'What is really the fundamental idea of the *Book of Changes*?' The monk answered, 'The fundamental idea of the *I Ching* can be expressed in one single word, resonance.' Mr. Yin then said, 'We are told that when the Copper Mountain collapsed in the west, the bell Ling Chung responded, by resonance, in the East. Would this be according to the principles of the *Book of Changes*?' The monk laughed and gave no answer to this question."[8]

The Einstein-Podolsky-Rosen (EPR) experiment illustrates the fundamental and acausal connection between particles seen in modern physics. Electrons have a property called spin and in the EPR experiment two electrons are created, one with spin "up" and the other spin "down." In quantum physics, these electrons are not in a fixed state of spin, but have probabilities that, if they are measured, the spin would be found to be either up or down. (Sixty percent of the time up, and forty percent of the time down, for example.) But with the electron pair, if one should be found to be up, the other automatically will be down. And this occurs no matter how great the separation between the two electrons.

The EPR experiment was, and still is, deeply disturbing to some physicists, Einstein among them. They argued that since information can travel only as fast as the speed of light, there is no way for the second electron to "know" that the first electron was measured and found to be in a particular state. The ability of the second electron to match, instantaneously, the measurement of the first electron—by being "up" when the other was "down," or vice versa—comes from what is called a "non-local" connection. Conventional cause and effect does not seem to be operating. Mysteriously, one part of the universe is intimately aware of what another part is doing. Here, in the field of ideas, there is resonance between East and West.

Chinese Medicine and the New Biology

The Philosophy of Organism East and West

> The gigantic historical paradox remains that although Chinese civiliza-
> tion could not spontaneously produce 'modern' natural science, natural
> science could not perfect itself without the characteristic philosophy of
> Chinese civilization.
>
> —Joseph Needham, Science and Civilization in China[9]

In the new biology, the universe is conceived as a hierarchy of organisms. Each whole, or organism, is composed of parts, which are in turn organisms at another level. Properties and characteristics emerge at each level of organization from the interactions and relationships between the parts. In this web-like world of scale, organisms gain identity as much from their role as parts of a greater whole as does the whole display characteristics derived from its parts.

Subatomic particles form atoms, which form molecules and crystals. Complex molecules organize into cells which merge into multicellular organisms. With complex organisms, mind emerges and individuals become parts in a system of social organization. Imagine the levels—higher and lower—in which you are embedded: the planetary ecosystem and society, organs, cells, and molecules.

These levels of organization and complexity evolve over time. Through the epochs of evolutionary time molecules emerged before cells, single-celled creatures before their multicellular progeny, and mentally challenged fish existed before cognitively developed primates. Seen in this way, evolution is a process of increasing complexity and rising levels of organization.

Alfred North Whitehead, the great philosopher of the organismic world view, pointed to the relationship between the part and the whole and the illusory tension between complementary facets of reality. For Whitehead, the universe was both eternal and transient, physical and mental, concrete and intangible: "The Universe is *many* because it is wholly and completely to be analyzed into many final actualities....The Universe is *one*, because of the universal immanence. There is thus a dualism in this contrast between the unity and multiplicity. Throughout the Universe there reigns the union of opposites which is the ground of dualism."[10]

The Eastern world view is also an organic one, with a hierarchy of levels and a dualism between the part and the whole that is resolved by a union of opposites. According to the Taoist Classic, the *Tao Te Ching*: "The way conceals itself in being nameless. It is the way alone that excels in bestowing and in accomplishing. The way begets one; one begets two; two begets three; three begets the myriad creatures. The myriad creatures carry on their backs the *yin* and embrace in their arms the *yang* and are the blending of the generative forces of the two."[11]

Like modern systems thinkers, the Neo-Confucians conceived of a hierarchy of levels of organization, each with unique characteristics. Li, the immanent and universal pattern of organization, shapes the qi at each level and in this way the microcosm reflects the macrocosm. The division between mind and matter that has often frustrated Western civilization bypassed the Chinese. Mind and other seemingly non-material phenomena like human values simply arise at the appropriate level of complexity and organization. As the great philosopher Chu Hsi described, mind is inherent in matter: "Cognition or apprehension is the essential pattern of the mind's existence, but that there is something in the world which can do this is what we may call the spirituality inherent in matter."[12]

Joseph Needham, who discussed the relationship between Chinese thought and Western organic materialism extensively in his mammoth *Science and Civilization in China* series, points to a technical term for "level of organization" in Neo-Confucian theory.[13] The existence of different levels of organization, each with characteristic properties, is seen in physics and in medicine. Large things, such as cars and rocks and pendulums, can be described by Newtonian equations of motion. On the other hand, small things, like atoms and subatomic particles, require quantum mechanical equations. Chemistry emerges from physics at yet another level of organization. Disease can be viewed at the level of the society, the person, and the molecule—and all three intricately interwoven levels offer valuable insights. Chinese medicine sets its gaze on the pattern of organization of the person, while conventional Western medicine is focused to a large extent on the level of the molecule.

Needham, in his titillating titration of ideas East against West, claims it was necessary that science went through the mechanical phase brought forth by Newton. But it was also necessary for the organic world view—brought to its greatest point of development by Alfred North Whitehead—to emerge in the twentieth century as a means of resolving the irreconcilable conflicts, whether vitalism versus mechanism or mind versus matter. He also makes a startling suggestion about the origin of the organic world view upon which the new biology is based.

Whitehead helped to perfect the organismic world view, but he did not invent it. Its origins can be traced back along a continuous thread of Western thought to an often forgotten figure in the history of Western science and philosophy, the great Baron Gottfried Wilhelm von Leibnitz (1646–1716). Leibnitz, a contemporary and arch-enemy of Newton, developed an organic philosophy based on "monads"— fundamental "organisms," not particles, of the universe—which like the Neo-Confucian world view kept spirit grounded in matter.

Leibnitz, Needham shows, was deeply interested in Chinese philosophy and science and made a study of Eastern thought through his contact with Jesuits and others who were at the time opening a dialogue with the East. Tracing this Eastern influence on Leibnitz's thinking, Needham raises a fascinating possibility: "Perhaps the theoretical foundations of the most modern 'European' natural science owe more to [great Chinese philosophers] such as Chuang Chou, Chou Tun-I, and Chu Hsi than the world has yet realized."[14]

The rivalry between Newton and Leibnitz reached its zenith over the calculus. The two men simultaneously invented this revolutionary mathematical method, but Newton used his position to bolster his own priority and attack the Baron's claim to originality and accomplishment. Perhaps the final irony for Newton—who as we have seen did not feel comfortable with the mechanical world view that he played such a large part in founding—is that his great rival Baron von Leibnitz was responsible for the conceptual germ that gave birth to the mechanically transcending organic world view. Leibnitz, it seems, had the very answer that Newton sought in his alchemical diversions.

From Particles to Processes

In the Chinese system, the Organs are discussed always with reference to their functions and to their relationships with the Fundamental Substances, other Organs, and other parts of the body. Indeed, it is only through these relationships that an organ can be defined.
    —Ted Kaptchuk, *The Web That Has No Weaver*[15]

All the systems concepts discussed…can be seen as different aspects of one great strand of systemic thinking, which we may call contextual thinking. There is another strand of equal importance….The second strand is process thinking….In systems science every structure is seen as the manifestation of underlying processes. Systems thinking is always process thinking.
    —Fritjof Capra, *The Web of Life*[16]

In both Chinese medicine and the new biology there is an emphasis on the web of relationships that link part and whole. Understanding parts, and the wholes they comprise, requires a sense of context, of framing the connections and relationships that shape a given level of organization. This contextual thinking has emerged most strongly in ecology, which by its very definition is the study of the relationships between organisms and their environment. Trees cannot be fully understood without accounting for the living and non-living systems they are intimately linked with. Endangered species cannot be protected without considering their habitat.

Systems thinking combines an emphasis on context with a shift from substance to activity. Western science began with a material bias, always looking at structure—searching in physical science for the fundamental "stuff" of the universe and moving, in biological science, down the ladder of the "stuff of life" from tissue to cell to molecule. Over time physical science has shifted its gaze from particle to process, from immutable things to dynamic events. As Needham put it: "This change of view, occupying four hundred years, may be characterized as the transition from Space and Matter as the fundamental notions, to Process conceived of as a complex of Activity with internal relations between its various factors."[17]

Mirroring the shift in physical science, the new biology sees complex living things as systems built up from a web of processes. In his book *The Web of Life: A New Scientific Understanding of Living Systems*, Fritjof Capra emphasizes that systems thinking is process thinking and that the structures in living systems arise from the patterns of organization of underlying processes. From the systems perspective, genetic information is set in the complex patterns of biochemical organization comprising a living system. The way in which genetic information is interpreted and utilized is shaped by the patterns of biochemical organization which are in turn shaped by an organism's relationship with its environment.

The processes at one level of organization are interlinked and embedded with those at higher and lower levels. We are not, as humans, ultimately selfish strands of DNA. We are a highly organized pattern of complex processes—involving both mental and physical phenomena—shaped by environmental influence in its broadest sense. These processes maintain, interpret, and copy our genetic information, and are at the same time direct reflections of our genetic self.[18]

This systems perspective, with its attention to levels of organization and its emphasis on processes, is having an impact in areas ranging from ecology to cancer. Ecologists study basic processes—such as the cycles of nutrients and water—that link living and non-living systems into a larger whole: the ecosystem. Leading-edge cancer researchers argue that tumors should not be seen as "things"—distinct entities separate from its host. Rather, cancer is a regulatory process gone astray, a complex system involving malignant cells and their milieu.

Western understanding of traditional Chinese medicine is challenged by the different approach used in the East. By the later part of the nineteenth century, Western medicine had acquired considerable anatomical knowledge. Together with aseptic surgical procedures and anesthetics, surgery became a successful and viable enterprise. Chinese medicine, by contrast—through, among other things, a cultural bias against dissection and surgery—had not developed such surgical skills and did not possess the same kind of detailed anatomical knowledge. In this light, the Chinese system was often seen as primitive and ineffectual.

While the Chinese achieved only a basic anatomical understanding, they were more interested in process than structure. Chinese medicine uses a process-centered description of the physiological and psychological landscape. The "organs" themselves are not defined anatomically, but in terms of functional groupings that include physical and mental processes. These mind-body "orbs" link the physical substrates usually thought of as organs in Western anatomy with other organs, parts of the body, basic substances, mental and emotional phenomena, and the meridian network.[19]

When minister Qi Bo, in conversation with the Yellow Emperor, describes the outer appearance of the liver, it is clear the "liver" is more than its anatomical namesake: "The liver causes utmost weariness and is the dwelling place of the soul, or spiritual part of man that ascends to Heaven. The liver influences the nails and is effective upon the muscles; it brings forth animal desires and vigor. The taste connected with the liver is sour and the color connected with the liver is green."[20]

This process-oriented and contextual view of the liver contrasts with an anatomically based perspective. The liver in Chinese medicine has a central function of "spreading and harmonizing." It is responsible for the free flow of qi, suggesting that a stagnation of qi anywhere in the body will involve the liver. Frustration and anger are psychological disharmonies involving the liver, which is also intimately linked to the gallbladder and the production of bile. The liver meridian connects the liver not only with the gallbladder but with the eyes. The liver has a close relationship to the nails and tendons and is the organ that stores the blood.

Functional, process-oriented understanding is also applied to therapy. Herbs and acupoints are described according to the psychosomatic processes they affect. There are herbs that calm the spirit, herbs that strengthen qi, blood, yin and yang, and herbs that dry dampness, affecting the fluid metabolism aspects of different organs. *Fu ling*, for example, a white, chalk-like, subterranean mushroom that grows at the base of coniferous trees, supports the body's water metabolism function, particularly that part attributed to the spleen.

The collection of herbs in a formula or an acupuncture point prescription describes and addresses a patient's unique pattern of disharmony. The functions of the herbs or points match the systemic dysfunctions of the person. Blood deficiency affecting the liver with blurry vision, dry eyes, and a touch of irritability—a pattern based on the liver's relationship to the blood, the eyes, and the emotions of irritability and anger—is matched by the "four things soup" augmented with the fruit of the matrimony vine (called *gou qi zi* in Chinese).

The four things soup is a base prescription for strengthening blood, while *gou qi zi*, a vibrant red and tasty berry, supports the yin aspect of the liver and kidneys and "brightens" the eyes in cases of blood deficiency. The third point of the liver meridian, *tai chong* or "great surge," also supports the liver yin and could be used as a part of a prescription to complement the herbal treatment.

The traditional Chinese system of medicine centers on five fundamental groups of processes, symbolically represented by the five phases. The earth phase, with its yin organ spleen, encompasses the digestive process. Metal, representing lung, includes the respiratory process, while wood, with its corresponding organ liver, describes an orb of functions embracing physiological and emotional regulation and the storage of blood. Water, with the yin organ kidney, encompasses water metabolism, storage of *jing*, and control of growth, reproduction, and development, while fire, with the heart, includes circulation.

In some cases, the yin organ's corresponding yang organ offers direct functional support. The stomach supports the spleen in the process of digestion, the gallbladder and liver are closely linked in the storage and secretion of bile, and the bladder works together with the kidney in water metabolism. In other cases the yin and yang organs are symbolically or "energetically" linked (in the sense of connection between meridians) as with the lung and large intestine and the heart and small intestine. The intestines are usually considered in the context of their role in the digestive process.[21]

In Chinese medicine, qi is synonymous with the functions and activities comprising these fundamental processes. Food is churned and "prepared" by the action of stomach qi. *Wei* or protective qi offers defense against invading pathogens and regulates the sweat glands. Heart qi moves the blood. Spleen qi keeps the organs in their proper place. And kidney qi transforms and eliminates fluids.

Qi is also the link between mind and body. In meditation, qi follows the concentration of the mind. By concentrating on one's hands, for example, qi will follow *yi* or consciousness. Because of the close relationship between qi and blood, blood flow to the hands will increase and the hands will become warmer. As a contemporary Chinese manual on healing exercise describes, through the special breathing exercise and meditation known as qi gong, mind and qi are brought together to nourish health: "In practicing qi gong, you must integrate the training of *yi*, your consciousness, with the training of qi, regulating your respiration. You must learn how to direct the movement of qi with your consciousness....Through conditioning, you will ultimately be able to lead or follow the movement of qi with *yi*."[22]

Emotions are intertwined with qi. According to the Yellow Emperor: "With anger the qi rises; with joy the qi becomes loose or moderate; with grief the qi disappears, with fear the qi descends...with thinking the qi knots or becomes stagnant."[23] These emotional patterns are correlated with the fundamental processes—anger with wood and hence liver, for example. (See Chapter 1.) The qi flowing in the liver meridian is a pattern of organizing "energy" intertwined with the emotions of frustration and anger as well as with the physiological functions associated with the liver "orb." Too much anger can affect the liver, and in a circular fashion, a poorly functioning liver suggests a predisposition to anger. In this way, the human mind-body system is a complex pattern of organization out of which arises the substantial body with its processes and structures—and the non-material mind. It is not simply that the mind affects the body and the body affects the mind, but that both arise as manifestations of the same organizing activity.

Searching for the Source

In conventional Western medicine and biology the brain is considered to be the control center of the body and mind is equated with the chemical events that take place in the brain. In Chinese medicine, the brain is considered a curious organ, the "sea of marrow," considered and treated largely in relation to the major "organs," particularly the kidneys. While the great Li Shi-zhen noted a connection between consciousness and the brain, Chinese medicine considers many aspects of mind in relation to other organs.[24] The heart is the storehouse of *shen*, or spirit. Mental agitation, clouded and disturbed thinking, and insomnia might be part of a heart disharmony. Depression and uncontrolled anger might be treated as a liver disharmony, while poor memory and declining mental capacity might reflect a declining kidney function and its failure to nourish the marrow. The ability to make decisions is dependent on a healthy gallbladder.[25]

The center or source of this system of psychological and physical processes in Chinese medicine is not the brain, but the "moving qi between the kidneys," an area in the abdomen between the kidneys and below the navel. The hara, as the fundamental pivot is called in Japanese, is the "energetic" source of the body. Here, the qi absorbed from breathing and eating combines with *jing* and prenatal qi from the kidneys to produce the basic energy that nourishes life.

In their book *Hara Diagnosis: Reflections on the Sea*, Kiiko Matsumoto and Stephen Birch describe the importance of this energetic center in Oriental medicine: "We see the hara as the place where many essential energetic functions occur. It is the residence of basic qi, that energy that precedes yin and yang, fire and water. It is the meditative center, the driving force of the pulse, the center of meridian circulation, and it plays a powerful role in classical nutrition theory."[26]

At first glance this Chinese view seems diametrically at odds with Western biology. Yet new biological research is beginning to offer support for the Chinese view that the brain is not necessarily synonymous with the mind, nor is it the clear command and control center of the body. Despite many years of working to map the mind in the brain, scientists find that the brain is "plastic." Areas of the brain responsible for a specific function can sometimes be damaged with no apparent effect.

After working for centuries to break the body into distinct and separate components, it is now appearing that boundaries are an illusion. Recent research demonstrates the intimate connection between the central nervous system, the immune system, and the endocrine system. The activity of the brain and nervous system, for example, is regulated by neuropeptides, chains of protein that are found throughout the body. These neuropeptides are so strongly connected to emotions that one scientist working in the area states flatly that emotions *are* neuropeptides. "Emotions," claims neuropeptide expert Candace Pert, "are neuropeptides attaching to receptors and stimulating an electrical change on neurons."[27]

It is fascinating that these biochemicals—strong correlates to emotion as they are—are found throughout the body and produced by everything from the spleen and stomach to the bone marrow and thymus. The mind, it appears, is not only "in" the brain, but distributed throughout the body. Emotions are intimately linked to the organs and the brain appears to be controlled by other parts of the body as much as it controls them. The brain is an important communications station, but it may not be *the* command and control center. As an article on the brain in *National Geographic* put it: "Some new truths are not as new as they seem. The flow of substances between our brain and body seems like a radical idea, but for 4,000 years Chinese medicine has said that control over the brain rests with the liver, heart, spleen, lungs, and kidneys."[28]

Proto-Cybernetics

For several months Wally was bothered by recurring "attacks." He experienced sudden, severe headaches accompanied by nausea and loose bowels. His eyes became itchy and sore, and for the rest of the day he lost any desire for food. A TCM "checkup" revealed a strong, wiry liver pulse and weak, slippery spleen pulse. Wally's tongue was red on the sides with thicker-than-normal fur toward the center. Diagnosis: a pattern of "liver invading spleen"—and to some extent stomach.

Wally responded well to herbal treatment. He was initially given a prescription based on the formula "free wanderer powder" (*xiao yao san*) with additions including tribulus (*bai ji li*), a thorny pea-sized fruit used to calm liver wind and improve headache, sore eyes, and itching. After several visits and numerous herbal "brews," Wally was as good as new. Relieved to feel better, he had no reservations about quitting his double Scotch with lunch habit. His TCM practitioner felt that the hot, damp quality of the liquor, taken in excess, may have been a precipitating factor in his condition, aggravating the liver and weakening the spleen.

Wally's pattern of liver invading spleen illustrates the system-based framework of Chinese medicine where basic processes are not considered only in isolation, but viewed in relation to each other. Of particular interest here is the fact that various relationships between organs and physiological processes are described in terms of positive and negative feedback. The insight into patterns of disharmony like "liver invading spleen" or "wood invading earth" arises from the negative feedback cycle of five-phase theory. While the five phases are merely one model of physiological interaction set out in the Chinese system—sometimes useful and sometimes not—they illustrate the proto-cybernetics developed by the ancient Chinese.

Cybernetics—the study of control and communication in living and non-living systems—is an important part of modern systems thinking. And an important part of cybernetics is the concept of feedback, the circular network of signals that makes possible the self-regulation and organization of a system. Positive and negative feedback are found in everything from electronics and engineering to physiology. Negative feedback—like that used in thermostatic control—offers stability, while positive feedback can provide the impetus for change and evolution.

Interesting examples of feedback abound. The ocean current El Niño, for example, periodically flows along the pacific coast of South America. El Niño has a dramatic effect on the climate over a large part of the globe. Scientists do not yet understand this phenomenon fully, but claim that it arises through a complex network of positive and negative feedback between oceanic and atmospheric processes.

Positive feedback is an important part of the growth and evolution of ecosystems. Through positive feedback an ecosystem can figuratively pull itself up by its own bootstraps. Plants are highly dependent on soil—which is not simply "dirt" but a complex system of living and non-living components. Plants fuel the biological processes that take place in the soil and provide structural elements, the organic matter of the soil. These processes and structural elements nourish and support the growth of plants. This positive feedback between soil and plants allows the system to generate itself, fostering the very conditions upon which it thrives.[29]

James Lovelock's hypothesis that the Earth is a complex self-regulated system—Gaia theory—envisions the global environment being shaped by a network of interactions between living and non-living systems. Through feedback, living organisms help to produce, on a global scale, the very conditions upon which their life depends.

The Chinese were not only the first to conceive of the idea of feedback, but were also the first to invent a cybernetic machine: the south-pointing carriage. This fascinating contraption was a horse-drawn, two-wheeled wagon complete with differential gears and an "immortal," a figure from Chinese mythology, with an outstretched hand always pointing south. Using negative feedback, the driver could maintain a fixed direction of travel without a compass.[30]

The emergence of the concepts of positive and negative feedback was a natural evolution of the Chinese world view. The ancient Chinese universe was not built from linear cause and effect relationships (where A causes B, which causes C, etc.). Rather, theirs was a world of net-like interconnection, where things were connected rather than caused. In the kinds of complex, interacting systems now the object of investigation in systems science (where A affects B, B affects C and then C affects A) cause and effect blur, and the network of interactions determines the behavior of the whole. To the Chinese, the universe and its myriad contents was just such a system.

The Chinese went beyond simply breaking the universe up into five fundamental "processes" of earth, metal, water, wood, and fire. The five phases were arranged cyclically, creating a system with positive and negative feedback—the cycles of creation and control. Earth creates metal, metal creates water, water creates wood, wood creates fire, and fire creates earth to complete the cycle. Negative feedback stops the system from unending increase, for wood controls earth, earth controls water, water controls fire, fire controls metal, and, finally, metal controls wood to complete the cycle.

The five-phases model was applied to a range of natural and social phenomena. In medicine, the feedback and interaction conceptualized in the five-phase creation and control cycles help physicians recognize patterns of disharmony involving relationships between physiological processes. Wally's "liver invading spleen" pattern, for example, is a pathology of wood over-controlling earth, a pattern commonly seen in the TCM clinic. This kind of systems perspective forms the backbone of Chinese diagnosis and therapy, enabling the practitioner to recognize patterns of disharmony and re-establish equilibrium in the system.

Feedback cycles are also used to formulate treatment. Since, for example, earth nourishes metal, a lung deficiency (recall that lung corresponds to metal) can be treated by tonifying earth.[31] Or, instead of treating a liver deficiency directly, a physician may choose to nourish the kidney, the "mother," which will in turn nourish her "son" the liver. In Wally's case, the liver was soothed and regulated and the spleen strengthened through herbal treatment to address a disharmony in the control cycle of negative feedback.

Health: A Multi-Level Problem

A century ago, Louis Pasteur and Robert Koch set the tone for scientific medicine. These medical pioneers showed that diseases had specific causes that when uncovered could lead to specific cures. For Pasteur and Koch this meant searching for disease-generating microscopic organisms, together with ways of treating and protecting people from these deadly scourges.

After stunning success in tackling infectious disease, this basic model was broadly applied to illness of all kinds, infectious and degenerative, acute and chronic. Research has led to improved understanding and better treatment of many diseases, but the search

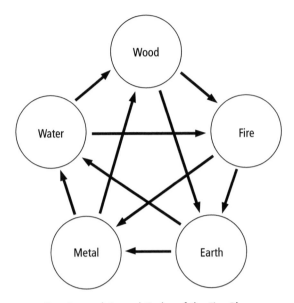

Creation and Control Cycles of the Five Phases

for specific causes has often floundered in a quagmire of complexity. Not all diseases are caused by microbes, making it necessary to search for causes in other areas.

Many researchers are focused on cause and cure at the molecular level. In this view, mental disorders are a problem of brain chemistry. Heart disease arises from faults in the molecular machinery that deal with fats, especially cholesterol metabolism. In its extreme, proponents of the molecular perspective argue that most non-infectious disease is simply "in the genes" and that the next medical revolution—gene therapy—will spell the end of sickness.[32]

Other researchers are exploring various features of individual behavior as the cause and cure, particularly with respect to the chronic, degenerative diseases that plague wealthy nations. In this view, health problems like hardening of the arteries are closely linked to the foods people eat, their level of activity, and the stress they experience. Dean Ornish, as has been previously discussed, has had spectacular success in reversing heart disease with his lifestyle modification program based on a diet comprised largely of vegetable-based foods, coupled with group support, appropriate exercise, and stress reduction.

Still others are focused on a level beyond that of the individual or the molecule. Many diseases, even infectious ones, emerge from broader social and environmental factors, such as poverty, nutrition, sanitation, community cohesion, and the growing number of toxins found in the modern environment. Andrew Pipe, a University of Ottawa cardiologist, notes that "poverty and childhood deprivation are distinct predictors of cardiovascular disease." Pipe laments that society can muster the resources to provide heart attack victims with paramedics, angiograms, and transplants, but so often neglects basic social needs that would have a much deeper effect on health. Even a year in a special educational support program, for example, can give inner city kids better opportunities—and better health.[33]

Public health researchers at Harvard University use the story of Roseto, Pennsylvania, to illustrate the powerful effect of community cohesion on health. The town was curiously blessed with an epidemic of good health. Even the heart attack rate was 40 percent below comparable towns where people ate the same foods, smoked, and exercised in the same way. The only thing that stood out about Roseto was its strong sense of community. As these community bonds eroded during the 1960s, the heart attack rate rose to a "normal" level.[34]

This powerful relationship between health and various personal, social, and environmental factors, together with the intractable nature of many illnesses like cancer, have encouraged some researchers to claim that the next revolution in medicine will be based on prevention, not cure. A *Scientific American* article, for example, pointed to a theoretically possible two-thirds reduction in cancer mortality with simple steps such as regular exercise, the ample consumption of fruits and vegetables, and the avoidance of tobacco and excessive alcohol consumption.[35] This emphasis on prevention resonates with Chinese medicine, which has for millennia noted that treating disease after it has already appeared is like starting to dig a well after becoming thirsty. (Eastern and Western perspectives on prevention are discussed in Chapter 6.)

The co-existence of different and powerful perspectives has created confusion about the cause of illness—and where to look for a cure. Was the captive polar bear that was cured of a behavioral problem with the popular antidepressant Prozac suffering from a chemical imbalance in the brain, or simply responding in a "normal" way to imprisonment in a city zoo? One newspaper reported that the growing rate of obesity amongst children—some 40 percent of 5 to 8 year olds in North America are now considered obese—was related to the fact that kids were watching more TV and playing more video games while taking part in less physical activity. But just to stifle confidence in a relationship between physical activity and weight, the paper reported on the same page a new Swedish study showing that weight problems were inherited. People cannot be blamed for their weight problems, the story suggested, it is simply something you are born with.[36]

Are health problems like obesity the fault of individual lifestyles or the result of faulty genes? Is heart disease a social problem, the result of defective molecular machinery, or the consequence of a rich diet and sedentary lifestyle? The answer is yes, all of the above.

From a systems perspective, these levels—molecular, individual, and social—are an embedded web. Molecules are organized into individuals, which themselves form societies. Individuals are shaped in part from the molecular template in the genetic material provided by their parents, and in part by the physical and social environment. While the individual plays a role in shaping society, so too the society shapes the individual. In this tightly woven web with no weaver, molecular patterns, lifestyle patterns, and social patterns can all be found with a relationship to health and disease.

At times, clear cause and effect relationships emerge from this interlaced nexus of organization. But such insights are limited and special cases. Indeed, there is no real reason to assume that every disease has a specific "cause." A central part of the new biology and medicine, then, is the challenge of overcoming several centuries of the method of breaking-things-down-into-pieces first articulated by Descartes. While Descartes' method has brought spectacular successes, its limitations are now clear and new, complementary approaches are needed.

Dean Ornish's multifactorial approach to heart disease acknowledges that many factors can influence the emergence of disease. And many factors can influence the healing process. Ornish's work shows us that psychological, social, and physical techniques can heal the person—and the disease. Stress reduction, group support, exercise, and dietary change can add up to a program with an effect greater than the sum of its parts.

The Cornell University nutritional scientist T. Colin Campbell argues that there is more to the relationship between diet and health than can be studied by looking only at single nutrients. He points to a "synergistic total diet effect" that may be hard to study, but is central to the ability of food to either prevent or cause disease. The starting point for nutritional research, according to Campbell, is the study of broader dietary patterns such as the relative proportion of foods of animal versus plant origin. The problem of fat, for example, is not just a question of fat. Lowering the amount of fat in the diet— a widely espoused goal—can be accomplished by using lower-fat animal products or by actually replacing many foods of animal origin with plant-based foods, resulting in different overall dietary patterns that may well have dramatically different consequences for health.[37]

The Power of Pattern

The concept of pattern has emerged as a powerful way of studying complex systems without breaking them into pieces. As biologist René Dubos suggested in the 1960s, humans are exceedingly complex, but do show patterns that can be studied in a scientific way. "Such patterns, however," warned Dubos, "can be recognized only if scientists devote to the study of man's responses to his environment the intellectual effort and technical skill they presently devote to the analysis of fragments isolated in a lifeless form."[38]

In the new biology the pattern of organization of a living system is distinct from its structure and defined as "the configuration of relationships among the system's components that determines the system's essential characteristics." Fritjof Capra uses the example of a bicycle to illustrate the distinction between pattern and structure. A bicycle's pattern of organization is the set of relationships among its components—wheels, pedals, frame, etc.—that combine to create an organized whole recognizable as a bicycle. Its structure is found in the actual physical components, made of specific metal or plastic in a specific way.[39]

Living systems, of course, are not constructed like a bicycle. They are self-organizing, able to repair themselves, and reproduce. Such patterns of organization have an evolutionary history, are dynamic rather than static, and are very sensitive to the surrounding environment.

One interesting example of the study of pattern in complex systems is fractal geometry. While some aspects of nature exhibit regular, defined geometrical shapes—such as a spherical tomato or cylindrical tree trunk—the forms of mountains, clouds, and trees, like much of nature, are more complex. Fractal geometry is a way of describing such complex, irregular patterns.

Fractal patterns repeat themselves on a series of scales. Break a piece from a head of cauliflower and it looks like the whole from which it came. Clouds and trees can be viewed from afar or with magnification to reveal the same pattern. In this way, the basic pattern of the whole is reflected in its parts or perhaps more correctly, there are not wholes but a hierarchy of scales. Many of the patterns seen in nature parallel fractal patterns generated by mathematicians.

Pattern is also a central concept in Chinese thought. Since the universe is conceived of as a vast web with no weaver, it is not possible to discern specific causes for particular actions. As Chuang Tsu describes, the body like the universe, is not a puppet responding to the tug on its strings but a self-organizing system: "It might seem as if there were a real Governor, but we find no trace of his being....But now the hundred parts of the human body...are all complete in their

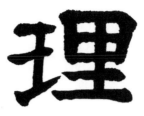

Li

places. Which should one prefer? Do you like them all equally? Or do you like some more than others? Are they all servants? Are these servants unable to control each other, but need another as ruler? Or do they become rulers and servants in turn? Is there any true ruler other than themselves?"[40]

The emphasis on pattern reached its zenith in the Neo-Confucian conception of *li*. *Li*, a character originally symbolizing the markings on jade, came to represent the organizing principle of the universe. Because of *li*, qi—the matter-energy—was shaped and the microcosm followed the macrocosm. *Li* was not an external law to be followed, but an innate, dynamic pattern that allowed things to follow their own nature as parts of a greater whole.

Pointing to the connection between *li* and modern organic philosophy, Needham goes as far as to suggest that *li* could prove a useful concept for modern science. There is not an ideal term to describe the order that appears at the various levels of organization, he claims, and *li*—the "pattern-principle" or "universal cosmic pattern, containing in itself all smaller and more limited patterns"—fits the bill.[41]

Pattern As a Healing Tool

The Chinese system of diagnosis and treatment is pattern-based. Like the fractal patterns studied by mathematicians, the pattern of the whole is reflected in the parts of the human body. The ear, radial pulse, and tongue, for example, all reflect the whole and are used to observe and guide the adjustment of the system's energetic configuration. By taking the pulse and observing the tongue, the Chinese physician discerns the state of the whole. Reflected in the ear is a miniature person, allowing the ear to be observed for signs of disharmony and treated with acupuncture to restore balance in distant, yet corresponding, parts.

The conceptual process of pattern recognition that leads to the choice of acupuncture points or herbal formula is in a sense the antithesis of the diagnostic process used in Western medicine. Western medicine takes a general problem and searches for a specific, underlying cause. A digestive complaint might be traced to a gallbladder problem or ulcer, for example. In Chinese medicine, the specific complaint or disease category is associated with a general pattern displayed by the patient. Single signs and symptoms themselves could be part of any of a number of patterns of disharmony. Each sign or symptom has meaning only in the context of the other information gathered by the physician.

Specific herbs or acupuncture points may be chosen to address a particular symptom, but it is the underlying pattern of disharmony that guides the therapeutic regimen. It is said in Chinese medicine that one disease has many treatments and that the same treatment can be used for different diseases. Advanced clinical manuals in Chinese medical specialties—like fu ke (gynecology) or nan ke (male urology)—describe the general patterns commonly observed for specific problems. Every TCM practitioner is familiar with these general patterns and so even new diseases like AIDS can be diagnosed and treated from within this same framework.

The eloquent exponent of Eastern medicine Ted Kaptchuk describes clearly this emphasis on pattern recognition: "The work of the Chinese physician...is to distinguish patterns...by recognizing the state of bodily disharmony within the domain of signs and symptoms. The process of Chinese medicine is the process of weaving together the elements and recognizing a pattern in myriad signs. For the Chinese, patterns are sufficient and are the ultimate guiding conception for diagnosis and treatment."[42]

In Chinese diagnosis, what is wrong? is not answered by describing a disease state, a part gone awry. It is answered by describing a pattern of disharmony of the mind-body system, the context of a part's misbehavior that provides the focus for therapeutic intervention. It is the pattern that is treated, not the disease, so that in restoring balance and harmony to the mind-body system the part regains its proper relationship to the whole. Healing takes place from within.

Specific health problems occur in the context of many different patterns. One clinical guidebook, for example, differentiates the problem of impotence into thirteen possible patterns ranging from deficient spleen with dampness to damp heat in the liver channel.[43] High blood pressure is commonly associated with five patterns, four involving the liver and kidney and one involving the spleen. These are only general tendencies observed in clinical practice and the pattern recognition process is highly individualized.[44]

This logical and systematic diagnostic approach leads to concrete ways of addressing disharmony. Dampness affecting the digestive system is resolved with herbs that help support the fluid metabolism aspect of digestion; lack of communication between the heart and kidney is treated by regulating the heart and kidney meridians with needles at *tai xi* (kidney 3) and *shen men* (Heart 7). Each treatment is formulated to suit the patient's precise signs and symptoms, and the herbal formula and/or point prescription are changed as the patient changes through the course of therapy.

Internal Milieu

A description of the body's "internal milieu" is an important part of pattern recognition. The Chinese attention to the internal milieu of the body—seen in the observation of damp and dry, hot and cold, and other qualities as internal conditions—mirrors the insights of the great nineteenth century physiologist Claude Bernard. Like the Chinese, Bernard recognized the interconnection between organism and environment. "Life is the result of a conflict which is not a struggle, but a close and harmonious cooperation between the external condition and the pre-established constitution of the organism," claimed Bernard just before his death in February 1878, "A living being is not an exception to the great natural harmony which causes things to adjust themselves to each other....it is a part of the universal harmony of things and life, let us say of an animal, is but a fragment of the total life of the universe."[45]

Bernard felt that the organism had an *internal* environment in addition to its external one. An essential condition of life is the ability of the organism to maintain a constant internal milieu in the face of changing external conditions. Many ideas in Chinese medicine are centered on this internal milieu. Patterns of disharmony such as damp heat in the lower burner describe a deviation from the healthy state of the internal environment. Herbs and acupuncture points are understood in terms of their impact on such pathological conditions. The herb Job's tears (*yi yi ren*) and the acupoint stomach 40 (*feng long* or bountiful bulge), for example, both help resolve dampness.

Energy and Organization

Chinese medicine uses the concept of qi to discuss the organization of the mind-body system in "energetic" terms. The new biology is also focused on the "energy" and organization of living systems. Ludwig von Bertalanffy, the pioneer of systems thinking, felt that the search for order and organization in living systems is "one of the fundamental tasks of biology." Von Bertalanffy was intrigued by the remarkable ability of living organisms to reach the same final state even when starting from different places. It is possible, for example, to get a complete organism from a single embryo, from two that have been fused, or even from a quarter of one that has been twice divided. This so-called "equifinality" of living organisms shows an underlying organization of the whole that is greater than the sum of the parts.

"Every healing process, every dynamic restitution following a disturbance, every return to the normal state after a clinical intervention," claimed von Bertalanffy, "is the reestablishment of an equifinal steady state." This "equifinal self-preservation of the organism" he equated with the "natural healing power" spoken of by old physicians.[46] In Chinese medicine, the natural healing power can be activated by threadlike needles inserted to restore the natural flow of qi.

Contemporary researchers are actively building on the work of von Bertalanffy, trying to understand the organizational, systems-level features of living organisms in informational and energetic terms. Lynn Trainor and his colleagues, for example, are using information fields to not only describe, but also predict the dynamic changes in the form of simple organisms. Other scientists are looking at the energetic, regulatory aspects of the organization and communication of living systems.

Some point to electromagnetic fields as regulatory and informational agents in living systems. In introducing a book on recent research findings, K.H. Li, for example, suggests that "There is evidence that it is the informational aspect of biological systems that characterizes the essential view of life." Li feels it is necessary to move past simply looking at biochemicals and look at how these are organized. He claims that electromagnetic fields play a key role in biochemical organization.[47]

The exploration of the energetic and informational aspects of biological organization is an exciting area of the new biology and as new concepts emerge, ancient Eastern ideas can be seen in a new light. New biology concepts will help in the understanding of acupuncture and mysterious Chinese concepts like qi. (The growing area of correspondence between Eastern and Western thinking about energy and organization in living systems is the subject of Chapter 9.)

Quality versus Quantity

Chinese medicine makes use of quality, while Western medicine strives to quantify, a seemingly inseparable gap between East and West. Chinese medicine attends to slippery pulses and damp spleens—things that must be felt and judged. As a modern TCM textbook puts it, the Chinese mind categorizes qualities, creating a complex network of qualitative correspondences between phenomena and relationships.[48] Metaphorical language borrowed from social and natural phenomena is used to describe the qualities of physiological and pathological processes. Dampness, heat, and wind can afflict the liver. The kidneys rule water, while the spleen governs blood. Tongues can be pale and swollen or red and thin and pulses can be wiry and slippery, floating or sinking.[49]

Western medicine concerns itself with blood pressure, the pH of urine, and the concentration of cholesterol in blood—things that can be measured and turned into numbers. In conventional Western science, qualities are subjective, vague, and even unreal. Observations must be turned into measurements that can be mathematically analyzed. Lord Kelvin, the nineteenth century scientist and inventor for whom the Kelvin temperature scale is named, expressed this Western preference for measurement clearly: "When you can measure what you are speaking of and express it in numbers you know that on which you are discoursing. But if you cannot measure it and express it in numbers, your knowledge is of a very meager and unsatisfactory kind."[50]

Emphasis on quantity has been of tremendous value in science. Despite the side effect of making the ordinary world of subjective quality somehow unreal, reducing things to numbers and predicting their behavior through mathematical equations is the foundation and the power of science. It can also be deeply satisfying and even beautiful.

There is now a hint in science and the new biology that at least a small crack in the doctrine of quantity is appearing. As scientists explore the complex processes that are the rule rather than the exception in the everyday world, there is a shift away from an exclusive emphasis on quantity.[51] The new mathematics of complex systems, for example, does not predict the precise course of system dynamics. Instead, it sets out qualitative features of a system's behavior, describing general patterns of organization that offer insight into the system.

Fritjof Capra feels that a truly comprehensive theory of living systems requires a synthesis of the study of quality and pattern now emerging in the new biology with the more conventional study of quantity and structure. While the study of quality and pattern is new to the scientific understanding of living systems, quality and pattern have formed the backbone of Chinese medicine for millennia.

A more flexible perspective is emerging in the new biology, one in which quality can be valuable and even "scientific." And while quantity is important, it can have limitations. When it comes to complex systems, restricting the scope of study to that which can be quantified makes it difficult to see the forest for the trees, a forest with many shapes and colors that can also be studied. As the new biology rediscovers the value of quality, the qualities used by Chinese physicians to help in the cure of their patients can be seen in a new light.

Final Thoughts

Joseph Needham and collaborator Gwei-djen Lu point to a paradox of Chinese medicine. The conceptual framework of Chinese medicine can be described as "medieval," yet it is also "subtle and sophisticated" with a strong sense of the wholeness, balance, and harmony of the mind and body. It may well be impossible to understand these "medieval" theories in terms of modern science, they claim, yet the Chinese have used these theories, often successfully, for thousands of years in their quest for health and healing.[52]

This paradox is resolved by the realization that while, from the point of view of conventional science, Chinese medicine seems primitive at times and perhaps inexplicable at others, it has many parallels to the new biology. Scientists are now struggling to overcome the limitations of conventional science in the study of complex systems. As they do so, a better understanding of the seemingly "medieval" theories of Chinese medicine is emerging. And at the same time there is the opportunity to learn from, and not just about, this ancient, yet contemporary and evolving, Eastern system of medicine.

6 | An Ounce of Prevention: Primary Medicine East and West

Modern medicine is based on science—and on powerful guiding ideas. One of the most powerful ideas is that of the magic bullet cure. A century ago, infectious diseases were found to have specific causes, and in time magic bullet cures—drugs that could kill the microbe without killing the patient—were also discovered. The excitement of this technological achievement permeated the popular imagination and generated optimism about the future during a time of unprecedented change. Life-saving drugs, automobiles, and electric lights were just the tip of an iceberg called "progress" that would shape a new civilization.

Yet as polio, typhoid, cholera, and smallpox faded into obscurity, a new set of plagues emerged. Heart disease, cancer, and stroke appeared as major killers, and chronic, degenerative conditions such as diabetes, obesity, and arthritis became the bane of life in modern industrial society. The response to this new pattern of sickness was based on two assumptions. Firstly, chronic, degenerative conditions were thought to be a natural consequence of aging and increasingly prevalent because people were living longer now that the infectious epidemics had been brought under control. This assumption—the inevitability of diabetes, heart disease, and the like—was joined by the assumption, or perhaps hope, that these health problems would succumb to the same strategy that had worked with their infectious predecessors. That is, with analytical science and enough research dollars spent, specific causes and magic bullet cures could be found that would banish the new diseases as effectively as the old.

Some progress has been made in coping with chronic degenerative disease. Still, the "war" is far from being won. Many cures do not qualify as magic bullets because of the severity and frequency of so-called "side effects." With vast sums of money and a spectacular array of technological wizardry many health problems can be managed. But few can be cured.

From the point of view of the new biology, the limitations of conventional approaches are rooted in the fallacy of these basic assumptions. Chronic degenerative disease represents a breakdown in a complex system. There is no fundamental reason to believe that such a breakdown can be reduced to a specific cause, nor that a specific, universal cure will be found. Complex systems may break down in the same way for different reasons, and similarly, may be restored in more than one way. Since every part affects the other, breakdown is a downwardly cascading process. So too, recovery can be enhanced by systemic interaction, allowing the system to figuratively pull itself up by its own bootstraps.

Imagine a tree with wilted leaves. Drought may have been a precipitating factor in the drooping problem, but excessive shading from neighboring trees and nutrient deficiency could have been exacerbating factors that increased the tree's susceptibility to wilt. While watering may well alleviate the droop, long-term soil building and reduced shading would improve the tree's resistance to drought. The leaves of a well-nourished, healthy tree would not wilt except in extremely dry conditions.

There is no fundamental reason to assume that chronic degenerative disease is inevitable—whether a consequence of aging or "in the genes." There is a growing realization that the newer "diseases of civilization" have a fundamental connection to the society in which they occur. By changing the social, environmental, and behavioral conditions that nurture disease to conditions that instead foster health, many of these diseases would not occur in the first place.

This powerful possibility of prevention is the great hope for the future, and also hints at a new hope for cure. Some researchers are now exploring—with considerable promise—the use of these same preventive strategies in the treatment of chronic, degenerative conditions.

The realization that prevention is the primary medicine strikes a chord with Chinese medicine. The attitude that it was possible to stay healthy and live to a ripe old age was pervasive among Taoists and a central idea in medical texts like the *Yellow Emperor's Classic of Internal Medicine*. Taoists obsessed with longevity developed many methods to achieve their goal: special exercises, breathing-meditation techniques, dietary proscriptions and prescriptions, and tonic herbs. The same methods, it was found, could be used in both the treatment of chronic disease and in its prevention. Ancient Chinese methods for health promotion such as qi gong and the use of herbs have traveled across time to the modern Chinese medical system, while striking a chord with the cultural milieu of the West.

Toward a Primary Medicine West

Yet it is certain that now as in the past the only real solution to any disease problem is prevention rather than cure, and that prevention demands both concerted social effort and personal discipline.

—René Dubos[1]

The most important medical advance in the nineteenth century was the discovery that infectious diseases were largely attributable to environmental conditions and could often be prevented by control of the influences which led to them; the most significant advance in the twentieth century is the recognition that the same is true of many non-communicable diseases.

—Thomas McKeown[2]

Human Health: The Broad Picture

The modern human, *Homo sapien*, has existed for about 100,000 years. Extraordinarily adapted to a wide variety of ecological niches, humans have lived for most of this time as gatherers and scroungers, eating a very diverse diet of plant foods—including seeds, nuts, fruits, tubers, berries, and greens—supplemented by the hunting and gathering of animal foods like grubs, shellfish, and game. These gathering groups evolved strategies to keep their numbers below the carrying capacity—the largest number of people that can survive on the resources of the region in which they live. As a result of the impact of industrial society there are fewer and fewer traditional cultures left, yet their ecologically sound ways of life are important examples to their "civilized" cousins who are now searching for a more sustainable society.[3]

Without idealizing the gathering lifestyle, it is far from the commonly preconceived picture of misery and constant struggle for existence. Even during times of drought, studies show that the indigenous Bushmen of Southern Africa, for example, lived comfortably while their agricultural neighbors went hungry. Despite the fact that the Bushmen lived in some of the harshest and most inhospitable desert territory in Africa, they spent only 15 hours a week gathering and preparing food, their children did not work, and their elderly were well-cared-for pillars of society. People in agricultural societies, by contrast, typically spend over 40 hours a week to obtain their food, while even those in modern industrialized nations still use up about 15 hours or more a week working to afford food and to prepare it.[4]

As long as they keep their numbers to sustainable levels to avoid pressure on the food supply, gathering people enjoy relatively good health. Their chief health concern is parasitic disease. Yet, about 10,000 years ago some gathering groups began to live a more settled existence with the help of domesticated plants and animals. And, as the pattern of living changed, so too did the pattern of sickness. It was agriculture that gave birth to civilization—and to the problem of epidemic infectious disease.

With the shift from hunting and gathering to agriculture, three factors combined to change the way people became sick. First, population increased. Farmers could grow enough food to feed themselves and others, and villages, towns, and even cities could be supported by the agricultural base of the surrounding area. The end result was more people, often concentrated in small areas. Without the cultural population controls of gathering people, population growth was held in check only by the limits of the food supply. This meant that people were often unable to get enough food and were very dependent on the vicissitudes of the weather. Since the agricultural diet was not as diverse as the gathering diet (peasant agriculturalists often relied heavily on a single crop, like potato or corn) and food was commonly in short supply, people were often poorly nourished (factor number two).

Large numbers of inadequately nourished people concentrated together in towns and cities combined with a third factor—poor sanitation—to create perfect conditions for the spread of infectious disease. Communicable disease was hardest on the children and good fortune was needed to make it through to adulthood. Indeed, the history of human civilization is a chronicle of plague and pestilence, from antiquity to the Middle Ages, and beyond. The European conquest of the Americas, for example, was shaped by infectious disease and the first contacts between New World and Old were devastating to indigenous South, Central, and North American people. The warrior Aztecs, weakened and demoralized by disease, were easily conquered by a minuscule Spanish force under Cortez and the first North American settlers found long deserted fields ready for farming.

It took another shift in the pattern of living to eliminate the threat of infectious disease, at least in some areas of the world. About 300 years ago, European people initiated another cultural transformation, this time from agriculture to industry. Agriculture itself underwent many improvements, making more food available, and the population of the blossoming industrial nations did not increase sufficiently to wipe out the benefit of higher productivity. By the nineteenth century, people were better fed, living conditions had improved in cities and towns, and the sanitation movement of the later part of that century greatly improved hygiene. This resulted in a marked decline in the threat of infectious disease, and by the time specific medical measures were developed to successfully treat infectious disease, the decline was already well underway.

While the shift from agriculture to industry helped break the pattern of infectious disease, it brought new hazards. Trains, cars, and even remote control television fostered a sedentary lifestyle; food was not only abundant, but rich and low in fiber; and the soil, air, and water became polluted with the discharges of industrial production. As infectious disease declined a new pattern of disease emerged: a new plague of "diseases of civilization" ranging from diabetes and obesity to heart disease and high blood pressure.

These diseases arise largely because people are poorly adapted to the stressful and toxic environment of industrial civilization with its sedentary living and rich food. We are stuck with stone-age genes in a computer-age world. The British medical historian Thomas McKeown classifies such "Western" illnesses as diseases of maladaptation. As he puts it, the human subspecies has existed for 60,000 years. It has been 10,000 years since the end of the gathering lifestyle and only 300 years since the advent of industrialization: "In these short intervals there has not been time for genetic adaptation, so that modern man is exposed to the hazards of industrial life with the genetic equipment of a hunter-gatherer."[5]

The problem of infectious disease was both created and improved by changing social and environmental conditions. So too the problem of chronic disease emerged from changing social and environmental conditions. The next major improvement in health will come, not from advances in the treatment of disease, but from prevention through a change in the pattern of living.

The Changing Face of Medicine

McKeown's thesis that many common diseases are rooted in the living pattern of industrialized nations is supported by research spanning almost a century. As far back as the 1920s Westerners working in foreign lands noticed that the people living there did not get sick in the same way as their fellow countrymen and women. Many diseases common in Europe and the United States were rare and uncommon in Africa and other areas. Chief among the explanations for this striking phenomenon was the dramatically different lifestyles of the people.

Medical pioneers such as Thomas "Peter" Cleave, who pointed to the value of dietary fiber at a time when many argued for its dangers, were sometimes thought of as eccentrics and their ideas often ignored, but they persisted. With the effort of individuals like Denis Burkitt—famous for the discovery of Burkitt's lymphoma—and Hugh Trowell, medical doctors who met while working in Africa, what began as vague anecdote gradually coalesced into more rigorous scientific evidence. Many studies showed that appendicitis, hemorrhoids, obesity, diabetes, and some types of cancer were intimately related to the "Western" lifestyle, particularly the "Western" diet. (The importance of the relationship between diet and health is the subject of Chapter 8.) While skeptics pointed out that people of different races may simply get sick in different ways because of their different genes, studies of migrant populations showed clearly that when people moved to new countries and adopted a new living pattern their disease profile changed to match that of their new home.

After gathering impressive evidence to support their claim, Burkitt, who died in 1993 at the age of eighty-two, and his colleague Trowell, who died four years earlier, proposed that the diseases so common in Western nations, and in other nations that shared their way of life, should be described as "Western." Burkitt pointed out in a book written just before his death that, while the term "Western" was not ideal because this same lifestyle and pattern of disease was shared by some non-Western peoples, it nonetheless expressed an important concept. There is a group of diseases which are common in the relatively wealthy and industrialized populations of the world. These diseases arise directly from a particular lifestyle, one that is at odds with the way of life to which humans have adapted through their evolutionary history, and as such are largely preventable. "This concept of Western diseases, which must be largely preventable once causative factors in the Western lifestyle are identified and then reduced or eliminated," wrote Burkitt, "must be one of the most, if not the most, important medical observations made in the last 30 years."[6]

While many in the health care community are not aware of this important medical observation and prevention is still not a priority, the face of medicine is changing—at least on the fringes. The Washington-based Physicians Committee for Responsible Medicine (PCRM), for example, is a prominent group championing the new view of health. Led by physician Neal Barnard, the PCRM actively promotes prevention, providing people with the information they need to make the lifestyle changes necessary to improve their health.

Barnard, who founded the PCRM in 1986, is enthusiastic about the potential of prevention and the value of those same preventive strategies in the treatment of disease. He points out that people have as much or more power than their physicians to influence their long-term health and he looks to a future when the physician's emphasis is shifted from treatment to prevention. "What I want to see in the future is a reduced demand for health care," says Barnard, "I want doctors to focus on people who already are healthy, and ask what they can do to maximize their health, because, hopefully, there won't be sick people coming to see them and they need something to do."[7]

Obesity: The War on Fat

The newfound knowledge that "Western" diseases are preventable is ground for tremendous optimism. Unfortunately, such optimism must be tempered by the reality of current trends. Obesity, the most apparent "Western" disease and a powerful indicator of more serious

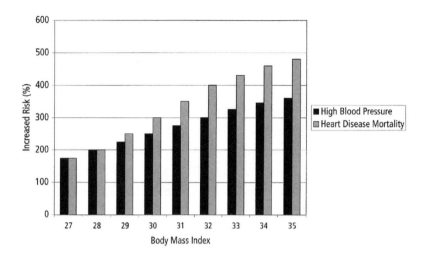

Obesity and Increased Risk of Cardiovascular Disease[8]

health problems, is on the rise around the world. Particularly troubling for future health is its rise among youth.

Scientists use something called the body mass index or BMI to indicate problems with body fat. The BMI accounts for the relationship between height and body weight, and values over twenty-five are linked with a gamut of health problems. (To calculate your BMI, take your weight in kilograms and divide it by the square of your height measured in meters. If you are not familiar with the metric system, take your weight in pounds and divide it by your height in inches squared, and finally multiply the result by 705.) Over half of adults living in the United States have a BMI above twenty-five.

The relationship between obesity and health problems is very strong. Those with a BMI over twenty-nine show a 110 percent increase in dying from all causes compared to those with BMIs below nineteen and a 360 percent increase in dying from heart disease in particular. A BMI of thirty-two and above increases the risk of dying from cancer by 110 percent. The risk of high blood pressure, arthritis, and gallstones also increases with weight. Most staggering is a whopping

2,660 percent increase in type II diabetes with a BMI over twenty-nine—which rises to 5,300 percent at a BMI over thirty-three—compared to BMIs of twenty-two to twenty-three.[9]

This troublesome tendency to gain weight is a response to a particular lifestyle pattern, something well illustrated by the Pima Indians of southern North America. Historically split into two groups—one in the state of Arizona, the other in Mexico—the Pima show with crystalline clarity the effect of lifestyle on health. Mexican Pimas are physically active, largely vegetarian, and thin. Their cousins in Arizona, by contrast, eat a typical rich American diet, and live a much more sedentary life. Their obesity rate is the highest in the world; diabetes is epidemic.

The physiological processes involved in weight control are extremely complex and still poorly understood. Fat itself is part of the body's hormonal system, manufacturing and responding to chemical messengers that travel throughout the body to regulate metabolism. The "set point" theory of weight control posits a complex system of feedback that keeps weight regulated, a system with certain built-in genetic tendencies that chooses a "set point" for an individual's weight based on environmental variables such as diet and lifestyle.

The set point is dependent on more than simply the number of calories consumed, a fact that explains the almost universal failure of "dieting" through calorie restriction. One of the many surprising findings of the China study led by Cornell University scientist Colin Campbell was the fact the Chinese take in more energy from their plate than the average American. The typical Chinese male consumes 2,641 calories daily, whereas his American counterpart manages only 2,360. While the Chinese consume, on average, 30 percent more calories than Americans (after adjustment for body weight), obesity is uncommon among the Chinese whose BMI for adult males averages 20.5 compared to the American 25.8.

Obesity and obesity-related disease are also fostered by the kind of food consumed. One culprit is fat, which is not metabolically managed in an effective way by the majority of people. The percentage of food energy derived from fat varies widely in the Chinese population because of significant regional variations in diet. Still, the Chinese figure of 6 to 24 percent, with an average of 15 percent, is strikingly different than the American average which approaches 40 percent. Even the recent recommendation of health authorities to reduce fat intake to 30 percent of total calories does not approach the high end of the Chinese range. Campbell found that "Western" diseases appear more frequently among Chinese people who eat the most fat compared to those who eat the least. Also significant is the fact that the Chinese consume most (90 percent) of their protein from plant sources, while most (69 percent) of the protein consumed by Americans is of animal origin.[10] Unfortunately, reports from China indicate that the traditional lifestyle and diet is changing and the problem of obesity is rearing its ugly head.

Another dietary culprit is refined carbohydrates—the processed grains and refined sugars that together with fat constitute the majority of calories consumed by the mythical "average" person in modern affluent culture. Refined grains and purified sugars have lost much of their nutritional value and are stripped of their fiber, a component of food once thought to be bad for health but now recognized as beneficial. With the growing recognition that excessive fat is a problem, there is concern among nutritionists that in some cases fat is simply being replaced with unhealthy carbohydrates. Evidence suggests that too many cakes, pastries, and even low-fat foods loaded with refined sweeteners can wreak havoc with metabolic processes.

The second "environmental" factor central to the problem of weight control is physical activity. Researchers compare the effect of a sedentary lifestyle on health to smoking a pack of cigarettes a day. Lack of exercise increases the risk of "Western" diseases, such as heart disease and colon cancer. Even "mental" diseases, like depression, are more common among those who fail to stimulate their metabolic processes through activity. A healthy activity level does not imply marathon running nor mountain climbing, but simply the equivalent of thirty minutes or more a day of brisk walking. Close to two-thirds of Americans get little or no exercise, and fewer than one-fifth take part in vigorous physical activity on a regular basis.

Cancer: Disease of Fear and Hope

The power of prevention as a defense against cancer has never been fully appreciated by the public at large.
—Scientific American, 1996[11]

Cancer is one of the most prominent features of the disease landscape—and perhaps the one that generates the most fear. In the 1970s, President Nixon declared war on cancer, responding to a popular hope that with enough money and effort cancer could be beaten. Yet after several decades and innumerable millions spent, the army is still floundering on the battlefield. Perhaps a flood-control metaphor is more apt. In some places floodwaters are receding, in others the water is unrelenting. With many fingers plugging the leaks, the dike has held—barely.

University of Chicago's John Bailar showed in a 1986 study looking at data from 1950 to 1982 that 40 years of research directed at finding the cure for cancer has not been able to reverse a slow, steady increase in death from the disease. In 1997, he followed up this study by looking at age-adjusted cancer mortality rates from 1970 to 1994. Bailar found that death from cancer increased steadily until 1991, then decreased slightly until 1994, the last year of his study. Mortality from some types of cancers, such as cervical and colorectal cancer, has declined, while death from others, such as cancer of the skin and brain, has increased. A reduction in death from childhood cancer by 50 percent since the 1970s deserves praise, claims Bailar. Unfortunately, children represent only a small fraction of cancer victims and most other declines have been due to reduced incidence or early detection, not better treatment.

New molecular biology-based treatments—much hyped like earlier approaches that did not live up to their promise—offer hope for the future. But Bailar is cautious: "In our view, prudence requires a skeptical view of the tacit assumption that marvelous new treatments for cancer are just waiting around the corner." And in light of these hard realities, the whole strategy toward cancer should be rethought: "A national commitment to the prevention of cancer, largely replacing reliance on hopes for universal cures, is now the way to go."[12]

The possibilities for prevention are stunning. Estimates by scientists not known for exaggeration show that at least two-thirds and maybe as much as 80 percent of cancer is preventable. Tobacco is responsible for about one-third of the cancer cases, while the other major culprit is diet, responsible for one-third or more cases of the disease. Also on the hit list are occupational and environmental exposure to radiation and chemicals, excessive alcohol consumption, and viruses. Key viruses are the papilloma virus and the hepatitis family—implicated in cervical and liver cancer, respectively. Genes are thought to be involved in less than 5 percent of cancer cases.[13]

Viral-related cancers are more important in the developing world, where infectious disease is still a problem, while diet and tobacco-related cancer dominates in industrialized regions. The challenge for developing countries and rapidly urbanizing nations like China is to conquer communicable disease, while maintaining healthy traditional diets and lifestyles. Unfortunately, tobacco companies, with profits capped by anti-smoking efforts and lawsuits in the United States, are working hard to create addicts through advertising around the world. And ironically, at a time when Americans are looking to traditional diets around the world—like that of the Japanese—as models of healthy eating, such diets are being abandoned in favor of "faster" food.

Another irony of the effort to understand and prevent cancer is the fact that cancer scientists now recommend a diet more in tune with the counterculture whole-food enthusiast than with the conventional four-food-groups nutritionist. The food choices recommended by *Scientific American* for people wanting to lower cancer risk sit in stark contradiction to the fare available in the modern supermarket and fast-food restaurant: "Their diet should be high in vegetables, fruits, and legumes (such as peas and beans) and low in red meat, saturated fat, salt, and sugar. Carbohydrates should be consumed as whole grains—whole-wheat bread and brown rice as opposed to white bread and rice, for example."[14]

Cancer is an exceedingly complex disease. The current understanding focuses on two events, initiation and promotion. Cancer is initiated when a cell is damaged by such things as radiation and chemicals, setting the stage for abnormal growth. Such events, however, are thought to take place constantly within the body and are in the vast majority of cases quickly dealt with by an elaborate regulatory system. Cancer is promoted when this recognition and repair function of the immune system is blocked from doing its work. The development of the disease is a gradual process that may take decades to unfold.

Toxins like those found in tobacco smoke are able to damage cells and at the same time promote cancer by impairing the immune system. The effects of diet are more subtle, involving the deleterious effects of some foods, like red meat, and the beneficial effects of others, like fruits and vegetables. Red meat, for example, is associated with excess iron intake, which is linked to an increased number of "free radicals"—highly reactive molecules that wreak molecular havoc in the body. Vegetables, in contrast, contain free radical scavengers called antioxidants, such as vitamins C and E. Too many fats of all kinds appear to weaken the immune system.

When it comes to this dreaded disease, nothing seems fair. Those with poor eating habits often live to ripe, old ages. Centenarians with a glass of port and cigar tout their decadence as the secret to long life. Some ardent exercisers and broccoli enthusiasts will get cancer. Problems with particular genes can confer a much greater risk of developing certain cancers, yet environmental factors interact with such genetic susceptibility to actually produce the disease.

Life is indeed a roulette wheel—where it will land nobody can say. Yet it is a wheel that can be heavily weighted in favor of health. As *Scientific American* puts it, if most people made at least two positive changes—such as exercising 20 minutes a day, eating leafy vegetables every day, or consuming red meat less than once a week—deaths due to cancer related to diet and lack of exercise could be cut by 25 percent.

From Prevention to Reversibility: The Case of Heart Disease

It is clear that "Western" diseases can be prevented. But once they have developed can they actually be reversed by the same changes needed for their prevention? This is an intriguing question with many implications for the future of medicine. And the answer appears to be yes, they can often be improved.

The PCRM points to several studies showing the outlook for people with cancer is greatly improved by dietary change. University of Arizona scientists found that colon cancer survivors have a reduced risk of recurrence when they increased the intake of dietary fiber. Women with breast cancer that had spread to other parts of the body reduced their risk of dying by 40 percent when they reduced monthly fat intake by 1,000 grams, the difference between the typical American diet and most traditional ways of eating. More needs to be learned about the ability of lifestyle change to assist in the survival of cancer, claim the PCRM, nevertheless, food can be one important tool in improving survival from cancer.[15]

Australia was the site of a novel study looking at Western disease prevention and reversibility. Like the Pima Indians of southern North America, the indigenous Aborigines of Australia are very susceptible to Western diseases, including obesity, diabetes, and heart disease. Some 60 percent of Aborigines living a Western lifestyle have a BMI topping twenty-five—the common cut-off level for marking problems with weight—and the diabetes rate is ten times that of Australians of European origin.

Working closely with a group of Aborigines in northwestern Australia, scientists studied the physiological changes induced by a seven-week return to their traditional hunter-gatherer lifestyle. This group of indigenous people had only recently been "Westernized" and some elders retain the tremendous skill and knowledge required to live entirely off the land. Most of the participants in the study were diabetics.

Samples of the food gathered by the group during the seven-week study were preserved with liquid nitrogen and flown back from the remote West Kimberley Region, offering insight into the nutritional profile of the traditional diet. Food gathering was a very energy-intensive activity and the food eaten was very low calorie, but nutrient dense. The participants were taking in only about 1200 calories per day and not surprisingly, between the physical activity and scarce calories they lost weight—an average of over 15 pounds.

The Aboriginal diet is remarkably diverse and included kangaroo, fish, yams, figs, honey, and a delicacy known as the witchetty grub. While high in animal foods and protein, the traditional diet is still extraordinarily low in fat. In fact, less than 15 percent of the calories come from fat because of the extreme leanness of wild animals. Even the fat profile is shifted away from the saturated toward the unsaturated variety and there are plenty of omega-3 fatty acids, fats that are thought to offer protection against atherosclerosis. The witchetty grub, for example, has a fat composition resembling olive oil, the oil commonly used in the Mediterranean diet. The wild plant foods are high in fiber, slowly digested, and higher in nutrient density than cultivated varieties.

Physiological assessment of the participants before and after the seven-week lifestyle change showed a dramatic improvement in their health. In addition to the marked weight loss, blood sugar levels dropped and insulin metabolism improved, demonstrating the reversibility of a diabetic condition. Risk factors for cardiovascular disease also improved: blood pressure decreased, as did cholesterol and triglyceride levels. This study shows that major lifestyle change can not only prevent, but even over a matter of weeks, can reverse Western disease.[16]

Dean Ornish is a pioneer in using lifestyle change to reverse Western disease. His comprehensive program of radical lifestyle change was designed specifically to reverse heart disease, but can also be used in its prevention, as well as in the treatment and prevention of other Western diseases. Ornish has found that the program is valuable as a weight-loss regimen, one that does not focus on calorie restriction, and he has also applied the program to autoimmune problems, such as rheumatoid arthritis. The Ornish program draws heavily on Eastern health ideas, bringing together stress reduction, exercise, group support, and dietary change—a major component of the program discussed in Chapter 8—to address the physical, mental, and even spiritual components of health.

Ornish argues against the no pain, no gain exercise philosophy, claiming that "moderate exercise is enough to provide you with almost all of the health and longevity benefits without most of the risks of more intense exercise." This means starting with 30 minutes a day of walking, and adding more when it is enjoyable. Fitness—your ability to exercise—is not equivalent to health, says Ornish, pointing to the fact that some physically fit athletes still die from heart attacks. But exercise is a central part of a comprehensive health program.

As part of his "stress management" package, Ornish makes use of stretching, breathing exercises, relaxation techniques, meditation, and visualization. Relaxation techniques, for example, help to break the cycle of tension so common in modern, industrial civilization. While tension allows a person overwhelmed by sensory overload to block such "stress," it brings life experience into the body in a way that leaves a permanent and deleterious record. The cycle of tension can be broken with mind-body exercises designed to bring about a state of deep relaxation. Meditation enhances the mental facet of relaxation, stretching the physical component, while breathing acts as a bridge between them.

While tension and stress impede circulation and disrupt digestion, research shows that meditation and relaxation techniques positively affect physiological processes. Ornish points to the psychological and even spiritual components of health: literally opening your heart requires figuratively opening your heart, a process aided by practices like meditation.

Research also shows that visualization—the guided use of mental images—affects physiological processes, and Ornish includes both "directed" and "receptive" visualization in his program, recommending they be done following meditation. He suggests that heart patients learn the exact location of blockages in their coronary arteries and develop a healing image of a healthy heart with a regular beat and unobstructed flow of blood. Patients create their own variations of the healing heart image, ranging from a machine tunneling though clogged arteries to a mild solvent eroding plaques.[17]

Beyond Blame

On the days that she must send unusually high numbers of wheezing children home from school, my sister has begun to take note of what the weather is like, which way the wind is blowing, how the air smells, and how labored her own breathing is. Perhaps it is once again time, we both agree, to look at the environment to understand what ails us.

—Sandra Steingraber,
Living Downstream: An Ecologist Looks at Cancer and the Environment[18]

Ingrid could remember being teased as a child, taunted with calls of "chubby" and "fatty" from the neighborhood bullies. Although she sometimes dreamed of what it would like to be thin, Ingrid had comfortably come to terms with her weight. Yet when told by her doctor that her cholesterol level was dangerously high, she decided to take action. With her mother suffering from heart disease, Ingrid's weight problem and high cholesterol level suggested that she too was at risk.

Several trips to the library and several weeks of reading suggested to Ingrid that she embark on a program of radical lifestyle change. Her doctor helped her develop a regimen of moderate exercise, starting with a morning walk around the neighborhood. She also signed up for a low-fat, natural foods cooking course, entering a new world of black beans, lentils, tofu, brown rice, and kale.

Ingrid quickly came to love the regular exercise. It helped her relax and created a sense of well-being that remained for the rest of the day. But the food was the hard part. Learning to buy and prepare completely new foods was a tremendous challenge. The jokes from her family and tantrums from her children when they were served tofu sandwiches on whole wheat bread instead of hamburgers were bad enough. The straw that broke the camel's back were the snide remarks thrown her way after she passed on the fried chicken—and later the chocolate layer cake—at the community picnic. Ingrid considered giving up, even after losing 10 pounds.

Ingrid's experience illustrates the profoundly social side of food. Food habits and preferences are personal only to a degree, reflecting the culture's culinary milieu. Australian Aborigines learn to appreciate the witchetty grub at an early age, while many American young people would scream at the sight of an insect in their food, preferring instead pizza, hamburgers, and fries. The Japanese have turned seaweed and raw fish into a high art form, while Texans have turned steak size into a matter of pride. Clearly, individuals cannot be blamed for what they eat and the effort to develop healthy eating patterns requires extensive education and social support, like that found in the Ornish program for the treatment of heart disease.

The same can be said about tobacco, a highly addictive substance that has, until recently in North America, been deliberately marketed to children. Smoking combines a social element with a physiological addiction that is hard to beat. Even exercise patterns are more than individual traits. While children can become physically active simply by walking to school, many parents are concerned about their children's safety and some suburbs do not even have sidewalks. In the warmer months of the year, pollution levels in many cities become particularly hazardous and health authorities advise that outdoor exercise is dangerous.

This brings up another side of health—pollution—important to the prevention of disease and something over which individuals have little control. With industrialization the environment has been profoundly

But They do!

altered. Thousands of new chemicals have been invented, some of which are now spread around the world and can be found even on the remotest mountain—and in the human body. Noise and light are ubiquitous in the urban environment. Even the electromagnetic environment has been dramatically altered. Greater amounts of ultraviolet light now penetrate the atmosphere because of a human-generated depletion in the protective ozone layer; background radiation levels have increased after atomic testing and the growth of nuclear technology; and the electromagnetic energy from electric devices such as cellular phones and power lines permeates homes and communities.[19]

The toll on human health of these dramatic and recent changes remains largely unaccounted. On one side there are the obvious acute tragedies, such as the chemical plant disaster in Bhopal or the nuclear meltdown in Chernobyl, and on the other, the long-term impact of chronic low-level exposure to pollution in its myriad forms. This is a problem of great complexity, for which science has no easy answer. Humans are intimately linked to their environment and can adapt successfully to even harsh and hostile conditions. But how well can we adapt to 24-hour-a-day light and noise, synthetic chemical toxins, greater levels of ultraviolet light, and air pollution?

Rachel Carson proclaimed that our fate was connected to the animals' and as animals around the globe suffer—the birds that fall dead from the thick and acrid sky above Mexico City, the St. Lawrence beluga whales whose carcasses are officially classified as toxic waste, the impotent Florida alligators, and the tumor-filled fish of the Great Lakes—it is hard to imagine that humans are escaping the toxic deluge unscathed. Air pollution taxes the heart and lungs. Chemical toxins push our immune system to the limit and some act as hormone disrupters, interfering with the body's chemical communications.[20] Noise and light pollution cause physiological and psychological stress. Electromagnetic fields interfere with bioelectromagnetic systems now only barely defined.

Despite the clear possibilities, the effect of pollution on health is the subject of perennial debate. Some scientists suggest that less than 2 percent of human cancer is linked to pollution. The University of California's Bruce Ames, for example, argues that it is highly unlikely synthetic chemicals play any significant role in cancer because of the many natural toxins to which people are routinely exposed and for which they have evolved elaborate defense mechanisms. Others, such as poet and biologist Sandra Steingraber, counter by pointing to an impressive body of evidence linking cancer to environmental contamination. Dioxin, for example, is among the most carcinogenic of chemicals studied and can be found in human breast milk. Some toxins found in diesel exhaust are also extremely dangerous and as common as the cars and trucks that produce them.

The incessant debate over our impact on the biosphere and ultimately ourselves illustrates only the challenge of giving definitive answers to complex problems—and the intimate link between science and the technologies in question. While the exact toll may never be fully chronicled, there is no doubt that humans have critically fouled their nest, creating an environment inimical to health and damaging the planetary life-support systems upon which they depend. The search for health and the prevention of disease must go beyond a focus on individual lifestyles to include the social forces that shape behavior and broader human-environment issues.

Building the Well and Forging the Sword: Prevention in Eastern Medicine

To administer medicines to diseases which have already developed and to suppress revolts which have already developed is comparable to the behavior of those persons who begin to dig a well after they have become thirsty, and of those who begin to cast weapons after they have already engaged in battle. Would these actions not be too late?
　　　　　　　　—*The Yellow Emperor's Classic of Internal Medicine*[21]

Chinese medical theory emerged in a milieu of naturalistic thinking. Understanding the mind-body system required setting the human condition in the context of a greater whole—a cosmos whose forces and fluxes affected the course of events in the lives of emperor and peasant alike. Yet this did not mean that individuals were always at the whim of fate and could do nothing more than pay homage in the hope of appeasing the gods. It was possible to contemplate and understand the Tao, the Way underlying all things, and to balance yin and yang in one's favor.

For the individual, this meant paying attention to internal and external factors—and their relationship—and taking steps to maintain balance and harmony in the face of incessant change. This was a lifetime effort and for some, like the Taoists, a way of life. Taoism, a strange admixture of the magic of the Wu or Shaman and the nature study of the philosopher-recluse, had at its core the quest for longevity and ultimately immortality.

This was not an immortality of the soul—for the Chinese did not split mind and matter, soul and body—but a perfection of the whole, the substantial and the rarefied self in union. This was at once a spiritual and a scientific pursuit, for the Taoists were, like the scientist, grounded firmly in empirical reality, even if they kept one eye on the Immortals in Heaven. Only by studying natural and biological processes could the adept achieve radiant health and, ultimately, the grand prize of immortality.[22]

The Taoists developed an intriguing assortment of longevity practices and were confident in the ability of the individual to determine his/her destiny. According to an eighth century text: "The manuals of the immortals say: 'One's life-span depends upon oneself. If one can conserve the *jing* and obtain the qi, one may attain longevity without end.' And they also say: 'Maintain the form without harmful exertion, conserve the *jing* without harmful agitation, restore the mind to emotional tranquility and peace. That is how longevity can be obtained.' The fundamental root of the life-force and life-span is set in this Tao."[23]

Even the renowned scientist, philosopher, and skeptic Wang Chong expressed confidence that appropriate effort would bring health and a long life. Writing in the latter part of the first century, he made it clear that the human life span was rightly one hundred years and, while too skeptical to admit to the possibility of prolonging this biological allotment, he had no doubt this could be achieved together with good health in later years by taking the proper steps. For Wang Chong, this meant nourishing the qi, drinking wine to foster the appetite, protecting the senses from turmoil, guarding the *jing*, and using exercise and herbs to keep the body in good shape.[24]

The Taoist path to immortality was divided—sometimes not so sharply—into two branches, both alchemical but profoundly different. The outer alchemist experimented with metals, minerals, and other substances, searching for the secret of transmutation and the elixir of immortality. The inner or physiological alchemist, in contrast, strove for physiological transformation, working to perfect the body-mind through an assortment of methods. These methods not only preserved life, but could rejuvenate and even, according to the eighth century text quoted above, "heal all diseases."[25] As Needham writes: "Thus what the physiological alchemists were talking about essentially was rejuvenation, and they believed that by their techniques they could 'make all things new.' However we may judge their physiological theories now, there is no reason for doubting that under appropriate conditions they could perform miracles of restoring physical and mental health."[26]

Taoism had an important influence on Chinese medicine, and accordingly Chinese medicine is deeply infused with Taoist attitudes and many of their techniques. Many famous physicians were themselves practicing Taoists. The great Sun Si-miao, for example, spent much of his one hundred years as a Taoist hermit, preferring the mountains to the pretentiousness of academic medicine in the capital. Combining Confucian scholarship with Taoist alchemy and folk medicine, Sun compiled the renowned book *Qian Jin Yao Fang*—*Formulas Worth a Thousand Pieces of Gold*, publishing it in the year 652 when he was seventy years of age. In addition to listing 863 valuable herbal formulas, he discussed everything from medical ethics to the collection and preparation of herbs and included twenty-nine chapters on specialties such as gynecology and emergency medicine. In this last topic, he advocated the widespread use of what could be considered a "first-aid kit," recommending families keep on hand useful herbs, moxa, and a good book or two on emergency herbal treatment—both for home and for travel. (There was an assortment of such books already available by Sun's time, like the *Pocket-book of Medicines for Emergencies* compiled by physician and Taoist Ge Hong in the year 341.)

Sun, of course, included a section outlining the steps to prevention, covering all the basics: nutrition, sanitation, exercise, breathing methods, and sexual techniques for health and longevity.[27] His prevention-oriented thinking shines in this short passage from his famous book. Here he advocates the use of moxibustion to ward off illness. Modern acupuncture texts carry on this tradition, recommending points like foot three li (the 36th point of the stomach channel) as a prophylactic during influenza season. Sun Si-Miao: "After enjoying good health for ten days, it is advisable to employ moxibustion...in order to expel pathogenic factors. Every day it is necessary to harmonize the qi and nourish the body. But massage and tao yin exercise is best of all. In time of health do not forget danger. Always try to prevent the coming of disease beforehand."[28]

The idea that it was better to prevent than to react after something has begun can be traced to the earliest Chinese texts, including the *I Ching* and the *Tao Te Ching*. According to legend, physicians in this early age were paid to keep their patients healthy and were considered failures if their patients became ill. As a text dated to 120 B.C. put it: "A skillful doctor cures illness where there is no sign of disease and thus the disease never comes."[29] And about 400 years later: "The prescriptions of physicians are best given before any serious signs have appeared; then it will not be necessary to run after the disease when the patient is already dying."[30]

This attitude comes through strongly in the *Su Wen* or *Essential Questions*, the first part of the *Yellow Emperor's Classic of Internal Medicine*. The *Yellow Emperor's Classic* helped codify the basic principles and ideas of Chinese medicine, one of which was the ideal of prevention. Accordingly, "The sage does not cure the sick only when they are sick but prevents the illness from arising." In a later chapter, Minister Qi Bo compares the superior physician to his inferior colleague: "The superior physician helps before the early budding of the disease....The inferior physician begins to help when the disease has already developed; he helps when destruction has already set in."[31]

The Secrets of the Hygiene School Taoists

Hygiene is the science of health and disease prevention, as well as a term designating those conditions and practices conducive to health. This makes it an excellent description of the theories and practices of the hygiene school of Taoism, a body of ideas and procedures having a major influence on Chinese medicine and Chinese culture as a whole. The Taoists' perennial interest in and even obsession with health led to the early development of what is commonly considered as hygiene, together with an assortment of more esoteric health-giving methods that have only in recent decades become more familiar in the West.

Basic hygienic practices emerged early in Chinese civilization. Clean water was considered important and there was a preference for boiled water and cooked food, especially while traveling. (This, of course, reduced water-borne disease and the transmission of parasites through contaminated food.) Bathing and washing with soap were also common practices. The skeptic Wang did not disagree with the ritual handwash performed five times a day, the hot bath every five, or the hair wash every three—whether the scholar needed it or not—but he did attack the superstitious belief in auspicious and inauspicious days for such attention to personal hygiene.

In washing, the Chinese traditionally used special plants like the soap-pod tree mentioned by Li Shi-zhen in his grand work of natural history and medicinal agents. Such plants contained effective detergents, and were mixed with flour, perfumes, or beeswax and other fat-like substances to produce something akin to modern cleaners and soaps.

Familiarity with toilet etiquette helped avoid embarrassment in ancient China. One story tells of the great amusement afforded household servants by an uncouth army commander after the hapless soldier drank the washing water offered during his trip to the aristocratic lavatory. Another level of humor was reached when the ill-mannered gentleman then proceeded to eat one of the jujube dates placed in the lavatory to buffer olfactory assault.

Sun Si-miao himself noted that face and hand cleansers, washing and bathing beans, and clothes-cleaning agents were greatly valued by scholars, lamenting that recipes for these products were often kept secret by pharmacists. "Yet when the sages discovered anything, they always wanted it to be universally known," wrote Sun, "How could one hope to conceal such things from all the people and prevent the sagely Tao from spreading? That would be strangely contrary to the ideas of the great men of old."[32]

The Chinese used toothbrushes and tooth powder, as well as toilet silk and paper. (Only plain paper though, for there was a proscription against the use of paper adorned with the written word.) There is also a long history of the agricultural use of human waste in China and fumigators and exterminators were part of the ancient imperial staff. Needham suggests, in comparing basic hygienic practices in Occident and Orient, that it was not until the late nineteenth century, with the spread of indoor plumbing, that the West had the advantage in that area.

Yet Taoists were interested in much more than cleanliness. Taoism required commitment to a complete way of life, including prescriptions for every aspect of existence, culinary and sexual, mental and physical. It was necessary to regulate one's lifestyle and consciously adapt to the vicissitudes of nature, particularly those of climate. The second chapter of the *Su Wen* is titled "The Importance of Adjusting the Mind and Body to the Climatic Conditions of the Four Seasons," showing that the importance of these ideas carried over into the medical sphere. Climate was responsible for an important class of external pathogenic factors that were to be carefully guarded against and studied by the physician for their relationship to disease.

Internal pathogenic factors included the emotions and much attention was paid to state of mind. The Taoist enriched and fostered the mind and emotions, fastidiously avoiding excess and deliberately cultivating a calmness of mind untouched by worldly events. As a text dated 190 claims: "In order to nourish the shen, pleasure, anger, pity, happiness, cares, and anxieties must at all costs be moderated."[33]

The overriding idea was the need to flow with, as Needham describes, the natural patterns into which the universe of human and non-human nature spontaneously tends to organize itself.[34] In order to align herself with the pattern of cosmic flux, the Taoist practiced special methods designed to nourish the three treasures—*jing*, *qi*, and *shen*. Since breathing and eating were the two primary sources of qi, breathing exercises were used together with special diet and herbs to boost qi. The effort to maintain and boost qi was combined with other exercises and herbs designed to ensure the effective circulation of qi, which was susceptible to stagnation. *Jing* could be nourished by nutrition, while being carefully preserved by specific sexual practices. *Jing* and qi in turn nourished *shen*, which was protected by avoiding emotional distress and nourished by a meditative state of mind.

Qi Gong: Eastern Mind-Body Exercise

From Chinese pre-history emerged a spectrum of techniques involving breathing, meditation, visualization, self-massage, and gymnastics in various combinations. Breathing itself was a central focus of many early efforts to achieve longevity. Adepts practiced techniques like breath holding and slowing, with a underlying goal of "fetal" breathing. Echoing the essence of a much earlier Tang Dynasty

(618–907 A.D.) Chinese text, a modern tract on a formerly secret Korean Taoist breathing method explains: "A child in the womb 'breathes' through the umbilical cord and this energy enters the area of the *tantien*. The *tantien* breathing techniques recreate this passage of energy to the *tantien*, restoring the suppleness, health, and energy of youth to the body. Taoist hermits in the mountains of Korea live for literally hundreds of years and this is because the first effect of these techniques is to return the body to the health it had in youth."[35]

Breathing techniques were often combined with movement to produce a form of exercise quite unlike the idea of gymnastics in the West. These Taoist-inspired exercises were soft and supple, involving deep relaxation and mental quietness. Even "harder" muscle-strengthening exercises—often associated with the Buddhist tradition—still involved this internal aspect. Eastern exercises are mind-body disciplines: the mind actively guides the qi behind the movement and sometimes symbolic visualization is incorporated into the practice. The physical movements are designed with the body's energy centers and acupuncture meridians in mind, working to circulate qi, harmonize yin and yang, and build intrinsic mental and physical health.

In early times, the exercises were called "tao yin," which is variously translated as "guiding the breath while extending the limbs and trunk" or simply "mind-body exercise." Ancient artwork depicts men and women, old and young, carrying out forms like "bird stretching" and "bear rambling." Many exercises were in fact modeled after animals and ancient texts describe them being used in the treatment of disease. Today, the term qi gong, meaning qi or breathing exercise, is widely used to describe such practices, and there are hundreds of different forms and variations spanning a wide range of traditions— Confucian, Buddhist, and Taoist. Some have a more spiritual emphasis, others medical, and still others martial, making them collectively capable of cultivating the enlightened healer-warrior long idealized in the East.

Fang sung kung, or "relaxation breathing," is a basic form of medical qi gong, used in the treatment of chronic disease. This exercise emphasizes the practice of deep relaxation and mental quietness. It is practiced while lying on the back with a pillow holding the head for support. Breathing should be relaxed, narrow, steady, and smooth. Thinking of "quiet" while inhaling and "relax" while exhaling, the entire body is gradually scanned and brought to a state of deep relaxation. The technique even has a poem to guide practice:

The Poem of Fang Sung Kung[36]

With a high pillow I lie on my bed;
I keep my body comfortable and relaxed.
I breathe in and out naturally.
And say the words quiet and relax silently.
I think of the word quiet as I inhale,
And the word relax as I exhale.
As I silently say the word relax,
I tell my muscles to relax.
First, I tell my legs and feet to become relaxed.
After repeating this three times to get my body at ease,
I tell all my organs and cavities to relax.
I keep my breathing rhythm steady, narrow and even
While focusing my attention on my abdomen.
As my mind enters into a state of mental quietness,
I enjoy this sleeplike but awake state of consciousness.
After I stay in this state for a short period of time,
I rub my face, get up, move around and feel fine.

Below is an excerpt of a tao yin set described in the eighth century. While relaxation breathing combines physical relaxation with a meditative state of mind, this set illustrates other interesting facets of Chinese healing exercise, such as saliva swallowing, stretching, and self-massage. Saliva was considered a valuable elixir by the Taoists. This exercise is performed while sitting cross-legged.

> *Step 1: Knock the teeth 36 times, then clasp the hands over the ears and thump the index fingers on the area where the neck and skull meet.*

> *Step 2: Leaning slightly forward to start, straighten the back while turning the head alternatively to the right and left, 24 times.*

> *Step 3. Creating saliva with the tongue, divide it into thirds, swallowing each in turn. This practice will allow one to walk through fire.*

> *Step 4. Massage the kidney area and lower back with both hands 36 times. The more this exercise is practiced, the better the result.*

> *Step 5. Joining the hands in front of the body, breathe five times. Then, interlace the fingers above the head with the palms up, followed by massaging the top of the head, 3 or 9 times. (This is an important acupuncture point, the meeting place of the yang vessels, called* bai hui *or Hundred Convergences.)*

> *Step 6. With the legs stretched forward, reach out with the hands like hooks to grab the soles of the feet, 12 times, then return to the cross-legged position.*[37]

The great Han dynasty surgeon Hua Tuo is credited with creating the Five Animal Frolics, a set of exercises imitating the movements of five animals. He taught the peril of too little exercise—and the danger of too much. In a famous quote, Hua Tuo compared the body to a door hinge, which was made of leather in ancient China. As long as the door was used the leather hinge would remain supple and strong, but if unused it would become rotten and weak. The classic passage is worth repeating:

> *Exercise brings about good digestion, causing the qi and blood to circulate. It is like a door-pivot never rotting. Therefore the ancient sages engaged in tao yin exercises by moving the head like a bear. Exercising the joints and twisting at the waist can slow the aging process. I have a method known as the five animal frolics—tiger, deer, monkey, bear, and crane. It can be used to get rid of diseases, and it is beneficial for all stiffness of the joints or ankles. When the body feels ill, one should do the exercises. After perspiring the body will feel light and the stomach will feel hungry.*[38]

The 100 Step Form, one modern variation of the ancient exercise, is composed of four sets of five steps of each of the five animals in the order described by Hua Tuo. There are twenty different animal-imitating movements in total, each with a poetic name. The clawed tiger, for example, climbs mountains and seeks prey, while the roving monkey picks fruit and looks at the moon. The entire set takes about ten minutes to complete and each of the five animals benefits one of the five yin organs.

Ken Cohen, a qi gong teacher and scholar, calls the five animal frolics a "complete qi gong system." Its ability to circulate qi and blood and improve health qualifies the set as medical qi gong; as the precursor of various animal-centered martial styles it can be considered martial qi gong; and since the set emphasizes a connection to nature the animal frolics are spiritual qi gong.

One of the greatest achievements of Chinese health exercise is t'ai chi chuan, the Supreme Ultimate Exercise. Its origin is uncertain, but legend points to an internal alchemist, the mountain Taoist Zhang San-feng, as the inventor. Zhang's legendary life of over 200 years during the Yuan and Ming dynasties, spanned the thirteenth, fourteenth, and even fifteenth centuries. Zhang, whose birthday on April 9, 1247, is celebrated by t'ai chi aficionados, is said to have conceived the exercise in a dream.

T'ai chi in its various forms is a set of elaborate and stylized movements, some of which imitate animals, such as the "golden pheasant standing on one leg." The movements of this simultaneously martial and medical, physical and mental, exercise embody the principles of Chinese philosophy, the *tai ji* or Supreme Ultimate manifest as yin and yang and the Eight Trigrams. According to the Classics of t'ai chi, the art rests on consciousness rather than muscular force, and according to Chinese medical theory repetitive twisting and stretching at the waist circulates qi in the governing vessel—a major acupuncture channel which runs up the midline of the back—and the kidney. Since kidney qi is the root of life, the exercise is able to promote health at its deepest level. "The mind is the commander; the qi, the flag; and the waist, the banner," say the Classics. "The mind leads and the body follows. The abdomen is relaxed, enabling the qi to permeate the bones."[39]

As a final note, it is interesting that Needham traces a thread of influence from East to West in the area of exercise. A Jesuit named Cibot wrote a book in 1779 describing Chinese-style gymnastics thinking they would be of interest to European medical specialists. While Cibot was not particularly keen on Chinese philosophy, he nonetheless sensed the Eastern system of exercise to be valuable in the treatment of disease. "[T]he postures of kung fu, if well directed," wrote Cibot, "should effect a salutary clearance in all those illnesses which arise from an embarrassed, retarded, or even interrupted, circulation."[40] Cibot's account, and perhaps also his enthusiasm, had a strong influence on the Swede Per Hendrik Ling, the father of modern physiotherapy.

Supernutrition: Food and Herbs for Longevity
Throughout Chinese history, the relationship between food and health was considered to be particularly strong, both in prevention and in cure. It was for this reason that Hu Si-hui, Imperial Dietician from 1314 to 1330, wrote *The Principles of Correct Diet*. The cover of the book shows two dieticians consulting with a patient, with the

motto "food cures various diseases" tucked in the righthand corner. Indeed, the line between food and herb, sustenance and medicine, is not clearly drawn—some foods are used as medicinal herbs and some medicinal herbs are used as food.

The ancient geographical work, *The Classic of Mountains and Rivers*, although reflecting a pre-rationalist tradition, lists sixty substances to be used in the prevention of disease. Although some are simply to be worn on the body, others are ingested, and the largest class is those credited with the general promotion of both mental and physical health. This practice of using herbs for boosting health was continued in the *Shen Nong Ben Cao*, the first herbal book in the tradition of rational medicine that evolved into the modern system of traditional Chinese medicine.

Although Shen Nong, the patron "saint" of herbal medicine and the Divine Husbandman credited with bringing agriculture to China, did not actually write *Shen Nong's Pharmacological Classic*, the book represents the origin of herbal medicine as now practiced. Shaped into its present form during the first several centuries A.D., the book is interesting in that it divides herbs into three categories. (Some scholars think this was done by the Taoist Tao Hong-jing when he edited it during the sixth century.) Superior herbs rejuvenated and nourished life, middle-grade herbs tonified and strengthened, while inferior herbs treated disease. Just like the superior physician, the most esteemed herbs were used to stop disease from occurring in the first place.[41]

A poem written sometime around the fifteenth century illustrates the use of herbs as longevity agents, the close connection between inner and outer alchemy, and the continuity of the Taoist quest for immortality. Many plants were used as health-building elixirs, while serving as subjects for proto-chemical study and agents for chemical transmutation. This is part of a collection of poems describing the natural history and alchemical value of what the unknown author describes as "dragon sprouts," an honorific name suggesting the herbs were esteemed plants making rejuvenation and a vibrant old age possible.

The Immortal's Palm Dragon Sprout—Author Unknown[42]

Growing near the frigid pool
And the cave where hermit prays,
This is gathered as a rule
In the early summer days
When it's fully ripe and rich.
Made into a sublimate,
To a powder it will switch:
Sulfur it will fix in state.
But this art is little known.
When it's eaten change occurs:
Hair will turn to darker tone,
Youthful looks the plant confers.

The Immortal's Palm Dragon Sprout is none other than *suan zao*, the wild Chinese jujube, the seed of which is a Chinese herb widely used today. The *Shen Nong Ben Cao* claims the fruit can lengthen life and many modern formulas contain *suan zao ren* as a useful anti-insomnia agent. Sour Jujube Tea, for example, features a fairly high dose of the jujube seed as its chief ingredient. The formula is prescribed in cases where yin and blood deficiency of the liver and heart have affected the patient's ability to sleep.

Supersex: The Spiritual Path of the Bedchamber

Most Taoists included supernutrition in their repertoire of longevity techniques—and many also included supersex. For the Taoist, sexual union was the road to both procreation and supreme spiritual achievement. While ordinary sex produced the former, the latter was the result of specific techniques taught in secret transmission between master and student. As an eighth century text reporting such confidential oral instructions states: "Thus all the old Taoist traditions say that if the semen is ejaculated it leads to other men, that is to say, a child is born, but if it is retained it leads to the man himself, that is to say, an immortal body is born."[43]

The Taoist approach to sex was always controversial in China, even among the adepts themselves. While attacks by staid, moralistic Confucianists and Buddhists eventually moderated the more public and openly enthusiastic practice of esoteric conjugation, such practices had spread from mountain temples to the villages and towns by the Ming dynasty. A tradition of celibacy did emerge in Taoism, but even these adepts—who considered their less proscriptive brethren as promiscuous and oversexed—practiced special "solo" techniques.

Despite the controversy the Taoist approach to sex was a healthy one, treading a path of balance between the all-to-common extremes of Dionysian hedonism and self-reproaching guilt. Man and woman were fire and water, yang and yin, and their coming together was natural and mutually enhancing. Sex, if used with thought and care, was a spiritually nourishing activity—and something that could make or break a regimen of longevity training. "The arts of the bedchamber constitute the climax of human emotions and touch the very hem of the Tao itself," claimed *The History of the Han Dynasty*'s author in the first century, "If such joys are moderate and well-ordered, peace and longevity will follow; but if people are deluded by them and have no care, illnesses will ensue, with serious damage to the nature and span of life."[44]

The earliest teachings on esoteric sex are associated with Peng Zi—a mythical figure who reportedly lived for hundreds of years through his mastery of sexual techniques—and a number of famed female Taoists, including the Chosen Girl, who is often found in conversation with the Yellow Emperor himself. The techniques taught by these Taoist Dr. Ruths were based on several ideas. One was a deep admiration for feminine characteristics and the need for a high level of female satisfaction. Especially in the bedchamber, the woman was thought to be superior to the man and the techniques of Taoist sex were designed to achieve a special level of female response—the "valley" orgasm—well beyond that achieved from "normal" procedures.

From the male perspective, sex was considered to be beneficial as long as sperm was lost only according to prescribed intervals which depended on age and state of health. Male techniques thus centered on the ability to prolong the sexual act using muscle control and other methods of preventing ejaculation. Men and women guided their sexual energy along the spine to nourish the brain and exchanged qi so that yin nourished yang, and yang nourished yin. These techniques involved the "energy" centers and meridians of the body and many required advanced meditation skills.

Healing could also be accomplished through sex, and books like the *Classic of the Plain Girl* offered prescriptions for specific ailments. For menstrual problems, for example, it suggests a woman lie comfortably relaxed on her side to receive the healing energy of her partner in two lovemaking sessions per day. Fifteen days constitute a course of treatment. Prescriptions were also provided for problems ranging from arthritis to weakness of the blood.

Ancient Practices for a Modern World

This discussion of prevention in ancient China and of the health-promoting techniques of Taoism has focused almost entirely on the past tense. Yet these ancient practices have survived intact, even undergoing a renaissance in recent decades. Chinese herbal shops, a prominent feature of North American Chinatowns, still busily cater to clients keen on many of the same longevity herbs used by ancients, often combined in formulas passed on through the generations. Qi gong in its myriad forms is now used as a therapeutic tool in Chinese hospitals and is being subjected to the scrutiny of scientific research. Dozens of books are available in English, together with courses in most major cities, making it ever more possible to learn and practice qi gong.

Exercises like tao yin, the five animal frolics, and t'ai chi are practiced and taught throughout the world. Even the most esoteric and secretive Taoist practices, like the sexual techniques, are now taught openly to Westerners. The Thai-born Mantak Chia, for example, offers courses through centers around the world, and has published a series of detailed books chronicling these ancient, living practices.

For a time, it appeared that Chinese medicine was on its way out. During the Nationalist era in China, traditional medicine was slated for destruction, only to be resurrected as a medicine of the people by Chairman Mao. Under Mao's leadership, other traditional practices did not fare so well, including those of Taoism. Yet turmoil in China has helped to spread Chinese medicine and Taoist-inspired practices around the world. Ironically, as global culture embraces the "virtual" reality of high technology, more and more people are grounding themselves with the ancient health-promoting techniques of the East.

Prevention East and West

The doctor of the future will give no medicine but will interest his patients in the care of the human frame, in diet, and in the cause and prevention of disease.

—Thomas Alva Edison

Experts at curing diseases are inferior to specialists who warn against diseases. Experts in the use of medicines are inferior to those who recommend proper diet.[45]

—Chen Zhi, Song Dynasty

What I want to see in the future is a reduced demand for health care. I want doctors to focus on people who are already healthy, and ask what they can do to maximize their health.

—Neal Barnard, President, PCRM[46]

It could be said that the ancient Chinese emphasized prevention simply because they were so poor at curing—and there is likely some truth in that idea. Transplants were not available for failing hearts and kidneys, while antibiotics able to effectively treat deadly infections had not yet been invented. Without the miracles of high technology medicine to rely on, staying healthy was all the more important.

The Chinese also approached the idea of prevention from another angle. The Taoist obsession with longevity generated a host of methods for improving and maintaining health, and a sense of confidence emerged in the ability of individual effort to make a significant difference in one's state of health. The ideas that "One's life-span depends upon oneself" and that it was possible to maintain good health even at an advanced age were powerful and pervasive throughout the eons of Chinese history. Such health did not result from luck, but from hard work.

Western medicine has come to appreciate the value of prevention from a different direction. While the Chinese system is strongly health oriented, the Western system is disease oriented. For close to a century, Western culture has been fascinated with high-tech, doctor-centered cures. Even the most prominent form of prevention, the vaccine, rests on technological achievement. Since this technological optimism was often combined with a sense of fatalism about disease—the feeling that getting sick is the result of bad luck, bad genes, or simply getting old—there was little room for thought of prevention. Perhaps Western medicine and culture has ignored prevention for so long simply because it was so good at curing, or at least thought it was.

The tide has turned. Research is now demonstrating that age-related decline can be significantly moderated by individual effort. Some decline with age is inevitable, but even very aged residents of retirement homes put on weight training regimens dramatically improve muscle strength and endurance. Similar research with mental "workouts" shows that psychological functions can be improved significantly—no matter what the age. Robert Kahn, a former professor of public health and at age eighty co-author of *Successful Aging*, chronicles the myths and possibilities of vital living in the later years of life. Describing research sponsored by the MacArthur Foundation, Kahn points out that mental decline is not inevitable nor as common as popularly believed, noting the brain's "remarkable and enduring capacity to make new connections, absorb new data and thus acquire new skills."

Ed started exercising at eighty-six; quoted at ninety-one he recounted: "Once I started, I felt stronger, full of action. The weight lifting helps my walking. I feel better, I sleep better, I eat better. It has changed my life." Researchers estimate that only 30 percent of aging characteristics can be attributed to heredity, and by age eighty genes have an almost negligible effect. Echoing the long-held Chinese sense that one can, in large part, determine one's own fate, Kahn states flatly: "MacArthur research provides very strong scientific evidence that we are, in large part, responsible for our own old age."[47]

As hope in magic-bullet cures for chronic disease wanes, research is chronicling the untapped potential for prevention. A medical specialist writing recently in *Scientific American* in response to an article on the lost war on cancer illustrates well this profound shift in thinking: "Until recently, there was little funding for studies of cancer prevention: curing cancer was seen as a quicker fix. Now that we know how effectively an established cancer can resist treatment, prevention is widely perceived as preferable. That it took scientists 23 years to reach this perception is unfortunate but understandable."[48]

It is interesting that one of the major hurdles to prevention-based health care is the invisibility of its success. While cure can bring fame for doctor and patient alike, prevention is imperceptible and even hard to prove. "It is…impossible to tell whether a healthy lifestyle warded off cancer in an individual," writes Harvard university professor Walter Willett and colleagues in *Scientific American*. "Conversely, successful treatment invariably becomes a landmark event. Moreover, the results of effective treatment become apparent quickly, whereas the impact of a prevention regime…may take years to emerge."[49]

The Chinese recognized this paradox of prevention and cure thousands of years ago. An intriguing discussion in the *Book of the Pheasant-Cap Master*—first penned during the third century B.C. and shaped into its present form during subsequent centuries—explores the theme of the superior and inferior doctor through a dialogue among two nobles and a general. The discussion revolves around a family of great physicians, and it is explained that one brother is really much more skilled than the other. He "treats" before symptoms appear, yet he is not known outside the family. The other brother— a great physician too, but no match for his sibling—works hard to treat already established diseases. Because of his success he is famous throughout the province. The moral of the story: effective cure brings fame, while successful prevention ensures only anonymity.

The ideal physician of ancient China bears a strong resemblance to the perfect doctor envisioned in the new biology and medicine: they were paid to keep their patients healthy, and considered failures in responding to disease. Neal Barnard, in a similar but modern vein, speaks enthusiastically about the possibilities of prevention, going as far as to suggest physicians switch to "treating" people when they are healthy rather than when they are sick. And the late Denis Burkitt argued that doctors need a new outlook: "How can it be cured?" must be changed to "How can this be prevented?"

Chinese medicine, with its systems-based conception of the mind-body, can perceive "imbalance" even without the presence of a defined and localized "disease." Chinese medicine is thus ideally suited for prevention. This is a result of its conceptual framework, a means of organizing signs and symptoms into a pattern of disharmony that can be addressed with acupuncture, herbs, diet, or exercise. These tools of the trade provide the means to both restore harmony when it has been lost and maintain harmony as a means of prevention.

Diet and herbs are most effectively used before problems develop. Qi gong can be part of a spiritual journey, a stress-management technique, or one part of a therapeutic regimen in the treatment of chronic disease. Even acupuncture and moxibustion can be used to boost immunity during flu season. The dual nature of these methods—their ability to be used in both the prevention and the treatment of disease—arises from their gentle and health-promoting quality.

Disease-oriented Western medicine has long ignored the gap between good health and disease. Exceptions like acute, infectious disease aside, people rarely wake up sick. Chronic illness tends to be a slow, gradual process with a significant period of time at the "subclinical" level before a specific biomedically definable disease appears. This is true of cancer. "The concept that people with cancer were healthy until a doctor told them that they've got an invasive lesion makes no sense at all," says Michael Sporn, professor at Dartmouth Medical School.[50] Sporn and a growing number of researchers are working to detect and treat cancer at its beginning rather than at its ending stage. These "chemoprevention" enthusiasts are looking to the preventive potential of many natural chemicals, like the dithiolthiones found in cabbage and broccoli, that will enable them to block the progression of the disease at its earliest stage.

Western medicine has traditionally focused on the heroic battle against well-established disease and many of its methods are correspondingly harsh and only used when their benefits outweigh their risks. The new medicine, however, shows a shift toward gentle and health-promoting methods that can be used for both treatment and prevention. Dean Ornish's heart disease program can be used either to reverse or prevent the disease, the difference being the degree to which the program must be followed. People who want to reverse serious heart disease must follow the program rigorously.

Many Westerners are now interested in traditional Chinese methods of preserving and restoring health. Longevity herbs such as *ling zhi* (reishi) and *dang gui* have become popular and ancient health exercises like t'ai chi are taught at community centers and practiced in parks throughout North America. This interest has emerged as a result of the strong resonance between Eastern and emerging Western ideas about health.

The idea that chronic disease is not inevitable, and that an individual can go a long way toward ensuring good health is a message that the PCRM is trying to get across and one with which the ancient mountain Taoists would have had little quarrel. The vegetarianism advocated by the PCRM, for example, emerges from the growing body of research demonstrating the contrast between the deleterious components of meat and the beneficial qualities of plant-based foods. Taoist vegetarianism too arose from the belief that meat contained factors deleterious to health. The confidence displayed by the dietary specialists of ancient China in the healing and preventive power of daily diet is now shared by modern nutritional experts. Scientists are studying the health-promoting chemicals found in plants with an enthusiasm rivaling the ancient Chinese enthusiasm for longevity plants. And Hua Tuo's words touting the benefit of exercise, both preventive and curative, are now echoed by researchers pointing to an exploding accumulation of studies demonstrating the value of exercise.

To Adapt or Not to Adapt

The reasonable man adapts himself to the world: the unreasonable one persists in trying to adapt the world to himself.
—George Bernard Shaw, *Reason*

As Thomas McKeown pointed out, the great plagues of the past were conquered largely by changing the environmental conditions that favored them. Poor sanitation and hygiene together with squalid housing and poor nutrition produced the perfect environment for infectious disease, and as this set of conditions changed for the better, so did the health of the people. McKeown also argued that the great plagues of the present—that collection of chronic health problems termed as "Western" disease—will be most successfully addressed by altering the conditions in which they thrive.

Humans have adapted to a remarkable diversity of conditions, and live everywhere from rainforest to desert, from the Arctic to the tropics. They are not well suited, however, for life in modern, industrialized civilization. Ironically, in our rush to create an easier life with technology, we have created an unnatural world out of touch with our essential selves and the ecological reality of the planet.

Two distinct approaches have emerged in response to this dilemma. On one side is the effort to adapt ourselves to this pathological environment of our own making by understanding how genes shape disease. From this perspective, since many diseases arise from genetic unsuitability to the modern environment, the solution is to alter and adapt human genes. On the other side is the idea that our "environment"—including our diet, lifestyle habits, and social patterns—should be adapted to suit our genetic selves.

Both trends can be found in agriculture. On one side is the effort to adapt our diet and agricultural systems to nature. Organic farmers, like the innovative market gardener Eliot Coleman, create agricultural systems from an ecological framework. Coleman's own success shows that by working with natural cycles bountiful harvests are possible. "Study the established balances of the natural world in order to learn how to nurture and enhance those balances for agricultural production," writes Coleman, "Pay attention to the existing framework of plant-pest relationships and learn how food production can be achieved through biological diplomacy rather than chemical warfare. The potential of such a new understanding is as yet undreamed of."[51]

Other thinkers go further, arguing that the human diet should be adapted to the cornucopia provided by nature. While some 30,000 species of plants are edible and 7,000 of these have been used throughout history, only twenty species comprise 90 percent and three species over 50 percent of the world's food supply. The majority of this food is grown in monoculture vulnerable to pests and disease, and heavily reliant on chemical fertilizer and pesticides. Our diets remain narrow because we cannot see past the few species discovered and nurtured by our forebears, claims Edward O. Wilson, renowned Harvard biologist, who argues that our diets, and modern agriculture, could be greatly enriched by "tens of thousands of unused plant species, many demonstrably superior to those in favor."

Wilson and others—notably the late agricultural pioneer and publisher Robert Rodale—have enthusiastically described many remarkable, but unfortunately ignored, super-plants that could provide the foundation of a more successful system of agriculture and a better human diet. Wilson, for example, highlights the winged bean (*Psophocarpus tetragonolobus*) as a "one-species supermarket." The plant's leaves can be compared to spinach, its pods resemble green beans, and it has edible and nutritious tubers. The soybean-like seeds can be eaten as is, used as flour, or processed into a coffee-like substitute. Winged beans grow like weeds, reaching almost 13 feet in only a matter of weeks. The winged bean is a nitrogen-fixing legume, enhances soil fertility, and requires little fertilizer. "With a small amount of genetic improvement through selective breeding," says Wilson, "the winged bean could raise the standard of living of millions of people in the poorest tropical countries."[52,53]

In contrast to its organic counterpart, mainstream "agri-business" is a type of food production based not on the understanding of ecological systems, but on the creation of an "efficient" industrial process. The actual growing of crops and raising of animals is an extension of a larger system in which food is transformed and transported large distances, with a large gap—in many senses of the word—between growers and consumers of food-stuffs. With the help of technology nature is shaped to fit an industrial model. Some potato varieties are chosen for how well they can be processed into French fries; tomatoes are bred and genetically altered for machine handling and long-distance transportation; and crops of all sorts are genetically altered to become insensitive to toxic weed killers by the very companies who manufacture the toxic chemicals.

While organic agriculture strives to work with natural systems, arguing that this is, in the long term, the most "efficient" approach, mainstream chemical-based agriculture has now turned to altering genes in its effort to create a more efficient system of farming.

Organic agriculture adapts to nature, chemical agriculture adapts nature to suit its own needs, resulting in an industrial system of food production that is often at odds with both ecological and human health.

With respect to the issue of human health and the prevention of disease, the question of adaptation, as in agriculture, looms large. One group of researchers is eagerly searching for the root of "Western" disease, tracing its origins in the environment of affluent civilization. Like-minded physicians are working to educate people about these findings and what they can do to improve their health. There is little fame and scant profit here, yet the preventive potential is enormous.

Other researchers eagerly search for the root of "Western" disease in the genetic code, hoping one day to successively alter the code in the effort to avoid disease. (Medicine is somewhat behind agriculture in the effort to manipulate genes. While genetically altered crops can be found in the marketplace, medical gene-altering is only in an early stage.) There is much fame and tremendous potential for profit here, yet the benefits are unproven and the ethical implications remain unresolved.

Genetic and environmental factors are intimately interlinked and there is benefit to be had from the understanding of both in the perennial search for health and the treatment of disease. Yet while the environmental factors related to "Western" disease are well understood and the preventive possibilities from even small changes known to be great, much of the scientific effort and public enthusiasm is now directed toward gene-altering technology. This strange emphasis arises in part from a distorted sense that environmental factors are not easily changed, while genes are. Nonetheless, a shift in thinking is now underway toward a Tao of health and healing implying that humans adapt their diet, lifestyle, and way of life to suit their true nature.

7 | The Mysterious Link Between Mind and Body: Holistic Health East and West

"Decades ago, physicians made an arbitrary separation between mind and body," wrote Jane Brody in a *New York Times* story on the growing popularity of complementary medicine, adding "and modern medicine is only now beginning to reintegrate them and more fully appreciate how they affect one another."[1] Brody reflects that while conventional medicine is returning to the realization that mind and body are not separate, isolated facets of human reality, other healing traditions never separated them in the first place and so take a more holistic approach to health.

The mind-body problem—the grand question about the nature of mind and its relationship to the body—has intrigued Western civilization from its earliest days. In the early days of science, Descartes struggled with the relationship between the soul and its container, the machine-like body, setting the stage for the modern attempt at resolving the problem. Since that time many great thinkers have wrestled with an understanding of mind and its relationship to the physical realm. The struggle continues.

Confusion over the body-mind problem is felt nowhere more strongly than in questions of sickness and health. The traditional boundary between mind and body is reflected in the structure of the health care system. Mental/emotional phenomena are delegated to psychology and psychiatry; physical problems are the domain of the specialties addressing various physiological and anatomical systems or disease categories. Yet such boundary lines are thin. Physical complaints often have a strong psychological connection, while mental/emotional disorders can have a strong physical component.

Some problems, like pain, sit solidly on the boundary line between the mental and the physical.

Over the past several decades, the thin, artificial line between mind and body has begun to dissolve and there is a growing sense that mind events affect physiological processes and vice versa. Movie-maker Woody Allen's famous line "I don't get angry, I just grow a tumor," is a more popular—and extreme—reflection of a dramatic shift in culture and science toward the recognition and study of mind-body interrelationships. The new biology is in part psychology.

While Western science and medicine is discovering—or perhaps re-discovering—the relationship between the physical and mental facets of existence, once again something new in the West is something old in the East. This is territory already mapped out by the Chinese, who did not even go as far as talking about the interaction between mind and body as if they could be considered isolated and distinct in the first place. For the Chinese, the mind and body are inseparable facets of an underlying "energy" event, a dynamic process with a more substantive aspect, the physical form, and a more ethereal one involving mind, emotion, and spirit.

In the Eastern way of thinking, mind events and anatomical substratum are interlinked by qi. Qi shapes simultaneously the material of the body and the emotions. Misbehaving qi can manifest as mental or physical disharmony, or both, a possibility that is inherent in the Chinese medical framework of organ systems which are considered "orbs" of both physiological and psychological processes. This basic orientation is central to Taoist practice, which is founded on the nourishment and care of the body. Only with a sound body can there be a sound mind and an adequate foundation for the transformative activity that is considered spiritual development in this unique Eastern religion.

Mind and Body in the West: A Search for Unity and Meaning

The Mind-Body Problem

"Am I my soul and body? Or can it be said that I am a soul and have a body? Or have I a soul and a body whilst myself being 'spirit'? Or is the I-concept perhaps an optical illusion?"
—C. A. Van Peursen, *Body, Soul, Spirit: A Survey of the Body-Mind Problem*[2]

Imagine a stroll through a park. There are trees, perhaps some elegant pines, a few stately elms, and plenty of grass. That is the world "out there." There is a body walking through the park complete with legs and arms, bones and muscles, eyes and ears, your body. There are also thoughts and feelings, perhaps a sense of satisfaction from a hard day's work mixed with anger at the behavior of a certain family member and even ideas about what to have for supper. And behind it all there is an awareness of the world out there, of the body as it walks, and of the thoughts continually arising and passing away.

In this potpourri of reality, where is the self? You probably don't identify your self with the world "out there"—with the trees, grass, and open sky—but the body is getting closer to home. Thoughts and feelings are certainly *your* thoughts and feelings, and most strongly of all there is the *I* in back of it all, that pure, clear awareness watching and experiencing.

Mind appears to be something distinct from the body and from the physical world "out there." But what is mind and what is its relationship to the body and to the outside, physical world? This basic question is the famous mind-body problem, the prickly thorn of philosophers and scientists through the centuries.

The Christian world has a tradition of dividing reality, setting God apart from man, spirit apart from body, heaven apart from earth. It was within this Christian milieu that René Descartes addressed the relationship between body and soul. The body for Descartes, as we have seen, was a machine, a complex but nonetheless mechanical contraption. The human mind was distinctly different, part of the spiritual world rather than the material.

While Descartes is usually credited with separating mind and body, he actually struggled to explain their close connection. Since, as ordinary experience shows, mind can affect the body and vice versa, one of the problems for Descartes was to explain how these distinctly different phenomena—mind and body—could still influence one another. He felt that the soul was joined to the body, but not through the brain, which connects the sense organs, or through the heart, which enables us to experience the passions. Instead, it is through "a certain very small gland"—the pineal gland—that body and soul unite. "Let us then conceive here that the soul has its principal seat in the little gland which exists in the middle of the brain," wrote the famous philosopher, "from whence it radiates forth through all the remainder of the body by means of the animal spirits, nerves, and even the blood, which, participating in the impressions of the spirits, can carry them by the arteries into all the members."[3]

Modern science and medicine does not accept that mind and body are different in kind. The lack of interest, until recently, in the mind-body relationship stems instead from the breaking-things-into-pieces and studying-them-in-isolation strategy that does originate with Descartes. From the point of view of science, material reality is the only reality. It can be measured and is subject to mathematical laws. To believe anything else is to accept mysticism and magic—to be, in a word, unscientific. The phenomenon of mind must be a part of this material reality.

The most extreme of "materialists" deny there is such a thing as mind, strange as this may sound. Humans can be described, they argue, in terms of sensory inputs and behavioral outputs. Less extreme materialists acknowledge the existence of thoughts and feelings, but consider them to be identical with brain events. A particular emotional experience *is* the activity of particular brain chemicals; a sudden flash of inspiration *is* the collective activity of neurons in a particular area of the brain. And no matter what the brand of materialism, consciousness—the ability to be self-aware—is still easier to deny than explain.

With the advent of the computer, the materialist approach to the mind-body problem grew in sophistication. Indeed, the conceptual link between the scientific understanding of the brain and the development of the computer is a close one. John von Neumann appears to have invented the computer and created a computer-based model of the brain at the same time.[4]

At least on a good day, the mind can solve problems and make and manipulate representations of the world, and, even on a bad day, has beliefs about things. While no simple machine can calculate and manipulate representations, the computer is able to do many impressive things of that sort. From the digital revolution a new model emerged, one built on the idea of mind as computer. The brain is envisioned as the hardware that runs a sophisticated software program bringing various mental faculties into being, especially those associated with intelligence.

Of Quanta and Self-Organization: Mind in the New Biology

In whatever form it is presented, I cannot accept the materialist view. And curiously enough, my objections are not based on the so-called "higher" mental abilities we possess, but on the "lower" ones. Not on the powers of understanding, reasoning, or choice, but on the modest functions of sensation, feeling, and emotion. To put it in a nutshell: the chess-playing computer Deep Thought, or an improved successor, may one day beat Kasparov, but it will not enjoy doing so.
—Zeno Vendler, University of California Philosophy Professor[5]
[Since Professor Vendler's comment, a computer has indeed beaten a chess master. It is not clear whether the computer enjoyed the experience.]

The mind-body problem continues to confound science. On one hand there can be no lament for the discarding of dualism—the position that mind and body are fundamentally different things. It is too difficult to describe mind and body as distinctly different and yet successfully explain the intimate relationship between them. On the other hand, the materialist position often goes too far, sometimes denying the reality and meaning of mental phenomena, and always tripping over the question of consciousness.

Descartes was enamored by the newfangled mechanical contraptions of his time and pointed to analogies between mechanical systems and the human body. He went too far in claiming that the human body *is* a machine. Modern scientists are enamored by the computer and have made useful analogies between the mind-brain and the computer. Some have gone too far in asserting that the mind-brain *is* a computer or, alternatively, in claiming that computers have minds (or will once programs and programmers rise to the challenge).

While some scientists continue to work with useful, but limited analogies, others have forged ahead into unexplored lands. What is needed is an approach that can offer meaning to mind and spirit, emotion and consciousness, while affirming the unity of underlying reality and teasing out the mysterious link between mind and body. While a complete theory of mind is a long way off, there is some intriguing research based on a fundamentally different conception of mind and body.

The mind equals brain equation is a starting point for challenge. The central nervous system and brain clearly play a central role in mental function, but this role is not so easily pinned down. Researchers became excited by the discovery that particular areas of the brain are closely related to particular mental functions. Yet if these areas are damaged other areas can sometimes take over those functions, suggesting a complex phenomena involving global coherence rather than simple mechanical correspondence.

While scientists typically study the body by breaking it up into its parts, recent discoveries are dissolving such human-imposed boundaries. The phenomenon of mind is closely linked to the brain, but the brain and mind are not so easily separated from the rest of the body. The brain and nervous system, the body's hormonal network—called the endocrine system—and the protective immune system, were all once studied largely in isolation, and now appear to form an interlinked network.

Peptides are small proteins used to carry information and control bodily processes. They are also involved in mental function. (We have already seen in Chapter 5 that certain neuropeptides are strong physical correlates of emotional experience.) It turns out that it is not so easy to think of each of the body's major systems in isolation. Some peptides involved in the brain and nervous system also play a role in the immune system, while endocrine-system peptides can be found in the brain. Neuroscientist Candace Pert was moved enough by the interdependence of the body's chemical information and control network to claim: "I can no longer make a strong distinction between the brain and the body."[6]

Another interesting challenge to the idea that our minds are literally in our heads is the emerging discipline of neurogastroenterology, a big-sounding name for the study of a semi-autonomous nervous system in the stomach and intestines. Scientists have pieced together a hitherto unrecognized "brain in the gut" which has all the same hardware as its more highly developed counterpart—the brain in the head. During embryological development primitive nerve tissue divides into two, one piece going on to form the central nervous system, the other becoming the intestinal nervous system. Later, the two nervous systems are coupled, offering a means of interaction.

The existence of an "intestinal brain" helps explain many curious phenomena, like the close relationship between emotions and intestinal activity. The intestinal brain even mirrors the wave patterns of the "head brain" during sleep. "Butterflies in the stomach" may be a metaphor since there are no real butterflies in the stomach, but the emotional experience is strongly associated with that area of the body.[7] Once again, we find an example of mental phenomena not located in the head.

The mind-body problem is closely related to our underlying world view and its resolution may well emerge from a shift in perception of reality. Classical science has given us a world view that separates the objective observer from a world made of hard, solid, material stuff.

At the same time, the mind is viewed as part of this same material world, identified with the physical operation of the brain.

Quantum physics has turned the classical view upside down and inside out. Some scientists argue that the quantum theory is only relevant for really small things the size of atoms and so is not useful for large things like people and their minds. But others have seriously considered what the quantum theory says about the question of mind and the nature of consciousness.

The Nobel prize-winning physicist Brian Josephson, for example has turned to explore questions of mind and consciousness. Josephson goes as far as to argue that nature's most subtle secrets cannot be probed with the scientific method as it now stands. The "complete development" of science, he argues, requires that conscious experience be accounted for. "Mind, in its subtler aspects especially, cannot be handled in conventional scientific terms," says Josephson, "Even if it is legitimate to equate the workings of the mind with the behavior of the brain, the question of what exactly the brain is presents grave difficulties, even in principle, if we inquire at a sufficiently subtle level."[8]

University of California physicist Henry Stapp has thought deeply about the meaning of quantum physics and how it can be applied to the understanding of mind. Several hundred years of effort has not resulted in any useful understanding of mind from the classical point of view, claims Stapp. The quantum theory, by contrast, describes the subtle properties of brain matter and offers a framework entirely compatible with the nature of consciousness.

In his "quantum theory of consciousness," Stapp combines the late, great German physicist Werner Heisenberg's approach to quantum physics with nineteenth century psychologist William James' approach to the mind. James argued that consciousness had a unitary quality incompatible with classical physics, while Heisenberg noted the difference between the essence and the actuality of the things in the world. Quantum theory describes things like electrons as probability waves. They do not have fully determined characteristics, but are in essence a set of tendencies to take on various states. There is, in quantum theory, a point where these tendencies manifest, with one of the possible characteristics or another coming into being. This is the point of observation, the point where consciousness becomes an integral part of reality.

The brain involves micro-chemical events at a quantum mechanical level. At the same time brain events are global in character, involving integrated patterns of cellular excitation. It follows, according to the Stapp model, that these patterns are quantum mechanical and a certain point is needed for a particular state to be "actualized." For Stapp, this choosing of one state over another is a conscious event, a "top-down control of brain process by subjective conscious experience."[9]

A more radical, while less exotic, approach to understanding mind has emerged from systems thinking. One of the leaders of systems biology is the Chilean neuroscientist Humberto Maturana. Working with colleagues like former student Francisco Varela, Maturana broke completely new ground in his systems approach to understanding the cognitive features of living systems. The Santiago theory, as it is called, suggests that mind cannot be reduced to specific chemical and physical features of the brain. Instead, cognition and consciousness—the process of acquiring knowledge and the ability to be self-aware—must be studied as phenomena of the organism as a whole and its interactions with its environment and social group.[10]

Cognition is the most fundamental of mental processes and something that all organisms—not just those with a highly developed nervous system—possess. Cognition is a process that emerges directly from the self-organization of living systems. Recall that the central feature of living systems is their continual dynamic self-creation. Life itself is an organized pattern, an integrated web of processes in a state of continuous activity. While conventional science has emphasized the structures of living things that emerge from these processes, systems scientists suggest that the organizational patterns and relationships must also be studied.

Cognition emerges from the interaction of the organism with its environment. The structure of a living system is in a state of continual transformation and its response to its environment is one of structural change. This is not a simple mechanical change in a part, but a globally coherent shift in the web of relationships. Recall that living systems are non-linear systems: tiny inputs can have significant consequences while large inputs can be without effect. This opens the way for complex responses and the possibility of learning and intelligence.

Responses to the environment are not automatic and mechanical. Each organism responds in a different way, its nature determining what features of the environment require notice and what constitutes an appropriate response. In this way, the organism in effect creates its own world. Cognition is not the creation of a simple one-to-one representation of the "outside" world, but a response that is internalized in the organism's pattern of organization and structure.

As organisms become more complex, the range of response and possibilities for interaction grow: emotions become part of the pattern of each cognitive event, an internal world of thought emerges, and that most mysterious of all mental processes, consciousness, appears. Maturana also approaches these higher mental functions from a systems perspective, this time centering on the interaction between organisms. Organisms use communications to order their behavior, and humans use language as a higher level of behavioral coordination, a communication about a communication. The objects of language are at the same time objects of mind, but their meaning is subjective and relational. Just as cognition "brings forth a world" for an organism, communication builds a web of relationships that "brings forth a world" that includes thoughts and even consciousness.

The Santiago theory of mind is a radical departure from conventional science. It does not locate the mind in the brain, nor does it see mind as separate from matter. Instead mind is seen as the very process of life itself, the shaping of dynamic, self-organizing systems by the web they are a part of. Emotions are not things, but a coloring of a unified cognitive process. And thoughts and consciousness emerge as a self-created world from self-creating systems. "The world everyone sees is not *the* world," claim Maturana and Varela, "but *a* world, which we bring forth with others....As we know how we know, we bring forth ourselves."[11]

Where Mind Meets Body in Health and Healing

The headline of a newspaper story describing yet another study on the link between mind and body was characteristically succinct: "Hostile feelings damage heart." In the study, Stanford University researchers had found that simply recalling anger-filled life experiences was enough to lower the pumping ability of the heart. Other research had indicated that hostile people were at an increased risk of heart disease and the new study supported this idea. Although the observed drop in pumping efficiency was small, the participants were only asked to *remember* angry incidents. A larger drop would be expected during the actual event itself, leading the study's chief scientist to suggest people with heart disease would benefit from the practice of anger management.

This is but one example of the growing body of research exploring the mind-body link. In the 1960s and '70s, scientists began to discover that the "parts" of the body—such as the central nervous system, the immune system, and the endocrine system—were very closely intertwined. This meant that various mental processes and behaviors could influence the immune system and could affect the way we get sick. Scientists coined the term psychoneuroimmunology, or psychoimmunology for short, to describe the study of the immune system-mind/brain link. By the 1990s, the discipline had coalesced and scientists became more confident in confirming a mind-immune system relationship. The results of a 1992 conference, for example, were described in the matter-of-fact manner typical of science: "Data presented has confirmed the longstanding perception that state of mind and behavioral patterns have an impact on health and disease resistance."[12]

One "pet" story told by mind-body researchers recounts a serendipitous discovery of mind-body interaction. University of Ohio researchers were using a high-fat, high-cholesterol diet to produce heart disease in rabbits. It worked well except for the fact that the rabbits in the lower set of cages were not afflicted with the disease to the same degree as were rabbits in the upper cages. This made no sense: the rabbits were in the same kind of cage, getting the same food and water, and were even of the same genetic stock, yet clearly there was a dramatic difference in their susceptibility to heart disease.

And then came a clue. One researcher realized that in the course of caring for the rabbits those in the lower cages were being handled by a bunny-loving technician who caressed and even talked to the furry charges. Intrigued, but skeptical of the possibility that human-rabbit interaction was causing such remarkable protection from heart disease, researchers repeated the experiment—twice. The results were unequivocal: a little tender loving care could buffer the bunnies from the heart-degenerating effects of a high-fat diet by a whopping 60 percent.[13]

This kind of pet-human affection can also have effects in the other direction. During the height of the Cuban Missile Crisis, President Kennedy asked that his dog be brought into his office. The dog sat on his lap and was petted affectionately by the President as aides and advisors scurried around him. After ten minutes he—the President—was rejuvenated and the dog returned to his usual quarters. Health-promoting experiences with animals are very common and research has confirmed that pets can be very beneficial for elderly and convalescent people. Pet programs are now used in hospitals and nursing homes.

Studies have also examined the relationship between personality and disease to see if certain kinds of people get sick in predictable ways. The Type A personality and its relationship to heart disease is now famous. This personality pattern includes aggressiveness, hostility, time-stress, and competitiveness, a profile that appears to make it more likely to be afflicted with heart disease. Hostility is considered to be a particularly hazardous aspect of the pattern.[14] A Type C personality has also been postulated and has been linked to an increased risk for cancer. This type of person does not express emotions well, especially anger. They are overly patient and socially conformist and, unlike the Type A who over-reacts to the slightest stress, the Type C feels helpless in the face of stress.

The concept of stress has been a center point for thinking about the mind-body relationship. In his classic 1977 book *Mind As Healer, Mind As Slayer*, Kenneth Pelletier claimed that up to 80 percent of all disease involves psychosomatic or stress-related factors.[15] For Pelletier, the term psychosomatic suggests a fundamental interaction between mind and body affecting everything to do with health.[16] The stress pioneer, Hans Selye, defined stress as "the nonspecific response of the organism to any pressure or demand."[17] Stress is an unavoidable part of life, but it is the failure to respond effectively to it that can lead to disharmony and disease.

Stress, of course, has become the universal malady. Practically everybody has it at one time or another and some people have it almost all of the time. It is also a very popular medical diagnosis. Unfortunately, stress is not a faddish catchall, but an intimate feature of contemporary life.

Maverick medical doctor Larry Dossey points out that despite the evidence that mind is an important part of the health equation, all this research has changed little. Even though many people feel science is building a radically new perspective where the mind has the power to shape physiological events, says Dossey, when scientists and physicians refer to "mind" or "psyche" they are really referring to brain activity. The materialist outlook in science is simply so strong that mind-body research is really brain-body research.

Dossey points to a growing body of more radical inquiry that cannot be reduced to the workings of the brain. Some 150 studies have examined whether prayer can affect living systems, including people, and evidence is emerging that it can. In one study, for example, hospitalized heart attack victims were divided into two groups; in addition to standard medical care, one group was prayed for, the other not. A difference was observed in the number of complications in the two groups, with the prayed-for patients doing much better than their not-prayed-for counterparts.

For Dossey, this kind of research not only demonstrates that consciousness can affect the body, but suggests that mind has a non-local character. The idea that consciousness can result in action-at-a-distance challenges our most basic notions of reality. "These studies are exceptionally relevant clinically because they suggest that consciousness can bring about remarkable changes in the course of human illness and can make the difference between life and death," claims Dossey, who teaches courses on prayer in medicine at a number of the nation's top medical schools.[18]

The influence of mind-body research has not all been positive. There is now an all-too-common tendency to blame people for their illnesses. If anger and outlook can precipitate health crises, perhaps the sick have brought on their own affliction by being too angry and too pessimistic? Such blame is misplaced. It is not easy to change ingrained emotional states, let alone change one's basic personality. There is also the whole question of cause and effect: Are emotions causes of disease or reflections of a pattern of disharmony that simultaneously affects every level of the person? And finally, it is useful to keep in mind that psychological and social factors are but one part of the host of influences that can generate ill-health.

Mind in the Clinic: Thinking Your Way to Health

Our patients come to see that science is confirming what has long been known, namely that each one of us has an important role to play in our own well-being. This role can be more effectively played if we can become conscious of and modify certain aspects of the way we live which can affect our health. These include our attitudes, thoughts, and beliefs; our emotions; our stance in relationship to society; and our behaviors.

—Jon Kabat-Zinn, *Full Catastrophe Living*[19]

Robert Alexander Schumann (1810–1856) was one of the nineteenth century's greatest composers. His music is still a favorite of music lovers and musicians alike. Despite the brightness and joy of his compositions, Schumann's life was cloaked with darkness and despair. Suffering from depression, he resigned his post as Düsseldorf's Town Music Director in 1854. A month later on a late February day, Schumann jumped into the icy Rhine River. Although he was rescued, he had himself committed to an asylum and died of self-induced starvation two years later.

Was Schumann's dark state of mind and suicide caused by problems with his brain chemistry? Surely he would have been helped by modern antidepressive drugs that would have altered his neurochemistry and possibly saved his live. Schumann was also plagued with troubles. His financial and familial challenges, hostile father-in-law, and combination of jealousy over his wife's flourishing career as a pianist and almost complete dependency on her all helped to foster his darker side. Perhaps he could also have been helped by modern social and psychological supports—a stark contrast to a nineteenth century asylum.[20]

This example of Schumann's tragic life illustrates that mental health problems can benefit from a combination of physical, psychological, and social therapies. Researchers are now exploring whether this is also true for physical health problems, and preliminary results are proving that this does indeed seem to be the case. Dean Ornish's program includes social and psychological "work," as well as special mental techniques of visualization. Other researchers are exploring whether psychological intervention can influence the survival of cancer patients.

In one study, breast cancer patients were divided into two groups. In addition to standard treatment, one group was given autogenic training (a special mind-body technique involving relaxation skills and mental imagery) and educational materials designed to help cope with their illness. The other group was not offered such special training. As evidenced by measurement of white blood cell count and other blood parameters, those in the specially trained group had stronger immune systems.[21] In a similar study, patients with malignant melanoma were divided into groups, one group being offered special stress-reduction training, health education, and group support. The results were spectacular: twenty-five out of thirty-seven patients in the control group survived to the five-year point widely used in cancer research, while thirty-four out of thirty-seven of those who had undergone the special training survived to the five-year mark.[22]

Since stress is a center point for thinking about the mind-body in relation to disease, many mind-body healing techniques focus on its antidote: relaxation. Relaxation is not necessarily something that can be easily achieved: it must be learned. Autogenic training is one example of a Western tradition of mind-body training that begins with relaxation. Developed in the 1930s by German psychiatrist Johannes Schultz, autogenic training is designed to systematically reintegrate mind and body. It is practiced in lying or sitting posture and begins with "self-induced" feelings of heaviness and warmth in the limbs.

The key to the method lies in the student's state of mind. Achievement comes from a meditative state of passive concentration, of letting things happen, rather than an active effort of will. The quiet, meditative mind and relaxed body together help to reintegrate the mind and body, or as Schultz called it, a "general psychobiologic reorganization" or "Umschaltung." Autogenic training is more than a relaxation technique. The complete system is composed of numerous levels, starting with skills that focus more on body phenomena, such as respiration and temperature, and moving to mind-based skills centered on visualization.[23]

The pioneer of stress management in the modern clinic is Jon Kabat-Zinn. His stress-reduction program is used in hospitals and clinics around the world and his book *Full Catastrophe Living* has brought this highly successful technique of "using the wisdom of your body and mind to face stress, pain and illness" to the broader public. The "full catastrophe" program—which can be used for coping with the "full catastrophe" of life, and not just for facing an immediate health crisis—makes use of relaxation and stretching exercises, but borrows its essential elements from a form of Buddhist meditation which emphasizes mindfulness.

The meditative state combines passive concentration with awareness, resulting in an attitude of "letting go" which fosters physical relaxation and peace of mind. It also creates a space for coping with the mental and physical dimensions of pain and illness. Stress is both something to react to and the reaction itself. Awareness can break the cycle by reasserting control over the reaction. Kabat-Zinn reports many successes with his program and numerous studies support the value of the approach.[24]

Body, Mind, and Spirit in the East

The World As a Continuum

> The Chinese never separated Spirit and Matter, and for them the world was a continuum passing from the void at one end to the grossest matter at the other.
>
> —Henri Maspero[25]

Bian Que is one of China's legendary healers. Living several hundred years before Christ, he is credited with being China's first physician and even with the authorship of the great work, the *Nan Jing* or *Classic of Difficulties*. While it is unlikely Bian Que wrote the *Nan Jing*—and some scholars even suggest that "Bian Que" was not a single person, but perhaps a family that went by that name—his fame has lived on through the thousands of years since his death.

According to the Historical Records, Bian Que traveled widely and adapted his treatments to the subtleties of each region and each patient. In a region where women were held in high regard, he successfully specialized in women's problems; in a region where the elderly were of high import, he treated eye and ear problems related to aging; and in another region where children were idolized, Bian Que naturally gravitated toward pediatrics.

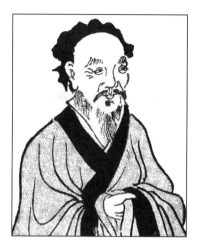

Bian Que

Once, Bian Que arrived in a kingdom just as a prince had died and his body was being prepared for burial. Sensing that the prince was actually still living but in a deep coma, Bian Que applied acupuncture, reviving the prince to consciousness. He then used herbs to bring the prince back to his usual vigor, a feat that earned him the reputation of being able to bring the dead back to life.[26]

One interesting legend involving the great physician bears directly on the Eastern conception of mind and body. Bian Que was at one time faced with two male patients—one of whom he diagnosed as weak-willed with strong qi, the other with strong will but weak qi. Because of these opposing characteristics, Bian Que decided upon a unique therapy: a transfer of the patients' hearts. The transplant went smoothly, but when the men returned to what they thought was their respective homes they were not recognized by their families. Their identity, spirit, self, was transferred along with their heart![27]

This shows the intimate connection between the body and the mind in Chinese thought. Mind and body were not seen as separate entities, even interacting ones, but as inseparable facets of a complete, living system. In this story, the Chinese sensed that as the heart was

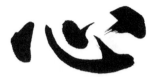

Xin

moved from one man to the other, so too their spirits were transferred and they suddenly found themselves unrecognizable to their families.

Xin is the Chinese word for both heart and mind, its character derived from the outline of the organ. In Chinese medical theory, the heart stores the *shen* or spirit and "mental" problems are often treated with reference to heart organ-system pathology. "It is impossible to say for sure that the classical Chinese scholars and practitioners made an explicit distinction between the heart and the mind," claim contemporary scholars Kiiko Matsumoto and Stephen Birch, "or if, depending on context, they understood implicit differences between them."[28]

This inseparability of the physical heart and the intangible mind is really a more specific example of a broader melding of the solid and substantial with the ethereal and immaterial. Human reality, for the Chinese, is set in the constant interplay of heavenly and earthly influences. Heaven, the yang, is spiritual, while earth, the yin, is material. Yet yin and yang are not individual entities, but relative qualities of a greater whole requiring their opposite to acquire meaning. As hot needs cold and heaven needs earth, the spirit needs a body for human reality to manifest.

Qi is central to this continuum concept. Qi is matter and energy, coalescing at times to create temporary forms while remaining rarefied at others; potentially substantial yet always susceptible to continual shaping by the inherent heavenly forces. While some traditions favored matter as the ultimate reality and others chose the material, the Chinese were unique in conceiving of a "spirituality inherent in matter." Not surprisingly, the Chinese thus viewed the various elements of the mental self in intimate link with the physical self.

The Mind-Body Model of The East

From a Western perspective the body is made up of stuff—molecules, cells, tissues, etc.—that can be subject to experimentation and examination. This is why the whole concept of the mind is so difficult—there is no stuff to take apart, measure, and analyze. For the Chinese mind presented no such problem because of an entirely different starting point. The body was not made of stuff, but of "energies" and fluids in continuous circulation. According to scholar Hidemi Ishida, "these fluids and energies are so essential to the body that the body is conceived as consisting basically of fluids; we may even say it *is* fluids."[29]

Mind, for the Chinese, is conceived of as a fluid circulating along with all the other fluids and energies. It is distinct from the body, but intimately intertwined with it as part of a larger whole. The mind is closely associated with the organs and considered to be resident in them. At birth, varying amounts of energy are apportioned to the organs, and it is from these differences that distinct personalities and character traits emerge. The art of Chinese "astrology," *ming shu*, or "the reckoning of fate," involves the interpretation of the heavenly stems and earthly branches at the time of birth. The stems and branches as calculated during each 2-hour period represent a distinct energetic pattern that influences human events, including personality.

Mind permeates the whole body. It is closely associated with blood and the meridians, and so is able to move freely throughout the body. Since mind is so intimately intertwined with the other energies and fluids coursing through the body, it is affected by the same influences and blockages.

Jing, the essence, is defined as "the substance that underlies all organic life."[30] It is the foundation of growth and development—the template of physiological process. But *jing* is also a foundation of the *shen*, the spirit, and the two are often combined as *jing-shen*, the most subtle life force. According to another scholar, Claude Larre, the combination *jing-shen* suggests a complementary interrelationship: essence provides a root for the spirit, enabling its expression, while spirit opens the richness of the essence for the highest experience of life.[31] Heaven contributes *jing* and *shen* to humanity, earth provides the structure and form.

Five aspects of mind are associated with the five phases and their accompanying organs. *Shen*, the spirit, is stored in the heart. There are two "souls": a material soul, the *po*, stored in the lungs, and a spiritual soul, the *hun*, stored in the liver. And finally there are *zhi*, the will, stored in the kidneys, and *yi*, intention or ideas, stored in the spleen.

Shen is the most ethereal energy; it exerts a governing influence on the other aspects of mind. According to Ted Kaptchuk, "Human consciousness indicates the presence of *shen*," which is "associated with the force of human personality, the ability to think, discriminate, and choose appropriately."[32]

The yin and yang souls, the material *po* and spiritual *hun*, can be compared with the idea of soul in the West. Unlike the West though, the Chinese conceive of the souls as finicky and only temporarily inhabiting a particular body. At death they leave to find another body, and might even leave earlier if not treated well. This is illustrated by a commentary on the *Tao Te Ching* written by the "Old Gentleman by the Riverside" sometime in the second century. In Chapter 10, the great Taoist Classic asks "Can you sustain the *hun* and *po*?" for which the Old Gentleman explains: "Sustaining the souls makes life possible. Joy and anger drive out the *hun*, sudden fright injures the *po*. *Hun* lives in the liver, *po* in the lungs. Therefore overindulgence in wine and delicious foods is dangerous, as it harms these organs. To quieten the *hun* one must maintain calm and strive for the Tao; to leave the *po* in peace is to lengthen one's years and attain longevity."[33]

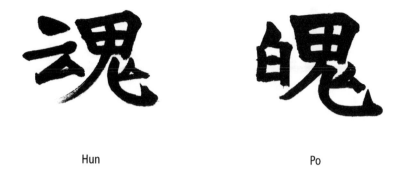

Hun   Po

The souls have a dynamic and active quality. The material soul, coming from and returning to earth, provides the impetus for physical form; the spiritual soul, coming from and returning to heaven, is the impetus for qi. As the Old Gentleman's commentary illustrates, the souls are affected by both physical and psychological events.

Will and intention are more specific aspects of the mind. *Zhi*, the will, is a character combining the idea of feet with mind, suggesting that the mind directs the feet into activity. According to the *Ling Shu*, "The function which fixes intention on things, we call the will."[34] Since the will is stored in the kidneys, it is that aspect of the mind that is in closest association with the *jing*-essence, also stored in the kidney.[35]

Yi, translated as "intention" or "ideas," is derived from a combination of the concept of spoken thought together with that of mind, suggesting "the intention someone expresses with words or sounds."[36] Together with will, intention controls the *jing* and *shen*, keeps the souls from leaving the body, smoothes the emotions, and even controls body heat. *Yi* is more yang and more closely associated with the mind compared to *zhi*, which is more yin and more closely associated with the body. The scholar Ishida contrast *yi* and *zhi* as "thinking mind" and "thinking body."[37]

This all adds up to a picture of the mind and its relationship to the body that is startlingly different from the conventional Western one.

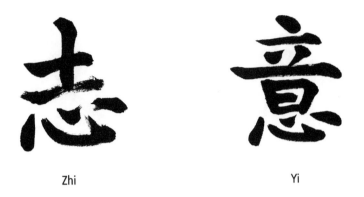

Zhi   Yi

The elements of mind exist together with the elements of body, both "elements" in the sense of distinct fluids and energies rather than as material components. While the various aspects of mind are associated with various organs, mind permeates the body as a whole and reflects its qualities and changes. In short, all events are mind-body events; human experience, for the Chinese, is a mind-body experience.

Emotions and the External Manifestation of Mind

Mind fills the entire body and when it is healthy its manifestations are evident in a number of ways. The eyes, in particular, reflect the radiance of mind. According to the *Ling Shu*, one of the two parts of the *Yellow Emperor's Classic*, the *shen* qi, the energy of the spirit, shines forth from the eyes, which are the messengers of the mind.[38] The *Guan Zi* or *Book of Master Guan*, a text dating to possibly the fourth century B.C. with many interesting chapters relevant to the understanding of mind, offers a clear statement of the mind's manifestation. From a chapter entitled "Ways of the Mind" we find: "The complete mind cannot stay hidden in the body. Rather, it takes shape and appears on the outside. It can be known from the complexion of the face."[39]

The chapter continues by pointing out that this externally radiating mind can be felt in addition to being seen. When mind in its exuberance fills the body and flows outward, this is as easy to recognize as one's own children. The external manifestation of mind creates an "energetic" interaction between people: that immediate intuitive sense about others that plays a strong role in shaping interpersonal relationships. Again, the *Guan Zi*: "When people meet someone whose appearance and mind are full of positive energy, they will feel happier than if they had met their own brother. On the other hand, when people meet someone with negative energy, they will feel more hurt than if they had been confronted with arms."[40]

The health of the mind is revealed in the health of the sense organs, both of which are a reflection of the health of various organ-energies. Healthy lung qi means a good sense of smell, for example, and strong kidney qi will result in excellent hearing. While the eyes are associated with the liver in particular, all body energies and aspects of mind are reflected in the parts of the eyes. The five yin organs, together with *zhi, yi, shen, hun,* and *po,* reveal themselves in the pupils, iris, veins, whites, and eyelids.

Another aspect of self more commonly associated with mind than with body is emotion. We have already explored the connection between emotion and the organs in Chinese medicine. Emotions are outer expressions of the inner mind, intimately connected to organ qi. As it says in the *Ling Shu,* when liver qi is deficient there is fear; when it is in excess, there is anger. Deficient heart qi can bring sorrow; excess can engender joy. According to the 2000-year *Record of Rites*: "Every human being has an inner nature which is made up from the qi of the blood together with the mind that resides therein. The mind manifests itself in a variety of emotions—joy and anger, sadness and happiness."[41]

Cultivating the Emotions and Calming the Mind

While inappropriate negative emotions are considered in Chinese medicine to be simultaneous causes and effects of organ imbalance, positive emotions and mental states reflect and support the balance of organ qi. The mind is not innately positive or negative but takes direction from the will and intention. It is also subject to the same excitations and blockages as the body and is particularly driven by the senses.

This explains the Taoist belief in the importance of purifying and strengthening the body. Only when the body is pure and qi can flow without obstruction can the emotions be stable and healthy. A modern Taoist master, Mantak Chia, explains this connection between the energy, qi, and the emotions, particularly with respect to the modern world: "The circulation of the life force energy is obstructed [by pollution and life in the "concrete jungle"] and the energy cannot flow efficiently or easily. When negative energy cannot be expelled from the body, it is trapped in the organs and in the membrane covering the organs...creating more negative emotional energy...."[42]

Another quote from the *Record of Rites* shows the importance of controlling sensual stimulation. The mind will follow a healthy and natural course if it is free from unhealthy influences. This quote is particularly interesting in this time of routine exposure to extreme violence and salacious imagery as everyday entertainment—and relevant to the subsequent debate over its effects, particularly on youth. The ears should never hear distressing sounds and the eyes should turn away from flustering sights, claims the ancient text, adding that vulgar music should not be allowed to affect the mind and that wild and degenerate qi should never be allowed to affect the body. It continues by concluding that such care is necessary for the mind and body to take a healthy direction: "Only then will ears, eyes, nose, mouth, and the mind together with the body naturally follow straightforward ways."[43]

There is a circular set of causes and effects between mind and body. By attending to the health and balance of the more bodily side of self, the mind will take a more natural and stable course. By cultivating the mind, the body will be healthier. The junction of the two is qi, the focus of all such "personal"—or spiritual—development work. Joseph Needham used the word ataraxia to describe this "peace of mind" and "emotional tranquility" cultivated by the ancient Chinese philosophers. He quotes the *Su Wen*, one of the two parts of the *Yellow Emperor's Classic*, to show the effect of the mind on the body and the benefits of deliberate mental cultivation: "When one feels naturally happy and free from self-seeking and upsetting personal desires or greedy ambitions, then the salutary qi of necessity responds and follows. Vitality thus guarding from within, how can diseases originate?"[44]

Even Buddhism—a tradition usually more concerned with mind than body—was strongly influenced by the mind-body model of the Chinese. The Indian Buddhist monk known as Bodhidharma, the founder of the Chinese Chan sect of Buddhism (known as Zen in its Japanese form) who lived during the fifth century, spoke clearly on the need to consider the development of both mind and body: "The spirit should be tranquil and alert, but the body should be strong and active," he claimed, "Without tranquility one cannot attain wisdom and transform into a Buddha; without health one cannot have good circulation and breathing. Hence the body should be properly exercised so that the muscles and tendons may be supple and the spirit will not then suffer from the misery of weakness."[45]

The Mind and Body in Medicine

Chinese medicine is mind-body medicine. Whether a patient's chief complaint is a mind problem or a body problem, both mental and physical signs and symptoms are included in the recognition of a pattern of disharmony. For example, a pattern of liver invading spleen, which involves both liver excess and spleen deficiency, is recognized by its combination of digestive disturbance and liver disharmony. One patient seeking treatment for a digestive problem may divulge emotional issues of irritability and frustration—typically considered liver signs—upon questioning by the practitioner, while another seeking help for excessive anger—a sign usually associated with the liver—might reveal a minor digestive complaint during examination. Both cases could fall into the same pattern of "liver invading spleen" depending on the overall set of signs and symptoms—some of which are emotional and others physical.

Like diagnosis, treatment simultaneously addresses the mind and the body as inseparable parts of a general pattern. While the two "liver invading spleen" cases above may well share the same general description, treatments will be adjusted to match the precise manifestations of the pattern in the individual. Yet no matter what the treatment strategy taken, it will focus on adjusting the qi—the bridge between mind and body.

Acupuncture and herbs address both mental-emotional and physical disharmony. As the *Spiritual Axis* claims, the acupuncture points are the places where *shen* and qi, spirit and energy, enter and leave. Some point names reflect this connection. There is the "spirit gate"—heart 7—on the inner crease of the wrist, a useful point for treating spirit disorders such as insomnia, irritability, poor memory, and even mania. Or there are the "door of the material soul (the *po*)" and the "house of the *shen*," the 42nd and 44th points on the bladder channel, respectively. Herbs too are discussed in terms of their physiological effects and their influence on emotional and even spiritual qualities.

A modern Chinese acupuncture text illustrates the general approach in treating "depressive syndromes."[46] Such problems, the text explains, can result from overthinking or the inability to achieve an important life goal. The resulting stagnation of qi affects the "free-flow" of the liver and can impair the spleen's activity of "transformation and transportation." As fluid metabolism becomes impaired, phlegm can appear, "misting" the heart and disturbing the shen. (Phlegm, in Chinese medicine, includes discharge from the lungs and sinuses as well as congested and congealed fluids affecting other organs and body parts.)

The pattern can be resolved by restoring the liver's free flow of qi, clearing phlegm, and harmonizing the spirit, for which three "back shu" points on the bladder meridian are chosen together with heart 7, the spirit gate, to calm the mind, and stomach 40, an important point for treating phlegm. (Back shu points are special points with a direct influence on particular organ systems.) The heart-shu complements heart 7 in harmonizing the mind, the spleen-shu strengthens digestive function and supports the treatment of phlegm, while the liver-shu treats stagnant qi.

Treatments can also be more creative and less "physical." Hua Tuo, the famous surgeon, once encountered a seriously ill official, and devised a novel cure—a sort of "shock" treatment. Hua Tuo felt that if he could stimulate the patient into a rage, cure would be ensured. After collecting an exorbitant fee, he left the patient with a rather nasty and belligerent note. The official became enraged and sick to his stomach, thereafter recovering from his illness.[47]

Mind and Body in East and West

Something New, Something Old

> spleenful adj. Ill-humored; peevish; irritable. [The spleen was once thought of as the seat of negative emotions.]
> —Dictionary Definition and Etymology[48]

The idea that mind and body are inextricably linked is new to modern science and medicine. But it is really nothing new. Pre-scientific European culture did not separate mind and body and the English language is still full of reference to this connection. The adjective spleenful, for example, originated from the idea that negative emotions concentrated in this organ. Perhaps the fact that such beliefs have declined for several centuries has played a role in the word's declining popularity.

On the other hand there are many other references to the mind-body connection still in common use, suggesting that such a connection is intuitively felt. Gall, for example, has specific meanings with respect to the liver and gallbladder, but also associations with emotions and states of mind. Common expressions link the intestines with fortitude and the stomach with nervousness and apprehension. And of course, the heart remains both the linguistic and pictorial symbol of romantic love.

As we explore scientifically the long-felt connection between mind and body, there is a common tendency to reduce the mental to the physical. Since mental events can be correlated with changes in brain chemistry, mental phenomena are often viewed as simply chemical events in a way that casts aspersions on their intrinsic meaning. The result of mind-body research should not be to devalue the meaning and intrinsic reality of human mental, emotional, and spiritual experience. It should be possible to view mind and body as intimately intertwined while maintaining the meaning and value of all aspects of human experience. It should be possible to affirm, for example, the long-felt intuition that romantic love is both a mind and a body event without replacing its mystery and power with the certainty of chemistry.

Here it is interesting to reflect on the Eastern view of the relationship between the mind and the body. Mind in the East is no more or less real than the body. Both emerge from the same source as expressions of qi—the body being more material and earthly, the mind more ethereal and heavenly. The health and structure of the bones, for example, is related to kidney qi, but so is fear. Emotional and mental events are rooted in the body. Everyday language describes psychological states in terms of the body's energetic center in the lower abdomen, the *hara* in Japanese. As Matsumoto and Birch point out, the expression "big hara" implies having an open mind, while "small hara" suggests narrow mindedness. The Japanese will denote anger by claiming "the hara stands up" and centeredness by "the hara is sitting."[49]

Physical reality—symbolized by earth—is shaped by the organizational quality of heaven, the spark of life in an organic, dynamic universe. The body's chemistry is shaped by mental, emotional, and spiritual experience, while mental, emotion, and spiritual experience is shaped by the body. The "spirituality inherent in matter" of the Chinese is a way of confirming the reality of the spirit without denying the reality of matter. It is an organic vision of the universe that is shared by some great Western thinkers, a profound vision that allows for spiritual experience in a world that has been viewed as dead for too long in the West.

Cause or Effect?

Much of the research on the mind-body problem is based on correlation. Mental depression following a traumatic life event is often found to be associated with a depressed immune system and increased incidence of illness, for example, and a dearth of social relationships is associated with poorer health. These kinds of correlations are very often interpreted in terms of cause and effect, another strong tendency in the Western mind-set.

Yet a closer look reveals that many such apparent cause and effect relationships are really a tangled web without a clearly delineated origin. A lack of social relationships, for example, may be a consequence of poor health, and not necessarily the cause of it. People with vibrant health will have the energy to maintain a strong social network; those who struggle on a daily basis with physical or mental health problems naturally cannot maintain the same social network. On the other hand, the feeling of isolation engendered by a lack of social support and connection to community can magnify life's stresses and strains, with negative ramifications for health. Cause and effect become chicken and egg in a downwardly cascading cycle.

Once again there is something to learn from the Chinese, who centered their gaze on the correlations themselves rather than searching for causes. Correlations suggest systemic patterns, and it is these patterns that form the reference point for understanding. In Chinese medicine, patterns are the theoretical and practical center of diagnosis and treatment. Anger, for example, is associated with a pattern of liver disharmony. Too much anger can affect liver qi detrimentally, but at the same time an anger problem suggests an already unhealthy liver. It is not that anger causes the liver problem, but that a liver disharmony is a simultaneous mind and body event.

Modern research parallels the Taoist view that balanced, healthy emotions, along with positive, healthy attitudes can go a long way in promoting health and maximizing "wellness." Mental health reflects into the physical dimension. But it is important to consider that negative emotional responses and negative attitudes are not under simple conscious control. Instructions to "control that temper," and "stop being so gloomy about life" imply that these kinds of personality traits are easily subject to will and intention. More realistically, professional assistance is often required to break out of entrenched and negative psychological states.

Psychological health can also be supported by physical means. The hygiene-school Taoists treated the body as a foundation for spiritual development, while simultaneously attending to the cultivation of mind. The cultivation of healthy attitudes and emotions is assisted by nutritional and other physically oriented support—such as exercise—while these same healthy states of mind exert a positive influence on physiological systems.

This kind of pattern thinking and appreciation of the circularity of causes and effects is important in the realm of healing. Many problems can be seen as primarily mental or primarily physical, and especially in acute situations may need to be addressed as such. But disharmony extends to both mind and body, something that is particularly apparent in the case of chronic illness. Whatever the problem, treatment, too, can involve both, and perhaps the more serious a chronic case, the more its treatment should involve both mind and body.

As an example, serious mental disorders like schizophrenia appear to have a physical basis. Researchers are now exploring genetic links; others are looking at nutritional factors, even reaching back to study maternal nutrition especially during the critical time of fetal development. From the Chinese point of view, serious mental disorders are often associated with a pattern of "phlegm misting the orifices of the heart." Treatment will be varied to suit an individual pattern, but will involve clearing phlegm. Western psychiatry with its use of drugs is, of course, also strongly centered on physical therapy. But just because the disease has a physical basis does not mean psychological factors are without importance in its development or treatment.

Heart disease is another interesting example. While primarily a primarily physical disease and primarily treated as such, a closer look reveals glimpses of mental, emotional, and even spiritual elements. Dean Ornish gathered together factors that could affect heart health and would be amenable to change, and combined them together into a comprehensive treatment program. While there is a physical component to the program, it also contains many mental, emotional, and even spiritual "therapies."

Ornish believes that in order to open the heart literally it must be opened figuratively. Socially focused work like group support and communication skills are combined with more personal mind-based practices like meditation and visualization. According to Ornish, for some program participants the more psychological component of the program is essential in order to successfully reverse heart disease. Ornish goes as far as to discuss the relationship between spirituality and healing.

By combining mental and physical therapies it is possible to create an upwardly cascading movement toward health, as each part affects the other in a positive way. Psychological and physiological integration can, of course, be extended beyond the realm of therapy. From a preventive, human development, and even spiritual perspective, approaches that integrate mind and body are more effective than those with a narrower focus.

In the West, we are learning that bringing a psychological component to physical training can enhance sports performance. For the Chinese, mind-body work reaches its zenith in qi gong, a unique exercise that derives its power from an intricate melding of the mental and physical. Qi gong is more than a means to get well: it is also a tool for prevention and spiritual development.

Toward a Synthesis of East and West

The Chinese model of mind and body is a rich and fascinating one in this time when the topic is so new in the West. Yet the psychology of the Chinese model is not particularly well developed. The Chinese themselves favor a social instead of an individual perspective, a cultural trait inherited from the socially oriented Confucianism of feudal bureaucracy and certainly supported by modern Communism. This tendency is also generally true of Eastern culture, both non-Chinese and non-Communist. Mental problems are often turned into body problems and the search for psychological understanding and personal development so popular in the West has little counterpart in the East.

A number of efforts have gone into filling this gap by combining Chinese pattern thinking and "energy" modeling with the more extensive Western understanding of emotion and personality. Some of these synthesists are Western medical doctors who have come to explore the Eastern healing arts, others are Westerners trained in Chinese medicine.

Traditional Chinese medicine practitioners Harriet Beinfield and Efrem Korngold, for example, have sketched such an East-West synthesis, taking the traditional five-phase system of earth, metal, water, wood, and fire and embellishing it with Western psychology. Since every medical system is intimately a product of the culture in which it is set, it is only natural, they argue, that Chinese medicine should be transformed and adapted as it takes hold in the West. "We are reinventing as well as recapitulating classical concepts in order to address the concerns of the people who walk through our clinic doors," they write in their book *Between Heaven and Earth*, noting that their patients "are curious about the origin and meaning of their difficulties and discomforts, suspecting that greater insight will enable them to avoid future problems."[50]

Leon Hammer, a Cornell University-educated psychiatrist argues that Chinese medicine has little to do with conventional Western medicine, but does have much common ground with Western psychology.

Both try to account for the whole person, attribute a significant role to the healer, and see symptoms as signs of an underlying problem. With his extensive training in a number of Western psychological traditions, Hammer embellishes the classical disharmonies of Chinese medicine with the richer features of personality and character set out in the West. He published his vision of the character qualities of Chinese "energy" patterns in a 1989 book, *Dragon Rises, Red Bird Flies.*

Like Hammer, Frenchman Yves Requena trained as a medical doctor and then went on to study and practice acupuncture. His East-West fusion appears in his book *Character and Health: The Relationship of Acupuncture and Psychology.* Requena makes use of both five phases and a six-fold division of yin and yang, combining them with a little-known Western tradition of systems-oriented therapy called diathetic medicine and a form of personality analysis used in Western psychology. Arguing that "Our most distinctive, individual behaviors are often in direct rapport with our biological activities," and that the "meridians are the junction of mind and body," he weaves character into the web of the East.[51]

These like-minded attempts to enrich Chinese thinking with Western insights illustrate the natural evolution of Chinese medicine as it sinks roots in the West. While a distinct Western version of this ancient Eastern medical art has not yet emerged, the mind-body model will undoubtedly be a focus of much dialogue and development in the future.

Locating the Mind

We have already touched on the curious question about the location of the mind. In the West, the mind is associated with the nervous system, particularly the brain. In the East, the brain is a "curious" organ, associated with the kidney organ-meridian system. The "energetic" center in the abdomen is the center of both body and mind, and elements of mind are distributed throughout the body.

According to the *Tao Te Ching,* the sage should put the mind in the energetic center in the abdomen below the navel and avoid excessive stimulation from the senses. According to the *T'ai Chi Classics*, "the mind directs the qi…[which] circulates freely, mobilizing the body so that it heeds the direction of the mind," adding, "The mind and the qi must be coordinated and blended…," and "The mind is the commander; the qi, the flag; and the waist, the banner."[52] In the Chinese tradition mind is something in and intimately linked with the body and its physiological processes. The link in that chain is qi.

Recent Western research offers a sense that this ancient perception of the mind being "in" the body, and of a relationship between mind and abdomen, may not be so strange. Neuropeptides closely associated with emotions can be produced throughout the body and the notion of a "second brain" in the abdomen, a primitive but primary collection of neurons and other brain hardware associated with the stomach and intestines, does offer new life to the expression "gut feeling." Whether or not the abdomen actually thinks, the "brain apparatus" in the gut is relatively independent from the brain in the skull. Some elements of mind appear to originate from outside the skull brain, and the abdomen may well be an important center point, a foundation of the mind-body forged over the course of human evolutionary history.

Chinese mind-body exercises and therapies working with the abdomen as a center and source clearly tap into this evolutionarily ancient pivot of physiological and nervous system activity. As we can see in this short excerpt from Taoist master Mantak Chia, this is another fascinating area of overlap between Chinese medicine and the new biology. Here Chia describes the abdomen-emotion link and the correlations between mind and body typical of Chinese medicine: "The small intestine is in charge of digesting emotions and food. Different contractions of this intestine correspond to undigested emotions. In Chinese medicine it is called 'the abdominal brain.' All the negative emotions are expressed in the small intestine by contraction and circumvolutions. Anger contracts the right side of the intestine near the liver. Worry affects the upper left side near the spleen. Impatience and anxiety affect the top. Sadness affects both

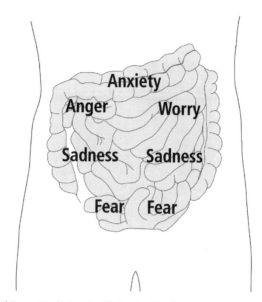

In Chinese Medicine the Abdominal Brain Stores Negative Emotions

lower lateral sides. Fear affects the deeper and lower abdominal areas."[53]

The West is in the middle of a shift in perception of self. Mind and body have long been considered as separate, isolated elements of who we are, and the mind is often equated with the brain's chemical and electrical activity. Now there is a glimpse that our physical and mental selves are intimately intertwined, not just in the brain but throughout the body. This new vision resonates strongly with some fundamental aspects of the Eastern perception of self. As deeper parallels emerge between East and West, dramatic shifts in the understanding of health and the strategies for healing are in store for the future.

8 | You Are What You Eat: The Role of Diet and Lifestyle in Health and Disease

Foods can have a surprising effect on many aspects of health.
—*Foods for Health*, a brochure of the Physicians Committee
for Responsible Medicine

The new biology takes a holistic perspective, searching for an understanding of health and disease at all levels of the complex mind-body system. At one level, there are patterns of molecular misbehavior that describe the microscopic pathology of disease. The heart, for example, can suffer when sticky deposits of fat and other molecules cover the surface of the arteries. These narrowed arteries can become hardened by calcium deposits and a build-up of fibrous tissue. From a molecular understanding of the processes, drugs can be developed to block or reduce such pathological molecular changes.

While disease can be described and treated at the molecular level, it can also be studied at the level of both person and society. We all have different eating habits and behavioral traits, patterns of living that affect our health. Such traits are widely shared elements of culture, and these common social patterns help to determine the disease profile of a society. Problems with the circulatory system, for example, occur much more frequently in societies where people combine a sedentary lifestyle with a diet characteristically high in animal fats and low in plant fiber. This kind of information can help develop strategies to prevent, and even reverse, disease of the circulatory system.

In the past several decades, research has demonstrated a powerful link between lifestyle and health. The potential for developing many so-called diseases of civilization—diabetes, heart disease, and the like—has a molecular basis, but it is a potential that is activated in large part by the environment—including a variety of personal and social factors. Considerable research is now directed toward the identification of these factors and the implications for prevention and treatment. Surprisingly, the power of dietary change is often as great as the highest of technology—and such changes are unquestionably cheaper than high-tech therapy. One heart specialist in a small northern community takes his patients home for cooking lessons, one example of the profound changes now underway.

While the idea that how we live and eat can profoundly affect our health has come as a surprise in the West, the Chinese have explored the importance and power of nutrition and lifestyle for millennia.[1] Taoists obsessed with longevity searched for ways of eating that would prolong life; physicians searched for links between factors in their patients' lives, such as their eating habits, and the patterns of disharmony they observed; and farmers and tradespeople searched for foods that could offers sustenance and health. Over time, an approach to nutrition was developed that, while different in many respects from its Western counterpart, comes to conclusions about the foundation of a healthy diet with a striking resonance to those of the new biology.

Nutrition in the East

In Chinese medicine, who we are determines what is most beneficial for us to eat. And what we eat is considered to affect the expression of who we are.

—Beinfield and Korngold, *Between Heaven and Earth*[2]

Of Taoists and Ancient Physicians

Taoism is a religion that believes in, among other things, the importance of cultivating mental and physical health. Taoists practiced mental and physical hygiene, special breathing exercises, gymnastics and meditation, and maintained a strict dietary regimen that included many special herbs. They were strong in their belief that, with effort, people could greatly improve on their chances of living a long and healthy life.

Sun I-khuei, a renowned physician of the Ming dynasty and a contemporary of Li Shi-zhen, echoed this ancient belief in claiming that "One cannot entirely attribute events to fate; on the contrary, man can act in such a way as to conquer Nature." In his book *The Mysterious Pearl Recovered Near the Red River*, Sun discusses the importance of moderation in all things and the value of diet in preserving health. He laments that many people do not pay enough attention to their health at an early enough stage.[3]

Diet was an important topic in the earliest medical texts. The Lady of Tai was buried in an elaborate tomb in 166 B.C. along with her son and many artifacts of her time. Manuscripts written on silk and bamboo and found in an excavation of the tomb, deal with a wide range of topics from yin-yang theory to astronomy. Some of the texts addressed medical subjects, among them a book on eating for long life and another on the therapeutic and preventive use of exercise.[4] Several hundred years later, *Prescriptions for Acute Diseases*, a third-century medical text, claimed that good health is primarily to be found in food and that it is not possible to stay healthy without eating well.[5]

Sun Si-miao, the great Tang dynasty physician and Taoist who lived from 581 to 682, wrote the *Thousand Ounces of Gold Classic*. Sun argued that the superior physician looks for the root cause of ill health and tries first to change the condition with food. Only when food fails should she prescribe herbs.

Sun described dietary treatments for a number of diseases, including enlarged thyroid (goiter), night blindness, and beriberi, a deficiency disease common in Asia and characterized by numbness and tingling of the limbs and wasting of the muscles. He treated goiter with seaweed and pork thyroid, night blindness with beef, pork, and lamb liver, and beriberi with rice bran, all approaches congruent with modern Western nutrition. Goiter can be improved with a diet high in

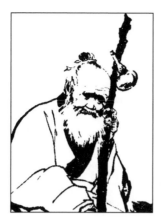

Sun Si-miao

iodine, an element found in seaweed; night blindness is helped by vitamin A, of which liver is a good source; and beriberi is linked to thiamine (vitamin B-1) deficiency, a vitamin found in high concentrations in rice bran.[6] (Beriberi is associated with a preference for highly refined grains, such as white rice, which are polished to remove the outer bran, an excellent source of thiamine.)

The Basic Healthy Diet

The nutritional recommendations of ancient physicians like Sun Si-miao were developed from the perspective of Chinese medicine. Chinese nutrition differs markedly from its Western counterpart. Westerners know that oranges are good for them because they contain large amounts of vitamin C and milk is healthy because it is high in calcium. The Chinese people, in contrast, may choose bitter melon (a cucumber-looking vegetable considered the "king" of bitter foods) to balance the heat and humidity of a summer day, or might eat small red beans (adzuki beans) to improve a damp constitution. While Western nutrition focuses on the molecular components of food, Chinese nutrition considers its qualities and macroscopic actions.

Individual balance is the focus of Chinese nutrition. There is not a rigid, universal approach to eating suitable for everyone. Rather,

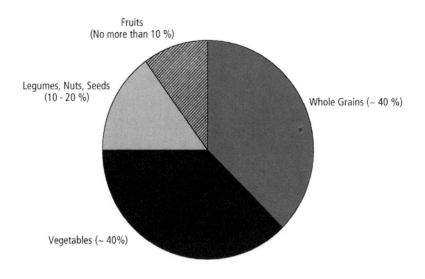

Fruits
(No more than 10 %)

Legumes, Nuts, Seeds
(10 - 20 %)

Whole Grains (~ 40 %)

Vegetables (~ 40%)

Basic Healthy Diet of Chinese Nutrition

there is a basic, healthy diet that must be adjusted to suit the person and environment, a flexible and evolving dietary regimen that will balance hot and cold, dryness and dampness, yin and yang. The basic healthy diet is built around generous helpings of whole grains and vegetables, with moderate amounts of legumes, fruits, and nuts and seeds. Animal products, if any, are eaten to supplement, not define, the meal. Food is usually lightly cooked, improving its digestibility without destroying its nutritive value.

According to Maoshing Ni, who practices and teaches Chinese medicine in California, the basic, healthy diet has equal portions of vegetables and whole grains, accounting for about 80 percent of food intake. Legumes, seeds, and nuts make up another 10 to 20 percent, with fruit comprising up to 10 percent. Animal products, if eaten, are to comprise no more than 10 percent of the diet. Ni also points to the usefulness of small quantities of sea vegetables such as nori, dulse, and kelp.[7]

The Five Flavors

In Chinese nutrition the basic, healthy diet must be adjusted to suit the individual and his or her environment and to accomplish this the Chinese describe foods in terms of their qualities and actions. Central to such a description are the five flavors of sour, salty, bitter, sweet, and spicy. The five flavors have five-phase correspondences linking each flavor with the various organ-meridian systems. The pungent or spicy flavor, corresponding to the metal phase, promotes the movement of qi and blood through its invigorating and dispersing nature. Many pungent foods, such as green onions and pepper, also warm the body. In contrast, salty foods, like seaweed and salt, tend to be cooling. Salty has a water phase correspondence and an affinity for the kidney. This flavor is softening and sedating.

Sour foods correspond to the wood phase and affect the liver channel. Sour foods like lemon and vinegar are obstructive and astringent. Bitter, the fire flavor, suggests both drying and heat clearing qualities. Bitter foods, like dandelion and bitter melon, are among the least popular of foods. The addictive sweet flavor has an affinity for the spleen and a correspondence to the earth phase. Sweet foods, like honey and yam, help to build blood and qi because of their tonifying and nurturing quality.

A healthy diet requires balance among the five flavors. The *Yellow Emperor's Classic* makes clear the benefits of a balanced diet: "[I]f people pay attention to the five flavors and mix them well, their bones will remain straight, their muscles will remain tender and young, their breath and blood will circulate freely, their pores will be fine in texture, and consequently, their breath and bones will be filled with the essence of life."[8]

Eating too much of any one flavor should be avoided. Too much sweet can damage the spleen, too much salt can injure the kidney, too much sour can stagnate the qi. According to the *Yellow Emperor's Classic,* sour in excess will cause the liver to produce too much saliva and will weaken the spleen; salt in excess will cause a decline in the health of the bones, weaken the muscles, and take away one's zest for life; sweet in excess will affect the balance of the kidney and produce fullness in the heart; bitter in excess will dry the spleen and affect the stomach; and pungent in excess will harm the muscles and spirit.

Many people are attracted to sweet foods, others are attracted to salty, sour, or spicy food—and most shun the bitter. These individual tendencies are a powerful diagnostic tool in Chinese medicine, offering an indication of the origin and location of disharmony. A patient with a sweet tooth bordering on addiction, for example, may be caught in an endless cycle of spleen disharmony. A malfunctioning spleen does a poor job of extracting qi from food, leading to lack of energy and a craving for sweet energy-giving foods. If the patient succumbs to his/her craving, the excessive consumption of sweet food will only aggravate the spleen disharmony.

Macroscopic Quality of Food

Flavor is one aspect of the macroscopic quality of food that helps describe its physiological impact. Another is temperature, a quality that has already been hinted at above. Some foods have a cooling quality, like salt and some salty foods; others are warming, including many pungent and spicy foods, like pepper and garlic. There is a continuum of temperature, from cold, cool, neutral, warm, and hot.

The quality of temperature ascribed to a food refers to its physiological effect. There are general signs and symptoms of heat in the body—including dark yellow urine, red face and eyes, affinity for cold, rapid pulse and red tongue—as well as indications of heat in particular organs. The same thing is true for cold, the presence of which is signaled by signs and symptoms like cold extremities, fear of cold, pale tongue, and slow pulse. Hot foods can be used to balance a cold environment, whether internal or external. A hearty beet soup with garlic, ginger, and a hint of chili can balance a cold, deficient constitution or buffer a cold Minnesota winter. Cool foods, in contrast, can balance heat. Mung bean soup with cucumber and lettuce salad provides a cooling repast appropriate for a scorching summer afternoon.

Chinese nutrition is also concerned with the physical temperature of food. Eating too many physically cold foods—such as ice cream straight from the refrigerator— will weaken the digestive system and can lead to a deficient and damp spleen. Overconsumption of cold and raw foods—which also tend to be cooling—is a culinary *faux pas* of Chinese nutrition.

Food also has an effect on the moisture level of the body. Some people are constitutionally dry or yin deficient, with signs and symptoms of dryness like dry stool, dry skin, and thirst, together with signs of heat in the case of yin deficiency, while others are damp. Pathogenic dampness is indicated by a lack of thirst, digestive disturbance, a heavy feeling in the limbs, and a thick tongue fur. Drying foods can help improve a damp condition and moistening foods will counteract dryness, but generally moistening foods such as honey, millet, and milk should be balanced with drying foods such as adzuki bean and corn.

Some foods are very moistening and their overconsumption can disrupt the spleen, causing congestion and stagnation with symptoms of dampness—a problem commonly seen in the Chinese medicine clinic. Too many sweet foods, too many raw or cold foods, and too many greasy, fatty foods—common features of the typical Western diet—can precipitate a damp condition by weakening the spleen and impeding its function of transformation and transportation.

Method of preparation affects the properties of food. A carrot, for example, though cooling when raw becomes more strengthening and warming when boiled or steamed. And baking with a little honey and dried ginger fashions an even warmer and more tonifying carrot.

Healthy spleen and stomach are essential to good digestion. According to the *Yellow Emperor's Classic*: "Ingested fluids enter the stomach. Here, they are churned and their qi is strained off. The qi is then carried to the spleen and further distributed by the spleen qi." The spleen is thus the root of qi and blood production; the stomach manages the intake and breakdown of food, so its partner the spleen can transform and transport the purest essence.[9]

The spleen and stomach are a temperamental pair: the spleen fears dampness, the stomach hates dryness, requiring careful attention to the balance of moisture in the diet. The stomach is also susceptible to heat, which can engender dryness. The perfect diet supports the spleen and stomach, providing nourishment for the other yin and yang organs. On balance, it is not too cold or too hot, too damp or too dry. The five flavors are mixed delicately together without a hint of excess. It is, in the midst of extremes, just right.

From Cucumber to Black Bean

Many foods are traditional folk remedies. Cucumber, for example, is cool and sweet, and affects the spleen, stomach, and large intestine. It acts to clear heat, quench thirst, and promote urination. Cucumber consumption will improve acne, it can be applied externally for burns, and it can help relieve hot eye inflammations.[10]

Corn is neutral, sweet, and acts on the stomach and large intestine. Like cucumber it promotes urination. It is also considered to benefit the heart. Corn, particularly the corn silk consumed as a tea, is traditionally used to improve the function of the gallbladder. Radish is cool, pungent, and sweet, influencing the lungs and stomach. It has a downward action and is used in cases of indigestion with stagnant food. Radish is traditionally thought to improve lung function, help prevent cold and flu, and can be eaten in cases of cough with phlegm.

Fresh ginger root is warm and pungent, and associated with the lungs, stomach, and spleen. Ginger acts to promote sweating, improve nausea, and counteract the common cold. As these examples suggest, there is not a clear line between food and medicine. A few slices of fresh ginger are often added to Chinese herbal formula because of ginger's harmonizing effect on the digestive system and sometimes—because of ginger's ability to counteract toxins—to buffer the side effects of potentially toxic herbs.

Another herb-cum-food is job's tears, a barley-looking grain that can be eaten like rice and is used as a medicinal herb. Job's tears is sweet, bland, and neutral, and associated with the spleen, lungs, and kidneys. It clears dampness, strengthens the spleen, and helps to stop diarrhea.

Among the fruits, grape is neutral, sweet, and sour, and is considered a blood and energy-nourishing food. It influences the lungs, spleen, and kidney, and is thought to stimulate urination and improve the tendons and bones. Raisins are recommended as a folk cure for anemia.

Longevity Foods East

The Chinese, in their quest for long life and immortality, were not content with simply eating to avoid disease. They searched for special superfoods that would nourish the mind and body and take health to new heights. The sixth century Chinese scholar Yan Zhi-tui attributed his good health in old age to eating kidney-nourishing foods: "I have been in the habit of eating kidney tonics throughout my life which is why I could still read fine print when seventy years old with no gray hair on my head."[11]

In Chinese physiology, the health of the kidney is related to the strength of the *jing*-essence, a primary determinant of long life. With age, the yin aspect of the body wanes and the kidneys decline, a tendency that can be counteracted with appropriate supplements. Kidney-nourishing foods include walnuts and mussels. Walnuts are a tonic to the kidney, especially its yang aspect. They are used to boost sexual energy. Mussels strengthen the liver and kidney, and are particularly good for the lower back.

Ling zhi, the spiritual mushroom, is perhaps the quintessential longevity food. This woody bracket fungus, *Ganoderma lucidum*, or reishi in Japanese, was used for over a thousand years by the time Li Shi-zhen wrote about it in his encyclopedic work on natural history. He praised its ability to improve memory and benefit the qi of the chest. With regular consumption of the herb, claimed Li, one would stay agile and live a long time.

Another revered longevity food is the soybean, long a staple of Asian cuisine. The soybean has been grown in China since at least the eleventh century B.C., and its origins are the subject of numerous legends, all a testament to its high esteem in Oriental culture. The soybean is commonly eaten in derivative foods, like soymilk, tofu, tempeh, and okara, the leftover pulp from the milk-making process. The Japanese often call tofu and even okara "honorable" in everyday speech and fuss over soyfoods like tofu and miso as Westerners would fine wines.[12] Many long-lived Japanese attribute their good health to the regular consumption of miso.

Nutrition in the New Biology

What our medical system can provide is much less important in determining our health than the lifestyle choices we make as individuals on a daily basis.
—Dean Ornish, *Dr. Dean Ornish's Program for Reversing Heart Disease*[13]

In conventional Western nutrition foods are described in terms of their components: fats, carbohydrates, and protein, fibrous indigestible material, and various vitamin and mineral compounds. A number of deficiency diseases can result from a lack of particular nutrients in the diet. A vitamin C-poor diet, for example, can cause scurvy, an illness characterized by bleeding and weakness and once common among sailors on long sea voyages whose daily fare lacked vitamin C-rich foods. From the perspective of the old biology, except for rare cases of extreme deficiency, nutrition has little to do with health and little relevance for medicine. Not surprisingly, physicians trained from within the conceptual milieu of the old biology have little or no education in nutrition.

A dramatic shift in thinking is now underway in the field of nutrition. From the perspective of the new biology, disease can be studied at other levels besides that of the molecule. Over the past several decades, powerful evidence has accumulated demonstrating that many "diseases of civilization" are intimately linked to the way people in industrial countries live and eat. These diseases are not simply the result of bad genes. While their mechanisms may involve genetic factors, they are activated in large part by environmental factors, including diet and lifestyle.

In the dietary realm, there is a general pattern of eating that increases the risk of illness. This is a diet high in fat, low in fiber, with a preponderance of animal protein and paucity of plant food. Such a diet contains too many bad things—such as cholesterol, fat, and refined carbohydrates—and too few good things—such as fiber and phyto-chemicals, various substances found in plant foods that protect against disease. One of the most startling discoveries of the twentieth century is the ability of lifestyle change, especially change in eating pattern, to not only prevent, but even reverse serious illness once it has developed.

Now We Are Kings

For the greater part of their existence humans have been scroungers, hunter-gatherers with an emphasis on the gathering. They ate a wide variety of fruits, nuts, roots, and other plant foods, supplemented with a wide assortment of lean animal food. With the coming of civilization this diet shifted to emphasize cultivated plants, particularly grains, but also legumes, vegetables, and fruits, again supplemented by animal foods such as meat, milk, and eggs. This "peasant diet" is characteristically low in fat, high in fiber, and largely plant-based, and the peasant life is an active, hard-working one. It was the kings, sultans, and emperors whose wealth allowed them to eat large quantities of animal products and live a sedentary lifestyle. These often gouty and obese lords gorged themselves on the richest foods in their lands and did little in the way of physical activity.

Several hundred years ago the feudal civilization of peasants and lords began to disappear in Europe. Some kings literally lost their heads and the emerging forces of democracy and industrialization brought profound changes to the way people lived. Democracy allowed ordinary people to become kings. They could own property, acquire wealth, and eat rich and succulent foods. Industrialism brought technologies that reduced the need for physical labor—automobiles that eliminated the need to walk, and more recently electronic devices to change channels on the television with the push of a button.

The peasants of yesterday are the kings of today, consumers wealthy enough to eat according to their desires and with little opportunity or need for physical activity. A largely plant-based high-fiber, lean diet has shifted to a high-fat, low-fiber diet emphasizing rich, sweet foods and animal products. Unfortunately, as we shall see, one of the side effects of this widespread opulence is widespread corpulence and a host of diseases that now plague the rich nations of the world.

Population Patterns

The British epidemiologist Thomas McKeown described the greatest medical advances of the nineteenth and twentieth centuries. (See Chapter 4.) In the nineteenth century, infectious diseases like smallpox and polio were brought under control largely by changing the environmental factors which had previously allowed them to flourish. In the twentieth century, argued McKeown, the greatest medical advance is the realization that the same thing is true for the chronic, noninfectious diseases that plague modern industrialized nations. That is, the prevalence of heart disease, cancer, diabetes, and other now common diseases is intimately linked to cultural factors and these factors could be altered as a means of prevention.

There is a distinct pattern of chronic, noninfectious disease found in wealthy nations. These are all diseases that were rare or uncommon before the twentieth century, and remain uncommon in areas of the world that do not share the lifestyle characteristic of wealthy nations. This pattern of disease includes gastrointestinal problems such as appendicitis, colon cancer, and hemorrhoids; cardiovascular illnesses such as coronary heart disease, high blood pressure, and varicose veins; cancers including breast, prostate, and lung; and other problems ranging from obesity, diabetes, and gallstones to dental cavities, gout, and multiple sclerosis.[14]

The scientists who study such things describe this distinct pattern as "diseases of civilization," "diseases of affluence" (although they afflict the rich and poor alike in the countries in question), or "Western diseases" (although it is a pattern no longer restricted to the West). Cornell University scientist Colin Campbell, a prominent researcher in the field, prefers the term "diseases of extravagance," noting that people pay extravagant amounts of money for the expensive causes (like animal protein) of diseases that cost extravagant amounts of money to cure.[15]

The idea that lifestyle, particularly diet, is a key factor in the emergence of such diseases arose with European and North American medical experts who traveled and worked in Africa and Asia. They became aware of the connection between how people lived and ate and the kinds of diseases that were common. In the 1920s and '30s British army doctor Robert McCarrison worked in India, finding among the hill tribes a very low occurrence of diseases common in Western nations. He believed this to be a result of the difference in diet, concluding that "The greatest single factor in the acquisition and maintenance of good health is perfectly constituted food." Canadian dentist Weston Price, also working in the 1930s, documented the changing pattern of disease in groups whose diet became Westernized. The work of these early pioneers was not widely accepted and they were often dismissed as eccentrics.

Evidence which began as a few twigs turned into a branch by the 1960s and '70s. Thomas Cleave, a Medical Officer with the British Royal Navy, gathered information from doctors around the world. He was intrigued by the fact that common Western diseases were uncommon in many parts of the world and came to the conclusion the underlying reason for this difference was lifestyle. British medical researcher Denis Burkitt picked up on Cleave's work and in the early

1970s published a number of papers on the relationship between diet and health. Thanks to Burkitt, scientists became interested in the idea that many common diseases were intimately related to diet and lifestyle. With Burkitt's 1981 book *Western Diseases: Their Emergence and Prevention*, co-authored with Hugh Trowell, a doctor who spent many years in Uganda with Burkitt, the branch had become a tree. Since that time, hundreds of researchers have sunk deep roots, producing thousands of studies providing overwhelming evidence that how you live largely determines how you will get sick.[16]

The Evidence

The characteristic shift in diet associated with Western diseases can be described in terms of its energy profile. In 1870, for example, the people of rural Wales took in 11 percent of their daily food energy from protein, 25 percent from fat, 4 percent from sugar and 60 percent from complex carbohydrates such as bread, potatoes, and oatmeal. One hundred years later, their descendants got 11 percent from protein, 42 percent from fat, 17 percent from sugar, and 30 percent from complex carbohydrates. The daily intake of fiber decreased dramatically from 65 to 21 grams per day, while cholesterol consumption skyrocketed from 139 mg per day to a whopping 517 mg per day. This same shift has occurred in the United States. Between 1860 and 1965, for example, the percentage of daily food energy from complex starch dropped from 53 percent to only 22 percent with a concurrent increase from 25 percent to 42 percent for fat.[17]

This profile is the result of a shift toward less plant food and more animal food. Fewer calories come from plant sources—grains, beans, and vegetables—and more calories come from animal products—meat, milk, eggs, butter, and the like. As a result people in Wales and the United States, as in other wealthy developed nations, eat more fat, more cholesterol, and less fiber. This dietary shift is accompanied by other cultural changes, like decreasing physical activity.

As diet and lifestyle change, Western diseases appear in a distinct pattern. Obesity is quick to emerge, followed by a dramatic rise in type

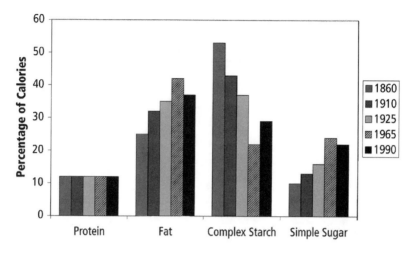

Changing American Diet 1860–1990[18]

II or adult-onset diabetes. Later, after the changes are established, there is also a rise in the number of cases of type I or insulin-dependent diabetes. In the cardiovascular realm, high blood pressure appears first, followed by an increase in stroke. Angina or chest pain becomes more common and over time the number of heart attacks increase, eventually becoming the major cause of death.[19]

Studies on the diet-health relationship come in many forms. The earliest research simply compared the prevalence of Western diseases in different areas of the world. In comparing the incidence of breast cancer in Japan, Spain, Israel, and the United States, for example, Japan, known for its healthy diet, has the lowest incidence of the feared disease and it is less common in Spain, with its diverse "Mediterranean" diet, than among Westernized Israelis or Americans.

Concern was quickly raised that differences in the incidence of disease may simply represent genetic variation between racial or ethnic groups. This led to the study of ethnic migrants, results demonstrating that when people move to a new country and adopt

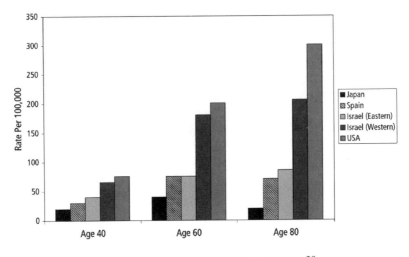

Age-Specific Breast Cancer Rates by Country[20]

new lifestyles, disease patterns change to match those of their new country. For example, Polynesians who emigrated to New Zealand develop Western diseases to the same extent as their neighbors of European heritage.

Another blow to the genetic variation theory was the observation that the prevalence of Western diseases follows lifestyle changes within a group. During the First and Second World Wars, for example, many nations were forced to enact strict austerity measures, and the subsequent shift to a simpler diet reduced the incidence of many common problems, including diabetes and heart disease. And of course, the shift to a pattern of Western diseases accompanies economic development and the Westernization of diet and lifestyle within a given genetic group.

Japan is an interesting case in point. The country isolated itself during the nineteenth century and maintained a feudal peasant society. Stimulated into change by a United States gunboat trade policy, it made a quantum leap from agriculture to industry and has never looked back. Perhaps because of the rapid change from peasant to factory worker, the Japanese people retained their traditional diet for many decades, a factor that places them among the longest-living of nations.

The Japanese have gradually adopted a richer diet. Between 1950 and 1975, for example, the percentage of calories from fat increased from 8 percent to 22 percent and carbohydrate consumption decreased from 78 percent to only 50 percent of total dietary calories.[21] And things have only become worse. According to Dean Ornish, animal fat consumption has risen by 800 percent in the last 25 years, obesity is becoming common, and cholesterol levels in Japanese boys—once among the lowest in the world—tops that of their United States counterparts by a startling 75 percent. "The time bomb is ticking," laments Ornish.[22]

Research in this field is both empowering and troubling. One interesting study was published by a British and New Zealand team in the *British Medical Journal* in 1994. They followed a group of 6,000 vegetarians and a control group of meat eaters for over 10 years, collecting data on the number and causes of death among the two groups. The team noted that a vegetarian diet had many positive health attributes and that previous research had pointed to a lower death rate among vegetarians. Yet these studies had failed to account for the fact that vegetarians are characteristically thin, non-smoking, and more well-off than the average citizen, factors that might have accounted for the results. (Being thin, non-smoking, and rich decreases one's chances of death from heart disease and cancer.) By following two large groups, the data could be analyzed to decide whether it was their diet or these "confounding" factors that caused any reduction in the number of deaths.

The study found a whopping 40 percent decrease in death from cancer and a 20 percent decrease in death from heart disease, numbers that did not change even when adjusted for lifestyle and social status. "The reduced cancer mortality seems largely due to diet and is not appreciably changed when other lifestyle-related variables are controlled for," concluded the scientists, and added: "The protective effects of diet (40 percent for cancer mortality and 20 percent for total mortality) are large."[23]

From Prevention to Reversibility

The idea that many of the diseases common in the world's wealthy nations can be prevented by lifestyle change is an exciting discovery. What are often taken to be inevitable consequences of genes or the aging process are clearly not so. Weight gain, high blood pressure, and the narrowing of coronary arteries are pathological changes that develop over many years in response to a particular way of life. With this newfound understanding it is possible to build a lifestyle program to prevent these kinds of changes, with the hope of creating healthier citizens in the future. Yet it is one thing to encourage prevention and quite another to successfully treat already-developed serious illness with lifestyle change. Can lifestyle modification, especially dietary change, actually heal?

Some of the pioneers of the new biology have explored the possibility of reversing disease with dietary and other lifestyle changes. Obesity, diabetes, and high blood pressure have all responded favorably to this low-tech medicine, but it is coronary heart disease, the most pervasive and dangerous of all Western diseases, that has captured the most attention. And the success has been spectacular.

Early studies of the 1960s and '70s were not very successful in altering the course of heart disease with lifestyle change. Critics charged that the changes used in these studies were too small. It was like looking for improvement in a group of smokers who switched from three to two-and-a-half packs a day. The change was not large enough.

An early success story was Nathan Pritikin, an American who literally ate himself out of heart disease. Faced with a serious heart problem, Pritikin scoured the available information and developed a lifestyle modification program for himself that included a diet based on traditional eating patterns in areas of the world where heart disease is extremely rare. His personal success grew into an intensive 25-day lifestyle program for people with heart disease. Research documented that 50 percent of type II diabetics no longer required insulin, 83 percent of participants taking drugs for high blood pressure were able to discontinue them, and 65 percent of patients taking medication for chest pain no longer required drugs. When Pritikin died—some 27 years after being diagnosed with coronary artery disease—an autopsy showed his arteries to be surprisingly healthy. According to the coroner: "The absence of developed atherosclerosis and the complete absence of its effects...are remarkable."[24]

Then came Dean Ornish—maverick cardiologist and medical pioneer. Ornish was unhappy with both conventional high-tech approaches and previous lifestyle studies for their failure to get to the core of the heart disease problem. He found that most heart disease patients treated with bypass surgery—described by Ornish as a procedure that "literally and figuratively *bypassed* the underlying causes of the problem"—simply continued to do the things that created the problem in the first place. He was aware of the many root factors involved in the illness—social and psychological elements, especially stress, diet, and exercise—and was also familiar through personal experience with the benefits of meditation and yoga. Ornish took a bold step and developed a comprehensive lifestyle program, combining stress reduction, dietary change, exercise, and group support.[25]

Ornish's patients changed their diet from the typical 40 percent of energy from fat to a "peasant" level of less than 10 percent. This was not a calorie-restricted regimen: patients ate as much fruit, grains, beans, and vegetables as they wanted, adding a small amount of supplementary egg whites and skim milk products. Meat, oil, nuts and seeds, and even avocado—a high fat fruit—were forbidden. Nor was it a case of simply restricting fat or cholesterol intake: the participants ate more vegetables and foods like beans and soy products that are not part of the typical American diet. This study increased its power by including a "control" group of patients who simply followed conventional guidelines for heart disease.

Results were unequivocal. Those patients who had radically changed their lifestyle reduced the frequency of their chest pain (angina) by 90 percent; patients in the control group showed a 165 percent increase. The radical lifestyle also reduced the severity of chest pain by 28 percent in contrast to a 39 percent rise found in the control group. Sophisticated high-tech measurements of the patient's arterial lesions showed that 82 percent of people following the radical change program had the course of their heart disease reversed. They did not just feel better: there were clear and objective physical changes. The level of improvement was also directly linked to how closely the program was followed.[26]

Longevity Foods West

Conventional nutrition is concerned with the basic components of food, the intake of which are essential for health. Vitamins and minerals, for example, need to be consumed in sufficient quantities—called recommended daily allowances (RDA)—to avoid deficiency. The overall diet must be designed to ensure adequate intake and shortfalls can be made up by consuming particular vitamins and minerals in the form of pills and capsules.

Over the past several decades new research has shown that the benefits of particular foods can go far beyond their vitamin and mineral content. The study of nutriceuticals—foods that have value in preventing and even treating disease—is burgeoning and generating widespread enthusiasm. For a long time, research about food has been mostly bad news. Cholesterol, for example, found in many common foods, is implicated in heart disease; too much fat can contribute to heart disease; and a high-fat diet is linked to cancer. Now the dark side of food is joined with a more positive prospect: many foods contain potent phytochemicals—naturally occurring molecules—that can improve health and prevent disease. Foods ranging from garlic and tea to carrots, blueberries, and broccoli are now being dissected in the laboratory to reveal a panoply of life-promoting biochemicals.

One interesting example of a food that has caught the attention of researchers is the soybean, that innocuous-looking bean-in-a-pod that has been a foundation of the Asian diet for centuries. The soybean and its many derivative foods—such as tofu, miso, tempeh, and soymilk—contain isoflavones, chemicals that have a hormone-like effect on the body. Genistein, a potent isoflavone found only in soybeans, has the ability to block the action of tumor-promoting agents. In the laboratory, genistein appears to hinder the growth of both prostrate and breast cancer cells. The soybean also contains daidzein, another cancer-fighting isoflavone, and protease inhibitors, phytic acid, and saponins, all complex plant chemicals that are being explored for their potential to reduce cancer risk. The benefit of eating soybeans is not restricted to cancer. It has also been shown to lower the cholesterol level in the blood. High blood cholesterol is considered a risk factor in the development of heart disease, suggesting soy might be a "heart-smart" food.[27]

Nutrition East and West: The Parallels

I began to wonder: What would happen if, instead of bypassing the problem, patients began to change what seemed to be the underlying causes *of their heart disease.*
—Dean Ornish, *Dr. Dean Ornish's Program for Reversing Heart Disease*[28]

The best physician looks for the root cause of disease. Then he first attempts to cure it with food. Only if food fails should he use drugs.
—Sun Si-miao, *Thousand Ducat Prescriptions, Tang Dynasty*

In the past several decades major changes have taken place in field of nutrition. Food is much more than a repository of various vitamin and mineral substances—it can be a primary cause of "Western" diseases and a veritable gold mine of potent phytochemicals useful in the prevention and treatment of disease. While nutrition is, in the old biology, largely irrelevant for medicine, it is, in the new biology, a foundation of health and healing.

The Basic Healthy Diet Revisited

With the rapid pace of research into the relationship between diet and health there is abundance of confusion. Many people sense that the standard American diet is unhealthy and are open to change. Yet with contradictory claims announced regularly in the popular press, it is hard to know what direction change should take. Part of the confusion lies in the emphasis on finding particular chemicals in food that represent the cause of disease. This molecular emphasis tends to obscure a perspective of the forest in the obsession with identifying trees.

Foods are composed of thousands of molecules, all with the potential to interact among themselves and with the thousands of molecules comprising the mind-body system. To make any sense, this molecular approach must be combined with a study of broader patterns in the relationship between food and health. And it is here, at the pattern level, that much less confusion reigns.

In their effort to study "Western" diseases, researchers like Cornell's Colin Campbell have noted a distinct dietary pattern associated with a high prevalence of Western diseases and another pattern where such diseases are much less common. As Campbell describes it, these diseases have "some very profound common causes." A rich diet containing a high proportion of animal foods, low in fiber and foods of plant origin, while high in fat and cholesterol, is this common cause. And the diet able to greatly reduce the risk of Western diseases is one that is low in animal products, fat, and cholesterol, while high in fiber and foods of plant origin.[29]

In light of the powerful evidence that food has a lot to do with health, governments have recently shifted their nutritional recommendations to favor a more plant-based eating pattern. In the United States, for example, the Department of Agriculture, which has issued "food guides" since 1916, now uses a food pyramid. Grains and complex carbohydrates, vegetables and fruits are the foundation of the pyramid, reflecting the fact that they are the foundation of a healthy diet. Dairy products and animal products are higher up on the pyramid, indicating that the quantity of these foods

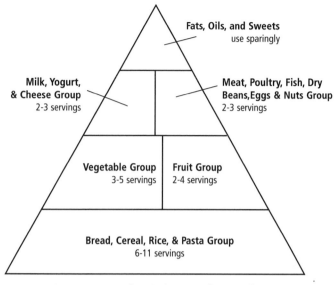

U.S. Department of Agriculture Food Pyramid

should be reduced in comparison to carbohydrates and vegetables. Fats, oils, and sweets are found at the top of the pyramid and should be used sparingly.

Government positions are inevitably subject to the fickle winds of politics and it is useful to turn to other sources of healthy eating wisdom. The Physicians Committee for Responsible Medicine (PCRM) points out that the government-issued Food Guide Pyramid suggests regular servings of meat and dairy products, reflecting a trade-off between health and agri-business interests. In response, the PCRM has developed its "New Four Food Groups": simply whole grains, vegetables, fruits, and legumes. In this recommended regimen, whole grains are given the most daily servings, legumes the least. The only known nutrient of concern in this entirely plant-based diet is vitamin B-12, which, although present in microorganism-transformed foods like miso and tempeh (B-12 is produced by bacteria and other microorganisms), can be obtained with a supplement.[30]

While this "new" way of eating—the standard fare of the world's agriculturalists for millennia—is a significant change in thinking from the nutrition of the old biology, it resonates strongly with the basic healthy diet of Chinese nutrition. In both systems, grains and vegetables form the bulk of the diet, supplemented by lesser amounts of legumes, fruits, nuts and seeds, and perhaps a small portion of animal-based food. The only minor difference is the recommendation in Chinese nutrition to eat an equal number of servings of vegetables as grains, while emerging Western guidelines suggest vegetable servings be less than grain servings. A minor point, but given the emerging recognition of the health benefits of vegetables, there may well be merit in this extra emphasis on vegetables.

The Complementary Nature of Nutrition East and West

There is considerable congruence between the basic healthy diet of new biology nutrition and that of Chinese nutrition, a confidence-generating fact in this time of often contradictory dietary claims. Yet a sticky point remains in the question of the extent to which animal products should be included in the diet. Some in the new Western nutrition, like the PCRM, suggest animal-based foods be completely shunned. The PCRM argues that a vegan diet—one that avoids meat, eggs, and dairy—can supply all known nutrients (except perhaps vitamin B-12). Dean Ornish, in his program for reversing heart disease, allows for a small amount of low-fat dairy and egg whites in an otherwise plant-based diet. In Chinese nutrition it is possible to find both an enthusiasm for the benefits of a plant-only diet and concern about possible deleterious effects of a diet completely devoid of animal products.

The Chinese tradition offers insight into the appropriateness of animal food in the diet through a system of constitutional typing emphasizing individual differences. For some people a complete abstinence from animal products can be beneficial; for others it may be useful to include supplementary foods of animal origin. This system combines an understanding of constitution with the properties of food to maintain individual balance.

There are a number of approaches used to categorize constitution. One approach is to work with three pairs of qualities: hot and cold, dry and damp, deficient and excessive. Symptoms of hot, cold, dry, and damp were discussed earlier in this chapter. Hot individuals counteract their constitutional tendency of overactivity by shifting the basic, healthy diet slightly in favor of cool and cold foods, reducing pungent and increasing bitter flavors. Cold constitutions, in contrast, need a warmer diet, with more sweet and pungent flavors, and less bitter. Dryness will benefit from a diet favoring moistening foods, while damp constitutional tendencies are moderated by increasing consumption of drying foods and avoiding foods with a dampening nature.

A deficient constitution is indicated by chronic tiredness, shortness of breath, passive personality, thin and pale appearance. The deficient constitution benefits from a greater quantity of strengthening foods, more sweet and less bitter flavors. The excessive constitution, with its non-stop energy, reddish complexion, loud voice, and boisterous personality, benefits from foods that promote the movement of blood and qi and a reduction in sweet and tonifying foods.[31]

By combining constitutional understanding with lifestyle and climate, a clearer picture of the role of animal products in the diet emerges. Strictly plant-based eating is widely considered beneficial for spiritual and intellectual pursuits, while the extra demands of a more physically strenuous lifestyle may be met with a small amount of animal food as a supplement to the basic, healthy diet. Damp constitutions—often with a tendency toward obesity— require a religious avoidance of excess fat and dairy products, foods that are dampness-generating. The richness of the Western diet is deleterious to those with damp constitutions and those with this pattern should eat few animal products.

A hot and dry constitution—deficient yin in the Chinese medical model—on the other hand, benefits from the moistening property of dairy products, as well as foods such as millet, clam, and barley. While deficient constitutions benefit from supplementary animal products, excess constitutions are poorly suited for the standard Western eating pattern and should strictly avoid a high-fat, low-fiber diet. A lighter vegetarian diet would even moderate their typically "Type-A" personalities.

Food As Medicine

In the Chinese tradition, there is no clear line between food and medicine. Many foods/herbs can end up either in a herbal prescription or on the dinner plate. These foods have physiological effects that can be harnessed for the prevention or treatment of disease. Adzuki bean, a small deep-red legume with a hearty taste, for example, has the ability to remove heat from the body and promote urination. It is used in prescriptions for edema and topically as a paste for hemorrhoids. As a folk remedy, it is used to promote milk production in nursing mothers. Overconsumption of adzuki beans can lead to dryness, but regular consumption is ideal for those with a damp constitution.

Job's tears, a barley-like grain whose properties were discussed previously, is a dampness-clearing herb and a common food. There is some interest in its possible anti-cancer properties, and when lightly roasted it is used as a digestive tonic. Job's tears is also a folk remedy for warts.

Recently, new biology nutrition has rekindled an interest in food as medicine, paralleling the Eastern enthusiasm for the healing power of food. The simple soybean, for example, is now thought to be much more than a good source of protein for animals or people too poor to afford meat. Soy and its derivative foods are a nutritious addition to a vegetarian diet as well as a rich source of powerful phytochemicals, plant molecules with surprisingly powerful physiological effects. Phyto-estrogens, for example, can affect the hormonal system and are postulated to have a preventive effect against some forms of cancer.

While Chinese nutrition is focused on the qualities of food and its effects on the mind-body system, Western nutrition is focused on the molecular constituents of food and their biological effects. Despite these differences, Western ideas about food resonate with those of the

East. The basic, healthy diet espoused by progressive Western organizations and Eastern nutrition are essentially one and the same. An awareness of the healing power of food, long part of Eastern culture, is now emerging from a scientific perspective in the West. It is possible to eat with confidence a diet that can help prevent and even reverse some of the common health problems of the modern world. As news reports chronicle newly discovered benefits of consuming various foods, it is interesting to reflect on this as a modern continuation of an ancient tradition.

9 | The Mystery of Qi: "Energy" in Chinese Medicine and the New Biology

Matter is Qi taking shape. Mountains forming, forests growing, rivers streaming, and creatures proliferating are all manifestations of Qi. In the human being, all functions of the body and mind are manifestations of Qi: sensing, cogitating, feeling, digesting, stirring, and propagating. Qi begets movement and heat. It is the fundamental mystery and miracle.

—Harriet Beinfield and Efrem Korngold,
Between Heaven and Earth: A Guide to Chinese Medicine[1]

One of the most extraordinary ideas in Chinese medicine is the notion of qi and its circulation through a series of channels in the body.[2] While qi is not a material substance that can be isolated and studied, it is of fundamental importance to medicine. By adjusting the circulation of qi at an acupuncture point the physician affects physiological functions, regulating and harmonizing the organism.

Qi remains a mystery. There is little correspondence in standard Western biology to either qi, the acupoints, or the complex system of channels through which qi flows. If acupuncture has any validity, say the skeptics, it may be through stimulation of the nervous system and consequent effect on various biologically active chemicals such as the endorphins, opiate-like molecules involved in pain response. Qi, according to this view, may simply be a long-held superstition or perhaps a crude metaphor for organizational and regulatory processes involving the nervous system. Yet the Western difficulty with qi may lie with the limitations of standard biology and medicine—for the new biology is offering glimpses of curious phenomena that are not without parallel to ancient Chinese ideas.

Qi in Chinese Medicine: Mystical Metaphor and Concrete Healing Tool

Cosmic Qi

Rather than using an alphabet, the Chinese language is composed of ideograms or characters built up from a set of basic symbols called radicals. The character for qi is a combination of the radical for vapor or gas and the rice or grain radical, symbolizing the fine essence drafting up from a pot of cooking grain. Qi is thus something ethereal and unseen, but known through its effects and consequences, like the saliva generated in a hungry person bending over a pot of aromatic rice.

Qi has a broad range of meanings, from simply gas and vapor to various cosmic and biological "energies." Cosmic qi, for example, played a central role in the formation of the universe. Out of the primal nothingness emerged space and time, and from them arose original qi. This qi separated into its heavy and light components, the light rising to become heaven, the heavy coalescing to become the earth. The qi of heaven and earth in turn produced yin and yang, their qi bringing forth the seasons and differentiated things of the world.

This ancient view of the universe reached its most sophisticated level during the great Neo-Confucian synthesis of Confucian, Taoist, and Buddhist ideas during the eleventh and twelfth centuries. Chu Hsi, a Neo-Confucian who lived from 1131 to 1200 and one of China's greatest thinkers, merged the concept of qi together with *li*, the cosmic principle of organization, to set out an organic philosophy of the universe. Chu Hsi envisioned a universe oscillating eternally between order and chaos, primal unity and differentiated diversity. In the beginning, swirling cosmic qi gathered speed, coalescing to form the earth and leaving lighter qi on the outside to form the heavens. Qi was shaped over time by the innate principle of organization, *li*, creating a patterned progression from primal chaos to ever higher levels of order.[3]

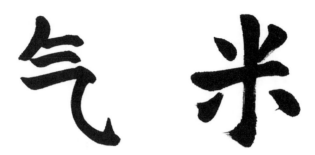

Vapor   Rice

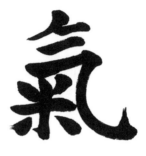

Qi

Qi: Matter, Energy, or Vital Force?

Qi is the basic stuff of the universe, neither matter nor energy, so fine and rarefied as to fill space. Joseph Needham, who felt qi best remained untranslated as a unique cultural concept, described it as matter-energy. It is a concept that finds its way into every aspect of Chinese science and culture, from medicine to art. The acupuncture needle regulates the patient's qi, a task aided by the practitioner's own qi connecting through the needle. The space of a master's landscape painting is bursting with qi that merges seamlessly with the qi of the rocks, mountains, and trees.

Scholar Paul Unschuld warns against the common interpretation of qi as "energy," suggesting instead that qi be rendered as "finest matter influence."[4] Qi often has this connotation of a force or "influence." In medicine, for example, there is damp qi—one of the six environmental qi or influences that can affect health—and pestilential qi—a disease agent present in epidemics.

Another scholar, Manfred Porkert, in contrast, argues that while not a precisely parallel concept, qi can be considered as "energy" in a general sense. He calls qi "configurational energy," an energy with a defined direction in space, structure, or quality. There are over ten fundamental types of qi described in medicine and more than twenty secondary types. Porkert describes thirty-two of them, such as heavenly or celestial qi, denoting the effect of the ever-changing cosmic pattern, and *wei* qi, the body's defensive energy.[5]

In the biological realm, qi is often translated as vital energy, suggesting a connection to the mysterious "vital force" of the vitalists. Yet there are essential differences between qi and the out-of-fashion idea of a vital force. In the West, the idea of a vital force was used to differentiate living systems from non-living matter. The Chinese world view, in contrast, does not draw a demarcation line between the living and non-living. Qi is used to describe physical as well as biological phenomena. While the physician can adjust the flow of qi in the human body, so too the practitioner of *feng shui*—literally "wind and water," an art without correspondence in the West but often translated as geomancy—works with the flow of qi in the earth to harmonize the human relationship with the environment. The Chinese universe is a living, organic one characterized by different forms and levels of organization and energy, *li* and qi.

Secondly, qi is not at heart a mysterious and unknowable philosophical concept like the vital force. As Ted Kaptchuk states: "For the Chinese, qi is not a metaphor; it is a real phenomenon that makes possible integrative descriptions of bodily changes. Diagnostic methods exist for determining its strength and motion, and there are specific treatments for supplementing its deficiency, draining its excess, and regulating its flow."[6] The physician can feel the qi arrive at a point being punctured; it is like a fish grabbing the fisher's hook. The patient's sense of fullness at the point and a radiating sensation along the channel show that the qi has been activated, offering confidence in the effect of treatment. The qi gong practitioner can feel the warmth generated by concentration on the sea of qi—the center and source located just below the navel—and can, in the exercise known as "qi ball," feel the static-electricity-like ball of qi between the hands.

Qi in the Physiological and Psychological Landscape

As we can see in the following passage from the *Yellow Emperor's Classic of Internal Medicine*, the ancient medical book written in the form of a dialogue between the Yellow Emperor and his minister Qi Bo, qi is a central concept in medicine:

> *The Yellow Emperor asked, "I heard all diseases are created by qi. With anger the qi rises; with joy the qi becomes loose or moderate; with grief the qi disappears, with fear the qi descends; with cold the qi shrinks; with heat the qi leaks; with fright the qi is disordered. With tiredness, the qi wilts; with thinking the qi becomes stagnant. These nine qi are not the same. What causes these diseases?"*
>
> *Qi Bo answered, "With anger the qi becomes counterflow.... With joy the qi becomes harmonized and the will becomes stronger. The* ying *and* wei *are able to flow through; therefore, the qi is loose or moderate....With heat, the skin tissues open, the* ying *and* wei *pass through, there is a great sweating. Therefore, the qi leaks. With fright the heart cannot perform its regal tasks. The* shen *cannot return. The thoughts and consciousness are not stable; therefore, the qi becomes disordered. With tiredness there is panting and sweating; the inside and outside are overcome; therefore, the qi wilts...."*[7]

This exchange between the Yellow Emperor and his minister eloquently illustrates the link in Chinese medicine between the emotions, qi, and physiological processes. Qi, as this passage shows, is of pivotal importance in the theoretical foundation and explanatory framework of Chinese medicine.

Qi in the body has five functions: it plays a protective role, activates, warms, transforms, and keeps things in place. As a protective force it provides defense against pathogens. In this sense, qi is called the "correct," the mobilizing force that resists invasion by outside agents and maintains health in the face of adverse environmental conditions. Chinese medicine describes disease as a struggle between the pathogen and correct qi, which must be debilitated before a pathogen can successfully take hold.

As a warming agent, qi is responsible for the maintenance of body temperature and the body's metabolic fire. Qi keeps the organs held in their proper place, prevents blood from spilling from the vessels, and checks the excessive flow of fluids such as sweat, tears, and urine from the body. Qi is also behind the transformative actions that take place in the body. Food is transformed into blood, for example, while ingested fluids are transformed into urine. As an activating agent, qi is reflected in the movement and activity inherent in everything from physiological functions to human growth and development.

Varieties of Qi

Manfred Porkert has discussed thirty-two distinct types of qi. Let us explore some of the most important ones, and set out a system-level model of qi in the human organism. A starting point is understanding the origins of true or genuine qi, the general designation for all the qi of the body.

Prenatal qi is inherited from one's parents. It is the root potential or basic constitution of an individual and is stored in the kidneys. The Taoists, in their great efforts to promote longevity, emphasized the importance of conserving and supporting the prenatal qi. Prenatal qi acts as the fundamental template for the functions and pattern of growth and development in the organism. When utilized and activated in this way it is known as original qi.

Original qi gushes forth from an area between the kidneys and below the navel. This is the root or source of life—the hara—so important in Eastern culture. Deep breathing combined with a relaxed concentration on the "sea of qi" below the navel is important in qi gong, the meditation-exercise used by ancient immortality-seeking adepts and modern health-seekers alike. As Qi Bo explains to the Yellow Emperor:

> *Each of the twelve meridians has a relationship to the source of the vital energies. The source of the vital energies is the root origin of the twelve meridians, it is the moving qi between the kidneys. This means that the source of the vital energies is fundamental to the five yin and six yang organs, the root of the twelve meridians, the gate of breathing. It is the source of the triple warmer.*[8]

"Thus," emphasize Kiiko Matsumoto and Stephen Birch, contemporary practitioners of Chinese medicine, "the abdomen is more than the physical center, the cavity in which the organs reside. It is the residence of the source of the body's energies, the energetic center from which life springs."[9] As Qi Bo describes, original qi is circulated throughout the body via the triple warmer, or sanjiao, one of the yang organ-meridian systems of Chinese medicine.

Grain qi is extracted from food by the transformative action of the spleen, while air qi is absorbed by the lungs from the air we breathe. Air qi, grain qi, and original qi combine to produce the true qi. The extraction of air qi from the respiratory processes and the circulation of qi and blood throughout the body are assisted by the ancestral qi of the chest. Ancestral qi, composed of air and grain qi, fosters the respiratory rhythm and harmonizes the heartbeat.

True qi is differentiated into its various forms according to function. True qi associated with the organs is called organ qi, the essence of each organ's physiological activity. Spleen qi, for example, is involved in the transformation and transportation of food. True qi flowing through the channels is called channel qi. The channels are the communication network of the body-mind, and channel qi the agent of information, acting to regulate and harmonize the organs.

Construction or nutritive (*ying*) qi is inseparable from the blood. As it says in the *Yellow Emperor's Classic*, "Construction qi secretes fluids, discharges them into the vessels, and turns them into blood, to nourish the limbs and supply the yin and yang organs."[10] Construction qi is involved in the transformation of food into blood, the movement of blood and the nourishment of the entire body.

Defensive (*wei*) qi, the complement of construction qi, flows outside of the vessels and offers protection against invading pathogens. Defensive qi nourishes the skin and it flows on the body exterior where it regulates sweating.

Original qi, stored in the kidneys, represents the pre-natal or inborn contribution to the qi that underlies physiological, emotional, and mental activity. Grain qi derived from eating and air qi acquired from breathing are the post-natal contribution. Proper nutrition and breathing are thus crucial components of good health, and why dietary habits and breathing exercises like qi gong are a foundation of prevention and therapy. Together, original, grain, and air qi form the true qi, which in its various forms—channel and organ qi, nutritive and defensive qi—regulates and harmonizes, nourishes and defends, allowing the mind-body in all its complexity to function in an integrated way.

Of Water-Works and Caves

The channels (also often called meridians) through which channel qi travels are the basis of acupuncture practice. Because of the integrating, regulating, and communicating function of channel qi, its adjustment special points along the channels can harmonize and restore patterns of disharmony. As described in the *Yellow Emperor's Classic*, channels are the conduits of qi and blood, making possible the balancing of yin and yang and the moistening of the joints and sinews.[11] Channel qi circulates through the body along a network of major and minor channels (the *jing-luo*), connecting the interior with the exterior, the yin organs with the yang organs, and the organs with the various parts of the body.

The Chinese character for channel is composed of the thread or string radical and the character *jing*, signifying the underground flow of water. The top line with three arrow heads of the character *jing* depicts the flow of water beneath the ground. *Jing* also connotes the threads in a fabric that give it form and, as a verb, to pass through or to direct. The channels are thus conduits directing the flow of qi.

The character for the acupoints suggests a cave, hole, or opening. It is a picture of a roof above, with a symbol meaning to divide below, implying a shelter created by the removal of earth. The character *shu*, with an implication of transportation or movement, is also used to designate a special set of acupuncture points, hinting at the energetic transmission between point and organ.

As explained in the *Yellow Emperor's Classic*, the acupoints are places where the vital qi enters and leaves. The points, channels, and organs form an integrated, interactive, and dynamic system. When a channel connects with its organ (when the spleen channel links with the spleen, for example) it enters and saturates or belongs to that organ, implying a strong, indivisible link. When a channel connects with a coupled organ (when the spleen channel connects with the paired organ of the spleen, the stomach, for example), it "spirally wraps" the organ, implying influence and interaction but with more distinction between channel and organ.[12] The continuous circulation of qi along a sequence of channels—starting at the lung and ending at the liver channel brings a collection of parts together into a harmonious whole.

Some scholars have pointed to the "circulation-mindedness" of the ancient Chinese, and suggest that their early conception of the circulation of blood and qi arose naturally in a society based on large-scale water-works. Chinese civilization had it origins in a rich agricultural area prone to flooding, and water-works were used to control water levels, irrigate crops, and provide transportation. The power and central authority of the Emperor arose from the need for a government that could organize and administer such large-scale efforts.

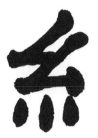

Thread

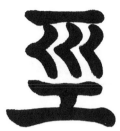

Underground Flow of Water

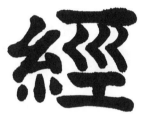

Acupuncture Channel

This culture of water-works contributed many water-based descriptions and metaphors to the medical field, creating a fertile ground for the idea of blood and qi circulating through the organism. (The Chinese notion of blood circulation predated the discovery of blood circulation by William Harvey in the seventeenth century.) The characters *jing* and *luo*, for example, used to denote the main channels and the secondary connecting channels, are also found in terms for large rivers and civic drains.[13] Each of the twelve main channels has five "transporting-*shu*" points rich with water metaphor: the well, spring, stream, river, and uniting points, the latter point name suggesting a river uniting with the sea. This use of water metaphors in the East can be compared to the machine analogies used in the West (see Chapter 3) and illustrates how important the cultural milieu is in shaping the understanding and interpretation of natural phenomena.

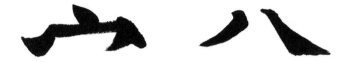

Roof   To Divide

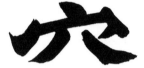

Acupuncture Point

Origins and Reality

Qi, the acupoints, and the channels—unique cultural concepts whose origins are obscured in the mists of time—are without direct or obvious parallels in Western biology and medicine, making it difficult for Western biomedicine to make sense of these distinctly Eastern ideas. Modern biomedical research on acupuncture has focused on various chemical changes produced by needling. There are also electrical correspondences to the acupuncture points. Point locators based on the difference in the electrical resistance of the skin between a point and its surrounding area have emerged from this kind of inquiry.[14] So while there appears to be some objective scientific measure of the points and their ability to produce biochemical changes, the channels are on shakier ground.[15]

In describing the points as real and the channels as the result of speculation, Manfred Porkert expresses a commonly held perspective:

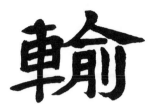

Shu

"[The detection of the conduits] by connecting the points is analogous to the way a subterranean water course reveals itself by springs sent up through 'punctures' in the earth's crust. The sensitive points provide the positive empirical and historically primary data on which the theory is based; the conduits, on the other hand, are only the result of systematic speculations."[16] Others have suggested that acupuncture developed empirically from the systematic stimulation of the body surface, perhaps as part of ritual demon exorcism practiced by the shamanistic tribes of pre-civilization China.[17]

Yet early texts written before the *Yellow Emperor's Classic* suggest that the concept of the channels existed before that of the points.[18] The texts describe various channels and their zones of influence without reference to points. Matsumoto and Birch point out that it is the internal, not the external or surface, trajectories of the twelve major channels that were classically considered to be the "main" channels. While the external trajectories are important for the practice of acupuncture, they were thought of as "branches." The internal meridians are the site of "the more important energetic exchanges and interactions," the surface branches merely "superficial extensions."[19]

This suggests a completely different origin for the Chinese concepts of qi circulation, points, and channels. Out of the timeless void of pre-history arose the spiritual practice/proto-science of Taoism. Taoists were interested in spiritual development, knowledge of the natural world, and immortality, for which they practiced both outer and inner alchemy. Outer alchemy was the search for the elixir of immortality; inner or physiological alchemy was a meditative process of transforming internal "energies" for spiritual development and immortality. This process of physiological alchemy involved the cultivation and circulation of qi and the interconversion of *jing*, qi, and *shen*, the three treasures.

The Taoists carefully cultivated their qi through diet and exercise, and developed many meditation-exercises to concentrate qi at specific sites and move it along designated routes. As Needham describes: "There were two ways of making it circulate. Concentrating the will to direct it to a particular place, such as the brain, or the site of some local malady, was termed *xing* qi. Visualizing its flow in thought was 'inner vision.'...The more passive way, of letting the qi take its normal course in circulating, was called re-casting it." He also quotes a Taoist text written before the tenth century: "Closing one's eyes, one has an inner vision of the five yin organs, one can clearly distinguish them, one knows the place of each...."[20]

The Taoists spent years practicing this kind of inner awareness, were familiar with their inner anatomy, and had some sense perception of this concentrated energy. Inner alchemy, so much a part of Taoism and Chinese civilization, likely played a key role in the discovery and elaboration of the channels and points upon which acupuncture is based. The techniques of inner alchemy were widely and continuously practiced and explain the mapping and importance of the inner trajectories of the channels. The discovery of subtle energy flows at the edge of interaction between mind and body arose in the course of systematic exploration of the inner environment by organized groups of men and women.

Energy and Organization in the New Biology

Previous chapters have explored the successful progression of biology from anatomy to molecular minutiae. While molecular biology has opened up a world of wondrous intricacy and described the molecular events involved in many diseases, questions remain about how all those molecules work together as performers in a perfectly choreographed ballet to form patterns at higher and higher levels of organization. How does the molecular dance become a cell and the cellular orchestra play together as an organ? And how do the organs in turn synchronize their performance as an organism?

Previous chapters have also explored the effort to understand this exquisite organization and order found in highly complex biological systems. The biological field (see Chapter 4) is one example of a provocative and useful idea, developed in order to understand pattern and form in living systems. Organisms such as starfish and salamanders, for example, can regenerate limbs, reforming parts to the specifications of their self and kind. The important idea here is information: the field provides the information necessary to successfully achieve such regeneration.

Other frontier scientists have turned their attention to problems of regulation and communication. The remarkable order and organization seen in living things requires information, but also a way to create order over space and time from such information. Behavioral patterns, for example, require organization over time; physical form requires organization over space. Liver cells must open communication channels to regulate their growth and function; they must whisper back and forth the messages necessary for group behavior, turning a haphazard crowd of cells into a functioning liver organ.

The conventional model of physiological integration is centered on the nervous and hormonal systems. The electrical signal used by the nervous system is the result of the flow of ions—molecules like sodium and potassium that are electrically charged—across nerve membranes. This nerve signal carries sensory information and integrates motor activities and is intricately linked to the hormonal system, a system of chemical messengers that flow through the body regulating physiological function. Without detracting from the importance of the nervous and hormonal systems, frontier scientists suggest that a complete description of physiological integration and the organization of living systems includes other phenomena that have been thus far undiscovered or perhaps overlooked.[21]

Electricity in Biology

Two researchers, both trained as medical doctors, have probed novel electrical features of biological systems. Swedish radiology professor Björn Nordenström, using both animal experiments and clinical research, has uncovered pathways of conduction for various ions in the blood vessels and lymphatic system. Nordenström hypothesizes that these complex macroscopic and microscopic networks of conduction—which he calls biologically closed electric circuits (BCEC)—are important for both structural and functional aspects of biological matter and they extend into all tissues of the body.

The BCEC system acts together with the mechanical pumping of the heart to provide a continuous circulation. "Without the two cooperating circulations we could certainly not live," claims Nordenström.[22] While the cell is electrically protected by its highly insulating membrane, there are membrane-spanning proteins that can transfer electrical current, allowing the BCEC system to act at the microscopic level and affect cellular function. Nordenström has used his research to develop an electrically based treatment for cancer.

American orthopedic surgeon and regeneration researcher Robert Becker explored for several decades the electrical properties associated with tissue injury and regeneration. Beginning work in the late 1950s, Becker was disturbed and frustrated by some of his patient's bone fractures that did not heal. He was intrigued by the ability of animals like the salamander to regenerate complete limbs and hoped that some basic animal research could shed light on the practical problems he faced as an orthopedic doctor.

After many laborious and painstaking experiments, Becker discovered that direct current (DC—current that flows in one direction) electricity was involved in the process of regeneration. In true regeneration, specialized cells like blood cells are turned into primitive or "undifferentiated" cells, which are in turn changed into differentiated ones like skin cells and bone cells according to the pattern required. (Every cell in the body has the same genetic information, but different parts of the DNA are "turned on" during embryological development to produce different types of cells. These are called "specialized" as compared with the unspecialized or primitive cells from which they originated.) This process, Becker found, was initiated and regulated by electrical current created in injured tissue.

Becker describes a direct current (DC) system of regulation that operates in addition to the electrical impulse of the nervous system. This current, considered by him to be a semiconducting phenomenon, is carried in the perineural cells found in close association with neurons in the brain and surrounding the cells of the peripheral nervous system. The perineural current, closely involved in the process of healing, is a more primitive but higher level of integration which serves to regulate and control the nerve impulse system.[23]

Whispering Cells

The experimental and theoretical research carried out by Ross Adey, working in Loma Linda, California, has led him to conclude that electromagnetic signals play a major role in cellular communications. Adey describes the signals traveling across cell membranes as the whispering of cells and claims that the study of the role of electromagnetic energy in living systems "is one of the most significant new scientific frontiers of this century, pointing the way to an understanding of the essence of living matter in physical mechanisms at the atomic level."[24]

Adey is interested in understanding the effects of weak electromagnetic fields on life, particularly their role in intercellular communications—the whispers between cells. He has developed a three-stage model for the effects of electromagnetic fields on cells. Firstly, electromagnetic fields and stimulating molecules like hormones can produce changes at the cell membrane surface, interacting with highly cooperative processes associated with calcium binding; secondly, proteins that stick all the way through the cell membrane—called transmembrane proteins—can transfer the signal to the cell interior; and thirdly, inside the cell these signals can produce changes in enzyme systems, organelles, and the cell nucleus. Adey concludes that the cell membrane surface is the key site of interaction between cells and electromagnetic signals. Even very weak fields can be amplified by highly cooperative biomolecular processes, processes that can only be understood using the most recent and sophisticated physical theories.[25]

Quantum Biology

The quantum theory is used to describe and predict properties of systems at the atomic level. The general feeling among scientists is that when dealing with really small things, like the parts of an atom, use the quantum theory, but when dealing with really big things, such as in biology, stick to so-called classical approaches, the basic methods that evolved from the work of Isaac Newton several hundred years ago. The Italian physicist Emilio Del Giudice challenges this view, arguing that the possibility of using the quantum theory to understand the organizational properties of systems of biological molecules has been overlooked.

Del Giudice's theory of super-radiance describes a coherent behavior of matter. Coherence is a way of saying a connection exists between seemingly separate parts. It is like an orchestra playing a Bach symphony, instead of several dozen musicians playing random notes on their instruments. The super-radiance model describes coherent states of interaction between systems of particles mutually coupled by an electromagnetic field. Del Giudice hopes that in the future this idea will provide a quantum-based framework for biology.

Del Giudice points to a new way of thinking. Instead of isolated particles only "knowing" each other through collisions and external forces (the classical notions applied to chemistry and biology), particles "move together as if performing a choral ballet, and are kept in phase by an [electromagnetic] field which arises from the same ballet."[26]

Del Giudice's model predicts long-range forces that may be important factors in biological self-organization. These forces, both attractive and repulsive, are highly dependent on the particular frequency of the system, resulting in a much more ordered biochemistry than the random model now used. The electromagnetic field in an area of coherence has the effect of ordering additional molecules within its sphere of influence, fitting them into patterns already set out by the same field. This could be described as a configurational energy, an ordering and organization of living matter in a way that is completely new to biology.

The late Herbert Fröhlich, a biophysicist who worked at the Oliver Lodge Laboratory in Liverpool, England, was a pioneer in the study of order and organization in living systems. He developed a theoretical framework for cooperativity in biological systems called "coherent excitations." Biomolecular systems are electrically polarized, and Fröhlich found that electric vibrations in a system of biomolecules could, through an input of energy, develop ordered (coherent) states.

Fröhlich has shown how this theory predicts a long-range selective interaction between enzyme—a workhorse protein molecule—and substrate—the substance upon which the enzyme acts. The enzyme and substrate are usually thought of in terms of a lock and key interaction: they are two molecules that fit together perfectly, like a lock and a key. One question that bothered Fröhlich was how the key could find the lock in the first place. The long-range selective interaction predicted by his theory explains the very effective chemical activity of enzymes by modifying the lock and key theory so that the key finds the lock more easily. The two molecules, by vibrating at the same frequency, "talk" the same language and the key can find its way by, in a way, seeing the light through the keyhole.[27]

Fröhlich has discussed the application of this theory to other biological questions such as the problem of cancer. Fröhlich describes cancer as a problem of growth control and suggests this control could rest in the excitation of a particular mode of vibration of the tissue.[28]

Experimental research has described a phenomenon known as ultra weak photon emission from living organisms—that is, living things have been found to give off very weak electromagnetic waves. The German scientist Fritz Popp has played a major role in the study of these "biophotons." Many scientists feel that biophotons simply *result* from the chemical processes of normal physiological activity, and as such, are nothing more than curious artifacts. Popp, in contrast, argues that biophotons are a *source* of physiological control, a part of the communication system within organisms. Biophotons play a role in the control and regulation of everything from cell differentiation and growth processes to enzymatic activity and immunological response.

The intensity of weak biological photon emission is very sensitive to all biological processes and environmental conditions. Popp interprets this as evidence for a coherent biophoton model—that is to say that the photons are not simply random and unimportant by-products of chemical reactions. He also points to experiments showing that DNA, the molecular blueprint of life, is the essential source and sink of biophotons. The double helix structure of the DNA might make it both a transmitter and receiver, a communications center for life signals.[29]

This brief sketch shows the effort on the part of frontier scientists to explore new ways of understanding the organizational and regulatory features of organisms. In some of this research electromagnetic energy plays a central role in the communications that make the parts work as a whole. While chemicals and chemical processes are building blocks for living systems, frontier scientists are offering glimpses of insight into their order and organization using concepts of information and coherence. The new biology is opening a window with a completely new view on the world of living things.

"Energy" and Organization in East and West: The Parallels

Acupuncture, with its concepts of qi, channels, and points, is an uncomfortable curiosity for conventional biology and medicine. Qi—a broad concept that links the organic and inorganic world into a dynamic, evolving world-event—remains a mystery, a fanciful theory or perhaps an imperfect metaphor. As a *Scientific American* editorial recently put it: "It is a lovely concept—and it is completely irreconcilable with empirical science."[30]

Yet, it may be that the West has been too quick to judge, too focused on narrow notions in biology and medicine that have held sway for several hundred years. As the new biology shows in its quest for understanding order and organization in living systems—something that has long remained as mysterious as qi—there are different windows through which life can be viewed, some of them opening toward new ideas with strong parallels to concepts from the East.

Parallels in the Physical Universe

The Chinese universe is an organic one with a resonance between microcosm and macrocosm. Qi is matter-energy, the basic stuff of the universe, shaped by *li*, the underlying force of organization. This is a universe having much in common with the organic philosophy of the new biology, a Western philosophy that even has hints of Chinese origins. (See Chapter 6.) The organic universe is an evolving multi-level pattern, with atoms, molecules, and crystals, cells, organisms, and galaxies.

Fritjof Capra, in *The Tao of Physics*, compares the Chinese concept of qi with the quantum field in modern physics. In quantum field theory, the idea of empty space is replaced by a dynamic energy field. Particles come into being when the field becomes particularly intense and localized, their interactions transferred as undulations in the field. Capra compares qi to the quantum field, as an ethereal and invisible form of matter pervading space and condensing to form the visible material world. The qi and the quantum field are at once the essence of material objects and the connection between objects found as waves.[31]

Capra quotes the eleventh century philosopher Chang Tsai, one of the great Neo-Confucian syncretists and an elder of Chu Hsi: "When the [qi] condenses, its visibility becomes apparent so that there are then the shapes of individual things. When it disperses, its visibility is no longer apparent and there are no shapes. At the time of its condensation, can one say otherwise than that this is but temporary? But at the time of its dispersing, can one hastily say that it is then non-existent?"[32]

Matter-energy, or qi, condenses to form the differentiated things of the world, but does not lose its underlying connection with the whole. This connection is the dynamic pattern, the vital rhythm, that animates the cosmos, a rhythm that pulses in both part and whole. Modern physics too looks for the underlying symmetry, or pattern of organization, in the field. This symmetry is the underlying reality; the particles, the things of the world, are its temporary manifestations.

Building Biological Bridges

Thousands of years ago the Taoist Masters discovered in their meditations the six sounds which were the correct frequencies to keep the organs in optimal condition by preventing and alleviating illness. They discovered that a healthy organ vibrates at a particular frequency.
—Taoist Master Mantak Chia[33]

Normal tissues and organs are subjected to a control...which prevents them from growing beyond their appropriate size, or of mutating. This control is absent in cancer. From a naive point of view of physics, thus, the cancer problem requires finding this control. Clearly it requires a long-range interaction between different cells, i.e., it must involve all, or most of the cells of a particular tissue or organ. It will be suggested, then, that the required control can rest in the excitation of a particular mode of vibration of the relevant tissue or organ.
—Biophysicist Herbert Fröhlich[34]

Chinese medicine, through its system of correspondence, is ripe with connections between seemingly unconnected things. The eyes and the emotion anger, for example, are linked to the liver. Often these connections can be interpreted through the channels. The liver channel, for example, courses through the eyes. (The liver channel travels from the inside of the big toe, up the leg, along the lower border of the ribs, to the throat and through the eyes, finally converging with other channels at the crown point of the head.)

At the same time, such connections reflect underlying patterns, patterns expressed in at least one way by the five phases. The emotion anger is part of a fundamental pattern that also involves the eyes, the liver, and the liver channel, a pattern connecting mind, body, and spirit. These energetic connections can be seen in the complex processes that take place during embryological development. Matsumoto and Birch, for example, have pointed to the links between embryological patterns of development and Chinese medicine energetics.[35] Qi makes possible the interconnections and underlying patterns described in Chinese medicine.

In the biological realm, qi is much less mysterious when viewed in the context of the new biology. Compare Manfred Porkert's translation of qi as a "configurational energy," for example, with Del Giudice's quantum biology, where biological molecules are ordered or configured within an area of coherence. Molecules perform their functional dance to a tune that they help to create; their interactions are not random events, but scenes in a dynamic and evolving play. As Fröhlich speculates in the quote above, this coherence or rhythmic organizing pattern—the qi—might extend from microscopic domains of coherence to the organ or tissue level.

There is a well-known Taoist exercise-meditation known as the six healing sounds in which specific sounds—often accompanied by guided imagery, vocalizations, and movement—are used to activate particular channels and harmonize the associated organs and mental-emotional states. Mantak Chia, a contemporary Taoist teacher, describes these sounds as "the correct frequencies to keep the organs in optimal condition by preventing and alleviating illness."[36] The Chinese were quite advanced in acoustics and the study of resonance, and the Taoists—in the course of their meditations and longevity questing—explored the physiological effect of acoustical resonance.

From the point of view of Western physiology breathing and eating are the foundation of metabolic activity. In Chinese medicine, grain qi and air qi are two of the three sources providing a foundation for the true qi. Grain qi is extracted from food, while air qi is absorbed in the course of breathing. The third foundation of true qi, the original qi, is more elusive. Stored in the kidneys, the original qi is the catalyst and template of physiological activity.

Matsumoto and Birch compare original qi—"an unobservable matrix or order from which all material things manifest, from which all other forms of qi derive"—with the ideas of the late physicist David Bohm.[37] Bohm was interested in the quantum theory, and struggled to come to terms with what it said about the world. He described empty space as an illusion: it was really an immense sea of energy containing an "implicate" or enfolded order. From this sea of energy, the explicate order, the things of the world, appear.

The original qi is a form of genetic information, and is closely associated with the *jing*, the essence of life that provides the foundation of constitution. Manfred Porkert describes *jing* as "unattached structive energy or structive potential," quoting the *Yellow Emperor's Classic*—"What life comes from is called *jing*, 'structive potential'"—and a later commentator—"What the first impulse of life comes from…"[38] Original qi is the active manifestation of this life potential, a projection of the information contained in the *jing*.

Here a comparison with the idea of the morphogenetic field and the work of Popp arises. Popp's biophoton model of a coherent electromagnetic wave projecting from the DNA describes an active manifestation of the basic template of life in Western science, the DNA. The biophoton is a source of physiological regulation and control involved with growth processes, among others. Like original qi, the biophoton represents an active manifestation of the information at the root of life: it is the catalyst and directing force, the "configurative energy."

The morphogenetic field—the biological field of information successfully describing and even predicting pattern formation in organisms (see Chapter 4)—also deserves comparison to original qi and *jing*. This field of organizing information is the implicate and unobservable matrix from which form and function unfolds. Like *jing*, it provides a "configurative potential" and is intimately linked to the genetic foundation of the individual. Like original qi—the configurative energy emerging from the configurative potential—it provides an unobservable but active matrix from which all structure and function arises.

Channel Qi and Microtubules: Linking Part and Whole

> *[T]ensegrity structures function as coupled harmonic oscillators. DNA, nuclei, cytoskeletal filaments, membrane ion channels and entire living cells and tissues exhibit characteristic resonant frequencies of vibration.*
>
> —Donald E. Ingber, Medical Doctor and Bioengineer[39]

Many interesting parallels exist between original qi and some of the ideas arising in the new biology. True qi and its specific forms of organ qi and channel qi also show parallels. Adey is exploring physical signals that play a role in intercellular communication, the previously unheard "whispers" that bring a collection of cells together into a functioning organ. Del Giudice's quantum biology points to a fundamental "coherence" in biomolecular systems, a long-range coordination of molecules that shapes and configures biochemical processes. This configurational energy—or perhaps qi—within a microscopic coherence domain may well extend, as Fröhlich suggests, all the way to the organ level. Together, a collection of coherent organ systems forms an organism buzzing with internal connections, a tuned multi-frequency network sensitive to the surrounding environment.

Frontier biophysical research clearly hints at an energetic system of physiological integration with parallels to the concepts of the channels and channel qi. This exciting and revolutionary vision points to a system of regulation and communication hitherto unknown to Western science, a system that the Chinese explored so long ago. Becker, for example, describes a bioelectromagnetic system of regulation that controls the nerve impulse network. As the result of his experiments on the electrical properties of the acupuncture system, he hypothesizes that the channels are conduits for very weak DC currents and the points are amplifiers in the network.

The greatest difficulty with Becker's model comes in considering the large amount of information needed to have a useful communication system. While the information carried in a DC system is limited, high frequencies have tremendous potential for information transfer. Fröhlich's ideas about high-frequency electric vibrations and Popp's biophoton model show that high frequency waves and vibrations can act as information-carriers, coordinating the activities of biological molecules and regulating biological activities at all levels. As science continues to unravel these bioelectromagnetic and bioinformational systems of regulation and control, we will understand more about the relationship of the part to the whole, shedding light on the great mystery of biological organization—and on the mystery of qi.

There are specific structures that can transmit informational signals throughout the cell—the microtubules. These mysterious and microscopic tube-like structures are built from protein, providing support and structure to the cell. The microtubules may function as conduits for bioelectromagnetic signals, and recent research demonstrates their ability to transmit mechanical forces and vibrations.

The microtubules and microfilaments that comprise the cell's skeleton link the outside of the cell to the inside—the cell surface to the nucleus. Scientists have found that they can affect the nucleus and alter cell functions by pushing and pulling on skeletal elements at the cell surface. Cells are aware of the shapes into which they are forced by their environment, and adjust their behaviors accordingly. Stretched cells, for example, respond by growing and dividing, since more are needed to fill the surrounding space.

Physician and scientist Donald Ingber, a professor at Harvard Medical School long interested in the mechanical properties of living systems, argues that studying the molecular machinery of living systems is not enough. We must also understand how all these molecules are put together. Ingber looks to common patterns in living and non-living nature for insights into the rules of self-assembly and biological organization. He is a pioneer in the study of "tensegrity," a system of organization that creates stable systems by a balance of tension and compression within a structure.[40]

Structures based on tensegrity are found widely in nature and can be observed at every level of biological organization. The bones act as compressive elements, while muscles and tendons provide tensile strength. Tensegrity helps stabilize large biomolecules like proteins and DNA, and cellular structure is stabilized by the tension and compression of microtubules and microfilaments. Even some of the properties of tissues can be explained from this mechanical analysis.

Through tensegrity, with the microtubules acting at the cellular level, small changes in one part of the cell initiate global changes in structure and function. This allows the cell to feel and react to its environment. According to Ingber, tensegrity explains the remarkable coordination of living systems. It offers an understanding of how the actions of even an arm movement—where skin is stretched, the extracellular matrix is pulled, cells are contorted, and the molecules that comprise the cell's basic framework are pulled—can occur so smoothly and continuously.

Tensegrity structures are also coupled harmonic oscillators, a physics term describing their ability to vibrate at characteristic frequencies in a coordinated way. Everything from DNA and microtubules to cells and tissues have their own vibrational frequency. The tensegrity network helps to spread forces to all parts of the interconnected system and to, as Ingber puts it, "couple, or 'tune,' the whole system mechanically as one." Perhaps it is not so mysterious that seemingly disparate parts are intimately connected, or that an acupuncture needle can heal by restoring balance at a distant site?

Final Thoughts

In the new biology, there is an emerging outline—the first glimpse of a new continent on the horizon—of channels and channel qi, features of the body that the Chinese have been aware of for several thousand years. The implications are profound. The molecular changes now associated with disease might be accurate descriptions of pathological processes, but this is not the only level at which the problem can be viewed. Molecules may misbehave because the choral ballet has lost its coordination, and there may a variety of underlying reasons for a particular misbehavior. Specific chemicals might restore molecular behavior—cure the disease—but cause further distortion in the energy and organization of the organism, manifesting as side effects.

As Del Giudice has suggested, while it is possible to influence living systems with chemicals—a major focus of conventional Western medicine—it is also possible to imagine changes induced via the electromagnetic field pattern of the system. Before this can happen, science must gain a better understanding of the regulation and communication that takes place in living systems. The dynamic interplay of health and disease must be explored at this "energetic" level, and therapies developed to restore the broken or distorted lines of communication.

Chinese medicine, with its major therapeutic techniques of herbal medicine and acupuncture, is a well-developed system of diagnosing and treating the organism at this energetic level. Specific diseases are set in the context of an underlying pattern of disharmony, a description of system-level changes that lead to a breakdown in regulation and coordination. Therapies balance the pattern and restore the system by focusing on the qi—the vibrational coordination that links part and whole—rather than the molecules themselves. As it delves more deeply into the energy and organization of living systems, Western science will have much opportunity to learn from and not just about this ancient system of healing.

Epilogue| The Future of Health and Healing

Toward a New System of Medicine

There are exciting times ahead in the field of medicine and health. The emerging understanding of the genetic basis of disease and the possibility of developing gene-based therapies, for example, may allow presently intractable illnesses to be successfully tackled. Other high profile, life-saving techniques like organ transplants will undoubtedly become cheaper and more effective.

Yet although these kinds of highly visible and much-hyped "high-tech" approaches to medicine will save individual lives, they will likely remain as insignificant determinants of the overall health and longevity of the population. More significant for the long-term health of the population are other, less high-tech discoveries like the relationship between mind and body, the importance of exercise, and the crucial role of nutrition. Although it turns out that these are not exactly new ideas, the rigorous investigative efforts of science are offering greater insights into these areas than ever before.

Research shows that it is not genes that largely determines one's fate when it comes to health and successful aging, but way of life. This means that some of the enthusiasm for high-tech approaches to medicine should be directed toward the tremendous possibilities of prevention. A portion of health care resources and effort needs to be shifted away from disease and toward preventive thinking and actions.

Another area of exploration with the potential to radically transform our understanding of human biology and the practice of medicine is bioelectromagnetics. While this fascinating frontier still represents only a fringe area of scientific endeavor, the study of the electromagnetic and "energetic" features of living systems is a new way of thinking about life. While the implications for conventional medicine can only be the subject of speculation at this time, it is clearly relevant in many ways to complementary medicine, particularly acupuncture and other so-called "energy"-based therapies.

This brings us to the question of complementary medicine, an area in which interest has exploded in recent decades. Despite the cautious and often overly critical position of some conventional physicians toward these "new" healing methods, their patients are eagerly exploring herbs and homeopathy, acupuncture and therapeutic touch. Clearly, an organized and rational integration of the conventional and complementary is needed in the long term to create the best possible medical system, one that is both cost effective and therapeutically effective.

The essence of the complementary approach to medicine is often missed. Complementary therapies can be more than alternatives to the conventional, simply substituting herbs for drugs, such as St. John's Wort for Prozac. Rather, they embody a complementary way of looking at the healing process, emphasizing the self-healing potential of the organism and using therapies that can stimulate and effect such a response. At times the focus must be on the disease and its elimination, while at others the constitution or "terrain" must be offered support so that healing can take place within. And there are times when both approaches must be combined. The ability to differentiate these needs must emerge from an integration of the conventional and complementary.

Integration is a challenging problem. On one hand, all things "natural" or "old and respectable" are not necessarily safe or effective. Herbs, for example, can in their extreme be as poisonous and toxic as pharmaceuticals when both are misused and abused. On the other hand, conventional medicine tends to be very critical of its complementary counterparts. Much of the criticism centers on the "double-blind, controlled study"—anything that does not pass this ultimate test, or has not yet been subjected to it, is dismissed as uncertain and possibly dangerous. (In this kind of study half of the patients receive a real treatment, and the other half—the control group—receive a sham treatment. Neither physician nor patient is aware of who gets what.) Yet from this same perspective much or even most of conventional medicine could similarly be placed in this category. Andrew Weil, the guru of complementary medicine, notes that the Office of Technology Assessment of the United States Congress found less than one-third of conventional medical procedures have been subject to rigorous testing.[1]

We must be very careful when we ask: "Has it been proven?" The legendary Albert Einstein was once asked for his thoughts on the issue of scientific proof. He replied that the problem was a very complex one and doubted he could be of much help.

Both conventional and complementary therapies need to be evaluated with the same care and critical eye. Yet there are many challenges when it comes to the question of testing. The "double-blind, controlled study," for example, is not well suited for Chinese medicine and acupuncture. At the very least the acupuncturist will know whether he/she is using a real, or a sham point. In Chinese medicine, therapy is individualized and the treatments—whether herbs or acupuncture—are changed over time in response to changes in the patient. Treating a group of people with the same disease in exactly the same way—as Western medical studies try to do—is a foreign idea.[2]

It is also important to be aware of the broader social forces that shape health. Wong and Wu, in their *History of Chinese Medicine*, quote from the *Ancient History*, which claimed the best physicians first attend to the diseases of the nation, then look after the diseases of the citizens. This is just as true today. In the effort to change medicine toward an emphasis on prevention, we should not forget to consider the close link between these diseases of the nation and the diseases of the citizen.

In the *Record of Rites*, an ancient Confucian Classic, there is a famous passage that talks of a time when the Great Tao prevailed, and laments that it is now "disused and eclipsed." In this golden age,

"Competent provision was made for the aged until their death, work for the able-bodied, and education for the young. Kindness and compassion was shown to widows, orphans, childless people, and those disabled by disease, so that all were looked after."[3] While some today would cringe at the socialist leanings of this ancient classic, there is no denying that health is a collective, community-based issue and that the health of individuals is intimately linked to the health of communities and the environment.

The Future Role of Chinese Medicine

Chinese medicine is one of the most prominent and fastest-growing systems of complementary care. It is a comprehensive and time-tested system of healing and with growing numbers of practitioners, it is increasingly accessible to Westerners. Chinese medicine and the Eastern body of knowledge represents an ancient and evolving insight into areas that are now the subject of scientific and medical interest, including the role of diet and exercise in the treatment and prevention of disease, the interrelation of mind and body, and the bioelectromagnetic system of the body. Many of its ideas and healing techniques will play a role in the integrated health care system of the future.

Chinese medicine offers two things. First are the various therapies, such as massage, acupuncture and moxibustion, and herbal medicine. With thousands of years of experience and development, there is much of value here. They are relatively gentle and safe, and largely geared toward support of the body's natural healing systems. Some, like acupuncture, are strikingly unique.

Secondly, Chinese medicine is more than the serendipitous discovery of certain herbs or special points on the body that can empirically treat disease. Usually overlooked is the fact that Chinese medicine offers a complementary conceptual framework for understanding and treating disease—a correlative system of assessing the state of the mind-body and rationally applying therapy.

This conceptual framework has some common ground with emerging systems theory. While systems theory approaches are only now entering medicine, Chinese medicine already offers a systems-based approach to diagnosis and therapy that can be used, tested, and even combined with conventional approaches. Chinese medicine with its framework of pattern recognition provides a complementary picture of "what is wrong" that offers understanding to both patient and physician and helps to guide treatment.

An ancient Chinese character for medicine depicts five bells representing the five tones. This image suggests that the purpose of medicine is to keep the body "in tune." Disharmony is disease and harmony is health; the job of the physician is to bring the pitch of the various types of qi into accord. While Western scientific medicine focuses on the finest elements of disease, Chinese medicine attends to the rhythmic pattern of the whole.

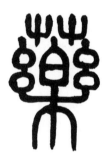

Yao: The ancient character for medicine

Western medical knowledge is based on studies involving large numbers of people. Unique individual responses are easily washed out in the statistics. Chinese medicine, in contrast, is highly individualistic: treatments are based on a personal and idiosyncratic pattern profile and are shifted during the course of therapy to reflect the changing state of the patient. Chinese medicine offers a means to observe and manipulate the "system" of the patient; Western medicine observes and treats the parts that are diseased as a group phenomenon. Even more success could arise from a combination of the two approaches.

According to Chinese medicine, the same "disease" can arise from different patterns of disharmony and furthermore, therapy should be directed at the pattern, not the disease. This insight of "one disease, many treatments" and the ability to classify patients accordingly could be one of the most useful contributions of Chinese medicine, one that has so far been almost completely overlooked.

The power of Chinese medicine can be seen in its use of herbs. The complex effects of complete plants on the human mind-body system cannot be completely reduced to that of one or several chemicals affecting one or several biochemical pathways. Plants are a not-so-easily-disentangled soup of "phyto"-chemicals, and when numerous plants are used together as they are in Chinese medicine, the complexity level becomes stunning. Effects unknown to individual plants can appear when they are used together, hinting at the complex synergy taking place in the soup. While it may be possible at some distant point in the future to fully understand such plant-human interactions from an analytical perspective, the Chinese systems approach already enables an effective use of plants and their combinations.

There is no telling exactly what the health care system of the future will look like. Yet, it would not be surprising if it contained elements of the old and the new, ancient acupuncture and herbs together with modern gene therapies and designer nutriceuticals. New therapies will also be joined by new ways of defining, understanding, and classifying disease, ways that might well contain some of the insights of Chinese systems-based pattern recognition.

The Personal Side of Health

What does all this mean for the individual with a health problem or simply with a desire to avoid disease? Most importantly is the insight of both modern medical science and ancient Chinese medicine that the power of individual action should not be underestimated. This does not mean that one's fate is completely in one's hands. Conscientious broccoli eaters and exercisers all die and some will die younger than a sibling fond of cigars and the TV remote control. Yet fate can be teased along in one's favor rather than tested, and the evidence is unequivocal as to the value of a preventive lifestyle for quality and quantity of life. Lifestyle intervention can also play an important role in the treatment and management of disease.

Both Western science and Chinese medicine offer important insights into the crucial role of nutrition, and the kinds of steps that are valuable in nurturing life through food. Exercise, if done properly, can be enriching and enjoyable. Western and Eastern styles of exercise, the hard and the soft, complement each other and both have value in a program of daily health maintenance. Eastern forms are also mind-body exercises, adding a new and increasingly popular dimension to the Western experience of life.

The increasing availability of complementary medicine has opened new avenues of exploration in the maintenance and restoration of health. Complementary approaches are most effectively used to stay healthy, and are extremely valuable in the treatment of chronic illness. Chinese herbs and acupressure massage, for example, can be used both as part of a wellness routine and in the treatment of disease. A skilled acupuncturist or Chinese herbalist can be called upon to restore health when it is lost or to fulfill the traditional role of keeping a patient from getting sick in the first place.

With complementary or conventional medicine alike, as with all things in life, a critical openness to possibilities and dangers can help to blaze a trail through the sometimes bewildering array of options and opportunity. When it comes to health and healing, balance is required between personal initiative and external intervention, as between complementary and conventional medical care. There are no hard and fast rules for achieving such a balance, but with so many options and opportunities so widely available, the prospects for health and healing have never been better.

Notes

Certain periodicals frequently cited in the notes have been identified by the following abbreviations:

Am. J. Acu.	*American Journal of Acupuncture*
BMJ	*British Medical Journal*
JHMAS	*Journal of the History of Medicine and Allied Sciences*
NEJM	*New England Journal of Medicine*
Proc. Nat. Ac. Sci. USA	*Proceedings of the National Academy of Sciences of the United States of America*
Sci. Am.	*Scientific American*

Introduction

1. Eisenberg et al., "Unconventional Medicine in the United States," *NEJM*, pp. 246–252.

2. The term "Western medicine" refers to "conventional," "mainstream," or "scientific" medicine based on the biomedical model, characterized by an analytical approach and technological intervention. This medical system is not the only approach to medicine in the West—others include homeopathy and chiropractic—but one that came to play a dominant role due to a host of political, social, and technical factors in the early part of the twentieth century. It is also no longer "Western" in that it is used extensively throughout the globe.

3. Reported on the Canadian Broadcasting Corporation (CBC) radio network, Oct. 28, 1996.

4. Schipper et al., "Shifting the Cancer Paradigm: Must We Kill to Cure?" *Journal of Clinical Oncology*, pp. 1149–1151.

5. Hall, "Herbs and the Brain," *Toronto Star*.

6. Oriental medicine, Chinese medicine, and TCM (Traditional Chinese Medicine) are used loosely and interchangeably to refer to an approach to healing that emerged in China in ancient times. This medical framework is characterized by a relational approach, therapies such as acupuncture, and a reverence for a theoretical tradition exemplified by the seminal work, *The Yellow Emperor's Classic of*

Internal Medicine. It was an elite system in a very heterogeneous medical milieu. At the same time, it was never exclusively Chinese, for other Asian peoples, such as the Koreans and Japanese, developed distinct traditions, nor was (or is) it a uniform and consistent body of theory and practice. There were strong sectarian tendencies supported by a tradition of apprenticeship and lineage.

What is today called Traditional Chinese Medicine (TCM) arose in modern communist China after a long period of decline in the "old-style" medicine in that country, resurrected within the ideology of dialectical materialism to serve, along with "Western" medicine, the health care needs of China. So modern "traditional" medicine in China is strongly influenced by both communism and science, bringing together sometimes contradictory schools of thought and purging elements incongruous with modern ideology.

Others have described a strongly Taoist "classical" Chinese medicine in terms of eight branches or categories of therapeutic intervention ranging from meditation and exercise to acupuncture and herbs. See, for example, J. Nagel, "Eight Branches of the Tao Healing Arts Before TCM," Empty Vessel, Vol. 5, No. 4, 1999, pp. 26–28.

7. Kaptchuk, "Oriental Medicine: Culture, History and Transformation." In *Introduction to Fundamentals of Chinese Medicine*, pp. xviii–xix.

8. Quoted in *Time Magazine*.

9. Krizmanic, "Medicine: Holistic in the Heartland," *Vegetarian Times*, p. 22.

10. Lau, trans., *Lao Tzu: Tao Te Ching*, p. 57.

11. Capra, *The Tao of Physics*, p. 126.

12. Anderson, "Gene Therapy," *Sci. Am.*, pp. 124–128.

13. Dossey, *Space, Time, and Medicine*, p. 7.

14. Ibid., pp. 63, 96.

15. Nicholson, personal communication.

16. Barnard, "Revolution in Diet and Medicine," *Spectrum*.

17. Ornish, quoted in *Time Magazine*.

18. Wong and Wu, *History of Chinese Medicine*, p. 54.

19. Lu, *Chinese System of Food Cures*, p. 5.

20. Steen, Letter to the Editors, *Sci. Am.*, p. 10.

21. Veith, trans., *Yellow Emperor's Classic of Internal Medicine*, p. 105.

22. Milburn, "Emerging Relationships Between the Paradigm of Oriental Medicine and the Frontiers of Western Biological Science," *Am. J. Acu.*, pp. 145–157.

23. Wiseman et al., *Fundamentals of Chinese Medicine*, p. 4.

24. Milburn, "Bioelectromagnetics: Implications for Oriental Medicine and Acupuncture," *Am. J. Acu.*, pp. 53–62.

Chapter 1

1. Quoted in Needham, *Science and Civilization in China*, Vol. 5, pre-text pages.

2. For an example of China's legacy of exploration see the brief biography of the great 16th century physician and naturalist Li Shi-zhen by Lu Gwei-djen. The reader interested in the Chinese study of natural phenomena is referred more generally to Joseph Needham's monumental works on Chinese science and civilization, *Science and Civilization in China*. Deng Ming-dao's *Chronicles of Tao*, an embellished account of a spiritual adept in China from the final days of the last dynasty (the Qing), is an entertaining presentation of the life of ascetic mountain Taoists.

3. Needham, *The Grand Titration: Science and Society in East and West*, p. 36.

4. The five phases play a prominent role in the history of Chinese medicine. For the interested reader, Matsumoto and Birch's *Five Elements and Ten Stems* offers insight into classical Chinese medical thought and the five phases, as well as their application to contemporary clinical practice. At the same time, the phases are by no means a critical facet of Chinese medicine's theoretical foundations. Indeed, TCM is commonly practiced with little practical reference to the concepts. Kaptchuk, in his *The Web That Has No Weaver*, sets out a lucid and critical discussion of the phases (pp. 343–357.) and argues for the supremacy of yin-yang theory: "The Five Phases correspondence can be helpful as a guide to clinical tendencies, but the test of veracity in Chinese medicine remains the pattern. Yin-Yang theory is more applicable in the clinic because it focuses on the idea that the totality determines relationships, correspondences, and patterns."

5. Needham, *The Grand Titration*, p. 23.

6. Chester van Huisen, personal communication.

7. Needham, *Science and Civilization in China*, Vol. 2, p. 577.

8. Ibid., pp. 68, 71.

9. Veith, trans., *The Yellow Emperor's Classic of Internal Medicine*, p. 12.

10. Quoted in *The 1994 Calendar of Chinese Medicine and Astrology*, Blue Poppy Press, Boulder, CO, 1994.

11. Kaptchuk, *The Web That Has No Weaver*, p. 52.

12. As Manfred Porkert points out in his erudite book, *The Theoretical Foundations of Chinese Medicine*, "Whereas in anatomy Western medicine, causal and analytic, primarily describes the aggregate carriers (or substrata) of effects, inductive synthetic Chinese medicine is primarily interested in the fabric of functional manifestations of the different body regions." And further, "The Chinese word *fei*,

'lungs,' for instance, calls to mind only coincidentally and vaguely most of the ideas someone with a Western education associates with the lungs." See page 107.

13. See Bennet, "Chinese Science: Theory and Practice," *Philosophy East and West*, p. 445; and Porkert, *The Theoretical Foundations of Chinese Medicine*, pp. 166–196.

14. Wiseman et al., *Fundamentals of Chinese Medicine*, p. 23.

15. Kaptchuk, *The Web That Has No Weaver*, p. 43.

16. Ibid., pp. 43, 44.

17. Ibid., p. 45.

18. Wiseman et al., op. cit., p. 66.

19. Ibid., p. 37.

20. Qiu, *Chinese Acupuncture and Moxibustion*, p. 31.

21. Ibid., p. 45.

22. Matsumoto and Birch, *Five Elements and Ten Stems*, p. 48

23. See, for example, Qiu, op. cit., pp. 393–407.

24. Needham, *Science and Civilization in China*, Vol. 2, p. 281.

25. Matsumoto and Birch, *Hara Diagnosis: Reflections on the Sea*, p. 39.

Chapter 2

1. Kaptchuk, *The Web That Has No Weaver*, p. 253.

2. That is to say he used a homophone, two different sets of Chinese characters representing Qing-zhu with each set having the same sound but a different meaning.

3. The books were likely written by Chen Shi-duo, one of Fu's students, sometime after his death. It was a common practice to attribute works to others, both as an honor to those such favored and as a means of encouraging interest in the book. *Women's Diseases According to Fu Qing-zhu* was not published officially until 1827, although copies had been in existence for some 150 years, causing some uncertainty over the author's identity. See Yang Shou-zhong and Liu Da-wei, trans., *Fu Qing-zhu's Gynecology*.

4. The other herbs in the formula are *tu si zi* (Semen Cuscutae), *shu di huang* (Radix Rehmanniae), *shan yao* (Radix Dioscoreae), *fu ling* (Sclerotium Poriae Cocos), and *jing jie* (Herba Schizonepetae). Fu Qing-zhu uses *tu si zi*, *bai shao*, and *dang gui* in highest dosages, and *fu ling*, *jing jie*, and *chai hu* in lowest dosages. Of course, formulas are used only as guides so that dosages and likely the herbs themselves would be modified to fit the patient.

5. Again, the clinical gazes of Chinese and Western medicines are not the same—they do not look for or see the same things. It is possible for Chinese medicine to see a pattern of disharmony where Western medicine gives a clean bill of health. It is also possible for the opposite to occur.

6. Menopausal symptoms are often encountered in the context of a kidney/liver yin deficiency pattern for which the formula Zhi Bai Di Huang Tang, another variation of Rehmannia Six, is often prescribed. Other common patterns include kidney yang deficiency, kidney yin and yang deficiency, and heart and spleen deficiency. The kidney is linked to reproductive processes in the correspondence system, and as part of the age-related decline of the kidneys the chong and ren vessels which link with the uterus and reproduction are no longer nourished. This accounts for the importance of the kidney in menopause-directed therapy.

7. Wiseman et al., *Fundamentals of Chinese Medicine*, p. 132.

8. The number of pulse types discussed ranges from twenty-four to thirty. Li Shi-zhen, in his *Bin Hu Mai Xue (The Pulse Studies of Bin Hu)*, discusses twenty-seven pulse states.

9. Wiseman et al., op. cit., p. 149.

10. Li, *Pulse Diagnosis*, p. 68.

11. Lu, "China's Greatest Naturalist: A Brief Biography of Li Shih-chen," *Am. J. Chin. Med.*, p. 36.

12. Wiseman et al., op. cit., p. 95.

13. Summer heat has been omitted for brevity. In addition to the six excesses there is "pestilential qi," a factor connected with contagious disease and not unlike the Western medical concept of viruses and bacteria.

14. Wiseman et al., op. cit., p. 103.

15. Traumas like snake bite, injury, and parasites are also listed as independent factors. There is also a class of miscellaneous factors that includes phlegm—a concept that embraces but has a broader meaning than the usual Western notion—and blood stagnation. See Wiseman et al.

16. There can be a general progression of disease from the exterior to the interior, formalized in the six stages of cold set out by Zhang Zhong-jing in the Han dynasty and the four stages of heat developed by Ye Tian-shi in the Qing. As the disease penetrates inwardly, patterns are generated that are partly exterior and partly interior.

17. This is an instance of yin being used to describe the nutritious fluid or substantial aspect of the body, a specific physiological characteristic.

18. There is some variation in the correspondence between the organs and regions of the tongue. The sides of the tongue correspond to the liver and

gallbladder in some systems, while others ascribe the liver to the left side and gallbladder to the right. See Maciocia, pp. 18–21.

19. Kaptchuk, *The Web That Has No Weaver*, p. 78.

20. Needham, *The Grand Titration*, p. 279; Bensky and Gamble, *Chinese Herbal Medicine: Materia Medica*, p. 6.

21. Bensky and Gamble's *Chinese Herbal Medicine: Materia Medica*, a standard English language reference, lists eighteen categories along with a number of subcategories.

22. A pattern of wind cold is an external attack by wind and cold pathogenic factors, with symptoms that would often be considered a "cold" or "flu" by Westerners. The treatment principle is to warm and relieve the surface, using herbs that induce sweating. If the wind cold pattern is not resolved with sweating, treatment may require harmonizing the ying and the *wei*, the nutritive qi and the protective qi, a special function that results from the combination of cinnamon twig and white peony root.

23. Bensky and Barolet, *Chinese Herbal Medicine: Formulas and Strategies*, p. 14.

24. See, for example, Kaptchuk, *The Web That Has No Weaver*, pp. 79, 80.

25. Qiu, *Chinese Acupuncture and Moxibustion*, p. 193.

26. Ibid., p. 260.

Chapter 3

1. For a popular description of his work by Ornish himself, see his *Dr. Dean Ornish's Program for Reversing Heart Disease*.

2. Needham, *The Grand Titration: Science and Society in East and West*, p. 245.

3. Needham discusses the Chinese contribution to the development of the mechanical clock in his *The Grand Titration*. A graph on page 278 shows the accuracy of the mechanical clock through the ages. It was not until the seventeenth century that the European clock matched the Chinese hydro-mechanical clock for accuracy. Since that time, in the form of quartz crystal and even atomic clocks, accuracy has increased by many orders of magnitude. Boorstin has a nice section on the technological and social dimensions of clock history in *The Discoverers*, with a plethora of references.

4. Boorstin, *The Discoverers*, p. 71.

5. Hooker, *Descartes*, pp. 155–157.

6. Ibid., p. 164.

7. La Mettrie, *Man a Machine*, pp. 93, 141.

8. Dobbs and Jacob, *Newton and the Culture of Newtonianism*, p. 55.

9. Ibid., p. 85.

10. Conrad et al., *The Western Medical Tradition*, p. 389.

11. See Magner, *A History of Medicine* and *A History of the Life Sciences*, for a discussion of Harvey and the iatromechanists.

12. Chinese alchemy also included an "inner" form concerned with the achievement of longevity through inner transformation using meditation and hygienic practices. This inner alchemy is still practiced today.

13. The importance of alchemy in Newton's life and work is an intriguing aspect of the history of science. See Dobbs and Jacob, *Newton and the Culture of Newtonianism*, for an introduction to and excellent discussion of Newton the alchemist.

14. Capra, *The Turning Point: Science, Society and the Rising Culture*, p. 107.

15. See Magner, *A History of Medicine*, pp. 231–239.

16. See Magner, *A History of the Life Sciences*, pp. 238–248.

17. Ibid., pp. 187–207.

18. Needham has discussed the Chinese use of inoculation against smallpox. One Chinese technique introduced smallpox via a cotton plug inserted in the nose. According to Wong and Wu's *History of Chinese Medicine* (p. 215), a mountain hermit inoculated the Emperor Chen Tsung's son sometime during the Emperor's reign from 998–1022 A.D.

19. See Conrad et al., *The Western Medical Tradition*, pp. 431–434, for a discussion of early European smallpox inoculation. Magner (*History of Medicine*, pp. 239–244) reports a death rate from inoculation at about one in 200 compared to one in six for naturally acquired smallpox, although the death rate from the pox could approach 40 percent during virulent epidemics.

20. Vaccination may have been greeted enthusiastically in China because of the long history of using inoculation there. It is also interesting that Li Shi-zhen described the use in China of a particular kind of cow-flea, ground and mixed with flour to form a pill, as a smallpox preventative. (Wong and Wu, *History of Chinese Medicine*, p. 216.)

21. See Magner, *A History of the Life Sciences*, pp. 273–295.

22. Payer, *Medicine and Culture: Varieties of Treatment in the United States, England, West Germany, and France*, pp. 67–70, 143–146.

23. Magner, *A History of Medicine*, pp. 218.

24. Magner, *A History of Medicine*, pp. 205, 263. The high mortality rate in the Vienna hospital was caused by the doctors' lack of hygiene in moving from the autopsy room to the maternity ward. This served as fertile ground for Ignaz

Philipp Semmelweis's work demonstrating the importance of medical hygiene. Unfortunately, Semmelweis was ridiculed at the time and met an untimely end in a mental hospital.

25. Wong and Wu note in their 1936 book, *History of Chinese Medicine* (p. 219), that the use of mercury as a syphilis treatment was popular in China, especially in the Ming dynasty, "but soon fell into utter disrepute on account of its unpleasant effects....And even to this day mercury is hated and detested by the general public as being the cause of unheard-of woes...." Cinnabaris, mercuric sulfide ore, is still used in Chinese herbal medicine.

26. See, for example, Magner, *A History of Medicine*, pp. 203–207.

27. Payer, op. cit., pp. 127, 128.

28. Although Chinese medicine, as with Western medicine, can be described as a historical progression of a coherent and evolving system of theory and practice, the reality is much more complex. Unschuld, in his *Medicine in China: A History of Ideas*, offers a glimpse of the complexity of medicine in China through the ages. While what is thought of as "Chinese medicine" today is credited—as is Hippocratic medicine—with throwing off the yoke of superstition and placing medicine on a rational footing, this never had the effect of reducing the popularity of "irrational" medicine.

29. Ania, *Homeopathy in Canada: A Synopsis*, pp. 4–10.

30. Conrad and Schneider, "Professionalization, Monopoly, and the Structure of Medical Practice," in Conrad and Kern, eds., *The Sociology of Health and Illness: Critical Perspectives*, p. 171; and Berliner, *Scientific Medicine Since Flexner*, pp. 30–56. Berliner notes also that the closing of many second-rate schools had the effect of limiting blacks, women, and lower class citizens access to medical education.

31. Magner, *History of Medicine*, pp. 346–347.

32. Anderson, *Gene Therapy*, pp. 124–125.

Chapter 4

1. This is a 1990 United Nations figure. The United States also ranked 24th for male and 20th for female life expectancy. Conrad and Kern, eds., *The Sociology of Health and Illness: Critical Perspectives*, p. 7.

2. Quoted in Sheldrake, *A New Science of Life*, p. 21.

3. Altieri, *Agroecology*, pp. 47–48.

4. The ecology of micro-flora and fauna in the gut is not well understood, nor is the relationship between these multifarious microbes and their human hosts. The Japanese have developed a "nutraceutical" product designed to feed beneficial nutrient-producing microbes and, since the idea was introduced by the great

Russian immunologist Élie Metchnikoff a century ago, people have been consuming live-culture yogurt in the hope of developing healthy populations of intestinal microbes. See René Dubos (*Man Adapting*, pp. 110–146) for a dated, but intriguing chapter on "The Indigenous Microbiota."

5. Aronowitz, "A Star Of Hope," *Discover*, pp. 26–28.

6. Dubos, *Mirage of Health*, Perennial Library, New York, 1959, p. 23.

7. The "medical heresy" was first discussed by biologist René Dubos and medical historian Thomas McKeown. See, for example, McKeown's papers in McLachlan and McKeown, eds., *Medical History and Medical Care*; and Dubos, *Man Adapting*, pp. 163–190. For a more recent discussion of the heresy see McKinlay and McKinlay's *Medical Measures and the Decline of Mortality*.

8. See McKinlay and McKinlay, "Medical Measures and the Decline of Mortality," in *The Sociology of Health and Illness*, p. 21.

9. Dubos, *Man Adapting*, p. 164.

10. Capra, *The Turning Point*, p. 129.

11. McKinlay and McKinlay, op. cit., p. 19.

12. Payer, *Medicine and Culture*, pp. 61–62.

13. Figure taken from Coburn et al., eds., *Health and Canadian Society: Sociological Perspectives*, p. 128.

14. McKinlay and McKinlay, op. cit., p. 19.

15. Conrad et al., eds., *The Western Medical Tradition: 800 B.C.–A.D. 1800*, p. 216.

16. Caldwell, *Prokaryotes at the Gate*, pp. 45–50.

17. Capra, *The Turning Point*, p. 133.

18. Golub, *The Limits of Medicine*, pp. 208–210.

19. Prigogine and Stengers, *Order Out of Chaos*, p. xxvii.

20. Quoted in Milburn and Oelbermann, *Electromagnetic Fields and Your Health*, p. 38, from Gould, "Nasty Little Facts," *Natural History*, February, 1985.

21. See Kuhn, *Structure of Scientific Revolutions*.

22. Dobbs and Jacob, *Newton and the Culture of Newtonianism*, pp. 24–27.

23. See Sheldrake, *Three Approaches to Biology: Part II. Vitalism*.

24. Sheldrake, *Three Approaches to Biology: Part III. Organicism*, p. 301.

25. See Capra's *The Web of Life* for an extensive and highly readable account of the history and basic ideas of systems biology.

26. Capra, *The Web of Life*, p. 158.

27. *Sci. Am.*, June 1995, p. 108.

28. Prigogine and Stengers, *Order Out of Chaos*, p. 175.

29. Lewontin et al., *Not In Our Genes*, pp. 12, 13; see also pp. 272–277.

30. Quoted in Capra, *The Web of Life*, p. 102.

31. It is interesting to note the vastly different interpretations of what the new biology says about the relationship between humans and the biosphere. Capra, for example, discusses the new biology in the context of the values of deep ecology, while Prigogine sets his own work in an almost anti-ecological framework of greater technological development and human domination of the planet. See Capra, *The Web of Life* and *The Turning Point*, and Goldsmith, "Superscience— Its Mythology and Legitimization," *The Ecologist*, 1982, pp. 228–241.

32. Capra, *The Web of Life*, p. 172.

33. See Milburn, "Emerging Relationships Between the Paradigm of Oriental Medicine and the Frontiers of Western Biological Science," *Am. J. Acu.*

34. See Sheldrake, *A New Science of Life and The Presence of the Past*.

35. Popp and Becker, *Electromagnetic Bioinformation*, p. iv.

36. See Milburn, op. cit. and "Bioelectromagnetics: Implications for Oriental Medicine and Acupuncture," *Am. J. Acu.*, for references and a summary of bioelectromagnetics research.

37. Ornish, *Dr. Dean Ornish's Program for Reversing Heart Disease*, pp. 12, 13.

38. Ibid., p. 26.

39. Quote from an electronic Reuters news article. See Bailar and Gornik, "Cancer Undefeated," *NEJM.*

40. Schipper et al., "Shifting the Cancer Paradigm," *Journal of Clinical Oncology*; and Schipper et al., "A New Biological Framework for Cancer Research," *The Lancet*.

Chapter 5

1. Needham, *The Grand Titration*, p. 320.

2. Beinfield and Korngold, *Between Heaven and Earth*, pp. 45–46.

3. Capra, *The Tao of Physics*, pp. 174–175.

4. Needham, *Science and Civilization*, Vol. 2, pp. 466–467.

5. Quoted in Capra, op. cit., p. 149.

6. Ibid., p. 291.

7. Capra, op. cit., p. 312.

8. Needham, *Science and Civilization*, Vol. 2, p. 304.

9. Ibid., p. 340.

10. Whitehead, *Adventures of Ideas*, pp. 192–193.

11. Lau, *Lao Tzu: Tao Te Ching*, pp. 102–103.

12. Translated by and quoted in Needham, *The Grand Titration*, p. 39.

13. See Needham, *Science and Civilization*, Vol. 2, p. 466. On p. 412 of the same volume, Needham footnotes a Neo-Confucian passage to illustrate this "was a world-outlook consonant with science," particularly the organic materialism of Whitehead.

14. Needham, *Science and Civilization*, Vol. 2, p. 505. Needham devotes an entire section to this fascinating relationship between Chu Hsi, Leibnitz, and organismic philosophy. He also presents a figure showing the title page of a work by Leibnitz on Chinese philosophy. See Vol. 2, pp. 496–505.

15. Kaptchuk, *The Web That Has No Weaver*, p. 53.

16. Capra, *The Web of Life*, p. 42.

17. Needham, *Time: The Refreshing River*, p. 198. Here Needham is discussing Whitehead.

See also Prigogine and Stengers, p. 287. Commenting on the study of elementary particles in physics Nobel laureate Prigogine and his colleague Stengers argue that it is difficult to talk about an elementary, isolated particle as a thing onto itself. They suggest instead a physics of processes.

18. As the father of systems thinking, Ludwig von Bertalanffy, put it: "As modern physics has dissolved matter into a set of vibrations, so modern biology is dissolving the rigid organic form into a stream of processes which produce an apparently persistent organic structure." (*Perspectives on General Systems Theory*, p. 99) Von Bertalanffy also notes that "the present understandable enthusiasm over molecular biology, therefore, should not mislead us to believe that an *organismic biology* dealing with the investigation of ordered and organized interactions in living systems, has become superfluous."

19. Manfred Porkert, in his scholarly interpretation of Chinese medicine, argues that the term orb is a useful equivalent to the Chinese term *"zang"* used to describe the yin organs. He also describes the difference in conceptual orientation of West and East: "Whereas in anatomy Western medicine, causal and analytic, primarily describes the aggregate carriers (or substrata) of effects, inductive synthetic Chinese medicine is primarily interested in the fabric of functional manifestations of the different body regions." See Manfred Porkert, *The Theoretical Foundations of Chinese Medicine*, p. 107.

20. Veith, trans., *The Yellow Emperor's Classic of Internal Medicine*, p. 139.

21. The "energetic" relationship between paired organs is used in diagnosis and therapy. There is a pattern, for example, of heart fire affecting the small intestine via the meridians. This is a damp heat pattern with heat in the heart and frequent, dark-colored urination conceptualized in terms of the heart-small intestine relationship. The connection between the lung and large intestine is used in the treatment of the common cold. Large intestine point 4, *he gu*, and large intestine point 11, *qu chi*, are used to treat the lung and reduce fever. The rationale for this choice is the hand yang ming meridian's (large intestine) "external-internal" relationship with hand tai yin (lung).

22. Chang, trans., *Knocking at the Gate of Life*, p. 42.

23. Matsumoto and Birch, *Hara Diagnosis*, p. 41.

24. Wiseman et al., *Fundamentals of Chinese Medicine*, pp. 88, 89; and Kaptchuk, *The Web That Has No Weaver*, p. 336.

25. See Beinfield and Korngold's book, *Between Heaven and Earth: A Guide to Chinese Medicine*, for a rich example of how far one can take the relationships between mind and body in Chinese medicine. They insightfully meld Western psychology with Chinese associative thinking and "energetic" understanding.

26. Matsumoto and Birch, op. cit., p. 86.

27. Swerdlow, *Quiet Miracles of the Brain*, p. 26.

28. Ibid., p. 26.

29. See Perry et al., "Bootstrapping in Ecosystems," *Bioscience*.

30. Temple, *The Genius of China*, pp. 62–64. Needham pointed out that the south-pointing carriage was not a completely cybernetic machine. It still required a driver as part of the feedback loop.

31. The Chinese did not search for rigorous "laws" of nature as did Western science and so the five-phase system in Chinese medicine should be seen as a flexible system, useful at times and not at others. Of course, it was sometimes applied perhaps over-enthusiastically and became a procrustean bed to which phenomena were made to fit. Nonetheless, the five-phase cycles are perhaps the first example of a self-regulating system with positive and negative feedback. See Kaptchuk, *The Web That Has No Weaver*, pp. 343–354, for an excellent discussion of the history and use of the five phases.

In their study of the five phases, Matsumoto and Birch point out that the five-phase system when applied to human biology was still an "open" system, in the sense that other "energies" were needed for completeness. Comparing the five phases to the eight trigrams, they note that: "Thus, the Five Elements system itself was not seen as all-inclusive. For the body to have a harmony of Yin and Yang the three energies represented by the three missing Trigrams need to be brought into the body." (Matsumoto and Birch, *Five Elements and Ten Stems*, p. 23)

Five-phase relationships are used in acupuncture with reference to the five shu points on the meridians. The five shu points are five points on each of the twelve meridians found below the knee and elbow given water-based (well, spring, stream, river, and sea) and five-phase correspondences. For example, in tonifying earth to strengthen metal as part of a lung treatment the point lung 9 could be used since it is the stream or earth point of lung. See Qiu, *Chinese Acupuncture and Moxibustion*, pp. 263–264.

32. Anderson, "Gene Therapy," *Sci. Am.*, p. 124.

33. Story in the *Kitchener-Waterloo Record*, Saturday, November 22, 1997.

34. Kawachi, Kennedy, and Lochner, *Long Live Community*, pp. 56–59.

35. Willett, Colditz, and Mueller, *Strategies for Minimizing Cancer Risk*, p. 95.

36. *The Toronto Star*, Friday, October 31, 1997.

37. Campbell, *Nutrients vs. Foods*, pp. 119–152.

38. Dubos, *Man Adapting*, p. 333.

39. Based on Capra, *The Web of Life*, pp. 157–159.

40. Needham, *Science and Civilization*, Vol. 2, pp. 52, 288, 289.

41. Needham, *Within the Four Seas*, p. 68, and *Science and Civilization*, Vol. 2, pp. 472–475.

42. Kaptchuk, *The Web That Has No Weaver*, p. 180.

43. Lin, *Handbook of TCM Urology*, pp. 117–135.

44. Kaptchuk, op. cit., pp. 323–324. See Kaptchuk's discussion on p. 321 regarding the relationship between Western diseases and Chinese patterns of disharmony.

One area of research in China is the integration of Chinese and Western medicine, and in this light Chinese physicians are studying the relationship between classical TCM patterns of disharmony and Western medical findings. For example, a 1995 paper in the Chinese Journal of Integrated Traditional and Western Medicine looked at patterns of deficiency-cold and deficiency-heat (yang and yin deficiency, respectively) and their relationship to plasma cortisol and its receptor. Cortisol is an important hormone produced by the adrenal gland and involved in carbohydrate metabolism. Researchers at Beijing Medical University found that Western medical measurements of cortisol and receptor strongly correlated with these Chinese patterns, in one case being elevated and in the other lowered from normal levels. (Z.F. Xie and G.Y. Zhang, "Effects of Plasma Cortisol and Its Receptor on Patients with Deficiency-Cold and Deficiency-Heat Syndromes," CJIM, 1995: 1(1), pp. 6–8.)

45. Bernard, *Phenomena of Life Common to Animals and Vegetables*, pp. 29, 48.

46. Von Bertalanffy, *Perspectives on General Systems Theory*, pp. 41, 45.

47. Li, *Electromagnetic Bioinformation*, p. iv.

48. Wiseman et al., *Fundamentals of Chinese Medicine*, p. ii.

49. Lu and Needham (*Celestial Lancets*, p. 8) point out that Chinese medical science was not completely without the use of measurement. Pulse rate is routinely measured in terms of respiration rate, and the length of the channels and bones and even the size and weight of organs were recorded by ancient physicians. Today, there is a trend toward a more analytical approach to traditional diagnostic techniques like the pulse and tongue, using mechanical and electronic technologies including the computer.

50. Quoted in Porter, *Cybernetics Simplified*, p. 34.

51. Prigogine and Stengers, *Order Out of Chaos*, p. 36.

52. Lu and Needham, *Celestial Lancets*, p. xx.

Chapter 6

1. Dubos, *Man Adapting*, p. 357.

2. McKeown, "A Basis for Health Strategies," *BMJ*, p. 595.

3. For an excellent account of traditional ecological wisdom, see P. Knudtson and D. Suzuki, *Wisdom of the Elders*, Stoddart, Toronto, 1992.

4. K. Arms and P.S. Camp, *Biology*, Holt, Rinehart and Winston, New York, 1979, p. 919.

5. McKeown, *BMJ*, p. 595.

6. Temple and Burkitt, eds., *Western Diseases: Their Dietary Prevention and Reversibility*, p. 11.

7. Quote from an interview published in *Spectrum*, #24 May/June 1992.

8. "Gaining on Fat," *Sci. Am.*, August 1996, p. 91.

9. Ibid., pp. 88–94.

10. Temple and Burkitt, op. cit., pp. 79–82.

11. Willett et al., *Sci. Am.*, p. 88.

12. Bailar and Gornick, "Cancer Undefeated," *NEJM*, pp. 1569–1574.

13. See Trichopoulos et al., "What Causes Cancer?" *Sci. Am.*, and Ames et al., "The Causes and Prevention of Cancer," *Proc. Nat. Ac. Sci. USA*.

14. Willet et al., "Strategies for Minimizing Cancer Risk," *Sci. Am.*, p. 90.

15. *Food Choices for Health*, Educational Material from the Physicians Committee for Responsible Medicine, Washington, D.C.

16. O'Dea, "The Therapeutic and Preventive Potential of the Hunter-Gatherer Lifestyle: Insights from Australian Aborigines," in Temple and Burkitt, eds., *Western Diseases*, pp. 349–380.

17. See Ornish, *Dr. Dean Ornish's Program for Reversing Heart Disease*, pp. 133–349.

18. Steingraber, *Living Downstream*, p. 188.

19. See Milburn and Oelbermann, *Electromagnetic Fields and Your Health*.

20. See Colborn et al., *Our Stolen Future*, for a lucid look at the present knowledge and threat of endocrine disrupting chemicals.

21. Veith, trans., *The Yellow Emperor's Classic of Internal Medicine*, p. 105.

22. While the methods of the scientist resonate with the Taoist interest in the natural world, the aims of the scientist have more in common with the Confucianist—both striving for heaven on earth through social transformation, the Confucianist through moral and ethical perfection, the scientist through technological progress.

23. Quoted in Needham, *Science and Civilization*, Vol. 5, p. 123.

24. Needham, op. cit., p. 137.

25. Ibid., p. 124.

26. Ibid., p. 47.

27. Porkert, *Chinese Medicine*, pp. 254–255.

28. Needham and Lu, "Hygiene and Preventive Medicine in Ancient China," *JHMAS*, p. 434.

29. Ibid., p. 433.

30. Ibid., p. 434.

31. Veith, op. cit., p. 220.

32. Needham and Lu, op. cit., pp. 460–461.

33. Ibid., p. 445.

34. Ibid., p. 445.

35. Ancient Chinese text quoted in Needham, *Science and Civilization*, Vol. 5, pp. 145–146; modern quote from Kitson, trans., *Sun-do: Taoist Secret Breathing Method*, p. viii.

36. Chang, trans., *Knocking at the Gate of Life*, p. 45.

37. Adapted from Needham, *Science and Civilization*, Vol. 5, pp. 158–159.

38. Needham, op. cit., p. 161.

39. Cheng and Smith, *T'ai-Chi: The "Supreme Ultimate" Exercise for Health, Sport, and Self-Defense*, p. 111.

40. Quoted in Needham, op. cit., p. 173.

41. See Bensky and Gamble, *Chinese Herbal Medicine: Materia Medica*, p. 5.

42. H.P. Yoke, B. Lim, and F. Morsingh, "Elixir Plants," in Nakayama and Sivin, eds., *Chinese Science*, p. 190.

43. Needham, op. cit., p. 209.

44. Ibid., p. 189.

45. Needham and Lu, op. cit., p. 448.

46. Quoted in an interview in *Spectrum*, Vol. 24, May/June 1992.

47. J. Brody, *The New York Times*, April 14, 1998.

48. Steen, letter to the editors, *Sci. Am.*, May 1994, p. 10.

49. Willett et al., "Strategies for Minimizing Cancer Risk," *Sci. Am.*, p. 89.

50. Quoted in sidebar, Greenwald, "Chemoprevention of Cancer," *Sci. Am.*, p. 99.

51. Coleman, *The New Organic Grower*, p. 169.

52. Wilson, *Biodiversity*, National Academy Press, Washington, 1988, p. 291.

53. There are many other agricultural and dietary changes that could dramatically enhance human and ecological health. The meat-centered diet of affluence, for example, is increasingly under fire for its deleterious effects, and shifting the diet so that meat is placed on the periphery, rather than in the center, of the meal would have far-reaching ecological and human health implications.

Chapter 7

1. J.E. Brody, "Alternative Medicine Makes Inroads," *The New York Times*, April 28, 1998.

2. Van Peursen, *Body, Soul, Spirit: A Survey of the Body-Mind Problem*, p. 8

3. Vesey, ed., *Body and Mind: Readings in Philosophy*, p. 47. See also in the same text (pp. 48–53), Descartes' correspondence with Princess Elizabeth, where she calls on him to explain his efforts at distinguishing mind from body while pointing to their unity. Princess Elizabeth remained unconvinced of his solution to the problem.

4. Capra, *The Web of Life*, p. 66.

5. Vendler, *The Mind-Body Problem*, p. 318.

6. Quoted in Capra, op. cit., p. 283.

7. Blakeslee, "Complex and Hidden Brain in Gut Makes Bellyaches and Butterflies," *The New York Times*.

8. Josephson, "The Elusivity of Nature and the Mind-Matter Problem," *The Interrelationship Between Mind and Matter*, p. 221.

9. Stapp, "A Quantum Theory of Consciousness," *The Interrelationship Between Mind and Matter*, p. 207. See also Fred Alan Wolf's book *Star Wave: Mind, Consciousness, and Quantum Physics* (Macmillan, New York, 1984) as another example of a physicist exploring the nature of mind and consciousness through quantum physics.

10. This description of a systems approach to mind is based on Capra's account in his book *The Web of Life* (see *The Web of Life*, chapters 10 and 11).

11. Capra, *The Web of Life*, p. 290

12. A. J. Husband, ed., *Psychoimmunology: CNS-Immune Interactions*, CRC Press, Boca Raton, 1993, quote from preface—no page given.

13. Dossey, *Space, Time and Medicine*, pp. 61–62.

14. Kabat-Zinn, *Full Catastrophe Living*, p. 212.

15. Pelletier, *Mind as Healer, Mind as Slayer*, p. 7.

16. Ibid., pp. 12, 13.

17. Kabat-Zinn, op. cit., p. 236.

18. Dossey, *The Interrelationship Between Mind and Matter*, p. 150.

19. Kabat-Zinn, op. cit., p. 198.

20. See Graham, *Philosophy of Mind*, pp. 142–152, for a discussion of the mind-body implications of Schumann's life and death.

21. Schedlowski et al., "The Effects of Psychological Intervention on Cortisol Levels and Leucocyte Numbers in the Peripheral Blood of Breast Cancer Patients," in *The Psychoimmunology of Cancer*, pp. 336–348.

22. Fawzy et al., "Short-term Psychiatric Intervention for Patients with Malignant Melanoma: Effects on Psychological State, Coping, and the Immune System," in *The Psychoimmunology of Cancer*, pp. 291–319.

23. See Pelletier's book, *Mind as Healer, Mind as Slayer*, for a detailed description of autogenic training.

24. Kabat-Zinn describes the use of meditation as a therapeutic tool in his book *Full Catastrophe Living*.

25. Quoted in Needham, *Science and Civilization in China*, Vol. 2, p. 153.

26. Porkert and Ullman, *Chinese Medicine*, pp. 245–249.

27. Matsumoto and Birch, *Hara Diagnosis*, pp. 36,37.

28. Ibid., p. 36.

29. Ishida, *Taoist Meditation and Longevity Techniques*, p. 45. This discussion is based on Ishida's presentation of the Oriental understanding of the mind-body relationship.

30. Kaptchuk, *The Web That Has No Weaver*, p. 43.

31. Larre and Rochat de la Vallée, *Rooted in Spirit: The Heart of Chinese Medicine*, p. 172.

32. Kaptchuk, op. cit., p. 45.

33. Needham, *Science and Civilization in China*, Vol. 5, pp. 133–134.

34. Ishida, op. cit., p. 53.

35. See Matsumoto and Birch, op. cit., p. 37; and Ishida, op. cit., pp. 52–54.

36. Matsumoto and Birch, op. cit., p. 37.

37. Ishida, op. cit., pp. 53, 55.

38. Ibid., p. 60.

39. Ibid., p. 57.

40. Ibid., p. 57.

41. Ibid., p. 61.

42. Chia, *Taoist Ways to Transform Stress into Vitality*, p. 73.

43. Ishida, op. cit., p. 62.

44. Needham and Lu, "Hygiene and Preventive Medicine in Ancient China," *JHMAS*, p. 445.

45. Wong and Wu, *History of Chinese Medicine*, pp. 72–73.

46. Qiu, ed., *Chinese Acupuncture and Moxibustion*, pp. 292–293.

47. Porkert and Ullman, *Chinese Medicine*, p. 249.

48. *Houghton Mifflin Canadian Dictionary of the English Language*, p. 1247.

49. Matsumoto and Birch, *Hara Diagnosis*, p. 11.

50. Beinfield and Korngold, *Between Heaven and Earth*, p. 131.

51. Requena, *Character and Health*, pp. 130, 182.

52. Cheng and Smith, *T'ai-Chi*, pp. 110, 111.

53. Chia and Chia, *Chi Nei Tsang: Internal Organs Massage*, p. 181.

Chapter 8

1. There is a Western tradition of insight into the influence of diet and lifestyle on health. Some 2,500 years ago Hippocrates claimed that: "Whoever gives these things (food) no consideration, and is ignorant of them, how can he understand the diseases of man?" For the most part these insights have been lost and ignored. Except for gross nutrient deficiencies, Western medicine has ignored the connection between diet and disease, a view demonstrated by the almost complete absence of nutritional training in Western medical schools.

2. Beinfield and Korngold, *Between Heaven and Earth*, p. 324.

3. Needham, J., *Science and Civilization*, Vol. 5, p. 46.

4. Ibid., pp. 136, 137.

5. Lu, *Chinese Foods for Longevity*, pp. 32–33.

6. Lu, *Chinese System of Food Cures*, p. 5.

7. Ni, *The Tao of Nutrition*, pp. 23–24.

8. Veith, trans., *The Yellow Emperor's Classic*, p. 109.

9. Wiseman et al., *Fundamentals of Chinese Medicine*, pp. 76–79.

10. Information on foods adapted from Henry Lu's *Chinese System of Food Cures* and Maoshing Ni's *The Tao of Nutrition*.

11. Lu, *Chinese Foods for Longevity*, p. 32.

12. Shurtleff and Aoyagi, *The Book of Tofu*, p. 62.

13. Ornish, *Dr. Dean Ornish's Program for Reversing Heart Disease*, p. 2.

14. Temple and Burkitt, *Western Diseases: Their Dietary Prevention and Reversibility*, pp. 15–25.

15. Ibid., p. 68.

16. Ibid., pp. 1–13.

17. Trowell and Burkitt, *Western Diseases: Their Emergence and Prevention*, p. 19; and Temple and Burkitt, op. cit., p. 248.

18. Temple and Burkitt, op. cit., p. 248.

19. Trowell and Burkitt, op. cit., pp. 431–432.

20. Ibid., p.275.

21. Ibid., p. 338.

22. Ornish, *Eat More, Weigh Less*, p. 53.

23. Thorogood et al., "Risk of Death from Cancer and Ischaemic Heart Disease in Meat and Non-meat eaters," *BMJ*, p. 1671.

24. Temple and Burkitt, op. cit., pp. 285, 292, 293.

25. Ornish, *Dr. Dean Ornish's Program for Reversing Heart Disease*, pp. 11–13.

26. Temple and Burkitt, op. cit., p. 296. An interesting side effect of the dietary change was noted by researchers: the healthy diet was also the least expensive.

27. Mindell, *Earl Mindell's Soy Miracle*, p. 40, 41.

28. Ornish, *Dr. Dean Ornish's Program for Reversing Heart Disease*, pp. 12–13.

29. Campbell, "The Dietary Causes of Degenerative Diseases," in *Western Diseases: Their Emergence and Prevention*, p. 69. In a description of his monumental China study, Campbell appeals to the need for synthesis and a broader view. As he puts it, "common causes cannot be fully understood by limiting investigations to the generalization of details of specific cause-effect relationships, a process that invites too much error, as has happened in this field too often in the past. Synthesis of detailed information into a larger picture is required."

30. *The New Four Food Groups For Optimal Nutrition*, PCRM, Washington, D.C. The PCRM works to debunk many of the nutritional myths that still linger. Protein, for example, immediately comes to many minds when the idea of a plant-based diet is considered. Yet it is actually difficult to get too little protein and most people eating a Western-type diet get more than enough. Iron is plentiful in a vegetarian diet and the excess of iron in a high-meat diet may actually be harmful. Calcium is plentiful in plant foods such as kale and sesame seeds, and evidence suggests that one factor responsible for calcium problems—like osteoporosis—is an excess of protein which increases calcium loss, rather than a deficiency of the nutrient in the diet. The World Health Organization RDA for calcium is about half that of Canada and the United States which are deliberately set high to compensate for the loss of calcium in high-protein diets. Ironically, eating less meat and dairy products might help prevent the calcium problems epidemic in wealthy nations.

31. The Ayurvedic tradition also uses a diet-according-to-constitution approach. For further exploration of the Chinese nutrition system of diet-according-to-constitution see Beinfield and Korngold's *Between Heaven and Earth* and Henry Lu's *Chinese System of Food Cures*.

Chapter 9

1. Beinfield and Korngold, *Between Heaven and Earth: A Guide to Chinese Medicine*, p. 30.

2. Qi is pronounced *chee*, and sometimes spelled chi.

3. See Needham, *Science and Civilization in China*, Vol. 2, pp. 455–505, and Mitukuni, "The Chinese Concept of Nature," in *Chinese Science*, Nakayama and Sivin, eds., pp. 76–89.

4. Unschuld, *Medicine in China*, p. 72.

5. Porkert, *The Theoretical Foundations of Chinese Medicine*, pp. 166–176.

6. Kaptchuk, *The Web That Has No Weaver*, p. 37.

7. Matsumoto and Birch, *Hara Diagnosis*, pp. 41, 42.

8. This is part of a passage from the Nan Jing, the *Classic of Difficulties*, a text that discusses unresolved issues found in the Huang Di Nei Jing. Matsumoto and Birch, *Hara Diagnosis*, p. 12.

9. Matsumoto and Birch, *Hara Diagnosis*, p. 12.

10. Wiseman et al., *Fundamentals of Chinese Medicine*, p. 24.

11. Ibid., p. 38.

12. For a discussion of the connection between organs and channels via the internal trajectories of the channels see Matsumoto and Birch, *Hara Diagnosis*, pp. 49–50.

13. See, for example, Unschuld, *Medicine in China*, pp. 81–82.

14. For a review of acupuncture research see G. Stux and B. Pomeranz, *Basics of Acupuncture*, Springer, Berlin, 1995, and S. Birch and R. Felt, *Understanding Acupuncture*, Churchill Livingstone, Edinburgh, 1999.

15. There are also electrical correspondences to the channels, but the channels do not correspond to either the nervous, lymphatic, or vascular systems. French researchers have demonstrated—using an injected radioactive tracer—pathways with a high degree of correspondence to the classically described channels. They found that the migration of the tracer did not follow the lymphatic or vascular system, and that patients with a specific organ problem showed a deviation from normal in the migration profile of the tracer. See "Etude des méridiens d'acupuncture par les traceurs radioactifs," *Bull. Acad. Natl. Med.*, 1985, 169, no. 7, pp. 1071–1075.

16. Porkert, *Theoretical Foundations*, pp. 197–198.

17. See, for example, Unschuld, *Medicine in China*, pp. 95–96.

18. Kaptchuk, op. cit., p. 108.

19. Matsumoto and Birch, op. cit., p. 50.

20. Needham, *Science and Civilization in China*, Vol. 5, p. 148. Needham also wonders "To what extent the later Taoist adepts pictured their qi as circulating along the tracts of the acupuncture physicians?" This question could really be inverted to ask to what extent were the acupuncture physicians concepts of the channels based on the discoveries of earlier Taoist adepts? It does seem clear from the technical details of Taoist practices described by contemporary masters that the routes of qi circulation and energy centers of inner alchemy correspond with those of the acupuncture

system. See, for example, the various publications of Mantak Chia, a contemporary Taoist master.

21. This section follows Milburn, "Emerging Relationships Between the Paradigm of Oriental Medicine and the Frontiers of Western Biological Science," and "Bioelectromagnetics: Implications for Oriental Medicine and Acupuncture," *Am. J. of Acu.*

22. Nordenström, *Frontier Perspectives*, p. 17.

23. See Becker and Selden, *The Body Electric*, for a popular account of Becker's decades of fascinating research.

24. Personal communication, 1992.

25. See Adey in *Physiological Reviews, Interaction of Electromagnetic Waves with Biological Systems*, and *ELF Electromagnetic Fields: The Question of Cancer*.

26. Del Giudice, *Frontier Perspectives*, pp. 20–21.

27. Fröhlich, ed., *Biological Coherence and Response to External Stimuli*, pp. 12–17.

28. Fröhlich, "Coherent Electric Vibrations in Biological Systems and the Cancer Problem," *IEEE Transactions on Microwave Theory and Techniques.*

29. Popp, "Biophotons and Their Regulatory Role in Cells," *Frontier Perspectives*, pp. 13–22.

30. Editorial, *Sci. Am.*, Jan., 1998, p. 6.

31. Capra, *The Tao of Physics*, pp. 236–237.

32. Ibid., p. 236.

33. Chia, *Taoist Ways To Transform Stress into Vitality*, p. 67.

34. Fröhlich, ed., *Biological Coherence and Response to External Stimuli*, p. 19.

35. Matsumoto and Birch, *Hara Diagnosis*, pp. 174–188.

36. Chia, *Taoist Ways to Transform Stress into Vitality*, p. 67.

37. Matsumoto and Birch, op. cit., p. 94.

38. Porkert, *Theoretical Foundations of Chinese Medicine*, p. 176.

39. Ingber, "The Architecture of Life," *Sci. Am.*, p. 56.

40. See Ingber, op. cit., pp. 48–57.

Epilogue

1. Lemley, "Why So Many Doctors Hate Andrew Weil," *Discover*, p. 59.

2. There are also many questions about the double-blind controlled study itself. This study design tries to separate the true effect of the treatment from a still mysterious

"placebo effect"—which is the name given to the improvement seen in many patients who are given the imitation therapy. The placebo effect is considered to be psychosomatic—the patients think they will get better, and their bodies follow. Some critics charge that complementary medicines are nothing more than placebos—expensive sugar-coated shams. Others, like Harvard's Herbert Benson, feel that we need to understand the placebo effect so that it can be used to enhance the practice of medicine. Still others claim that patients given imitation treatments get better for reasons other than the placebo effect and are very critical of the design of double-blind controlled trials. See Kienle and Kiene, "The Powerful Placebo Effect: Fact or Fiction?" *Clinical Epidemiology*, pp. 1311–1318.

3. Needham, *Science and Civilization in China*, Vol. 2, pp. 167–168.

Bibliography

Adey, W.R., "Biological Effects of Radio Frequency Electromagnetic Radiation," in *Interaction of Electromagnetic Waves with Biological Systems*, J.C. Li, ed., Plenum Press, New York, 1988, pp. 1–32.

————, "Electromagnetic Fields: Cell Membrane Amplification and Cancer Promotion," in *ELF Electromagnetic Fields: The Question of Cancer*, B.W. Wilson., R.G. Stevens, and L.E. Anderson, eds., Battelle Press, 1989.

————, "Tissue Interactions with Non-ionizing Electromagnetic Fields," *Physiological Reviews*, 1981, 61(2), pp. 435–411.

————, "Whispering Between Cells: Electromagnetic Fields and Regulatory Mechanisms in Tissue," *Frontier Perspectives*, Vol. 3, No. 2, 1993.

Altieri, M.A., *Agroecology: The Scientific Basis of Alternative Agriculture*, Westview Press, Boulder, 1987.

Ames, B.N., L.S. Gold, and W.C. Willett, "The Causes and Prevention of Cancer," *Proc. Nat. Acad. Sci. USA*, Vol. 92, June 1995, pp. 5258–5265.

Anderson, W.F., "Gene Therapy," in *Sci. Am.*, September, 1995, pp. 124–128.

Ania, F., "Homeopathy in Canada: A Synopsis," *Health and Homeopathy*, Vol. 1, No. 1, Fall 1995, pp. 4–10.

Aronowitz, P., "A Star of Hope," *Discover*, August 1994, pp. 24–26.

Ayala, F.J., "Biological Reductionism," in *Self-Organizing Systems: The Emergence of Order*, F.E. Yates, ed., Plenum, New York, 1987.

Bailar, J.C., and H.L. Gornik, "Cancer Undefeated," *NEJM*, Vol. 336, No. 22, 1997, pp. 1569–1574.

Barnard, N., "Revolution in Diet and Medicine," *Spectrum*, No. 24, May, 1992.

Becker, R.O., and G. Selden, *The Body Electric*, William Morrow, New York, 1985.

Beinfield, H., and E. Korngold, *Between Heaven and Earth: A Guide to Chinese Medicine*, Ballantine Books, New York, 1991.

Bennett, S., "Chinese Science: Theory and Practice," *Philosophy East and West*, Vol. 28, No. 4, 1978, pp. 439–453.

Bensky, D., and R. Barolet, *Chinese Herbal Medicine: Formulas and Strategies*, Eastland Press, Seattle, 1990.

————, and A. Gamble, *Chinese Herbal Medicine: Materia Medica*, Eastland Press, Seattle, 1986.

Berliner, H.S., "Scientific Medicine Since Flexner," in *Alternative Medicine*, J.W. Salmon, ed., Tavistock Publications, New York, 1984, pp. 30–56.

Bernard, C., *Phenomena of Life Common to Animals and Vegetables*, R.P. and M.A. Cook, Dundee, 1974.

Birch, S. and R. Felt, *Understanding Acupuncture*, Churchill Livingstone, Edinburgh, 1999.

Blakeslee, S., "Complex and Hidden Brain in Gut Makes Bellyaches and Butterflies," *The New York Times*, January 23, 1996.

Boorstin, D.J., *The Discoverers: A History of Man's Search to Know His World and Himself*, Random House, New York, 1983.

Caldwell, M., "Prokaryotes at the Gate," *Discover*, August 1994, pp. 45–50.

Campbell, T.C., "The Dietary Causes of Degenerative Diseases," in *Western Diseases: Their Dietary Prevention and Reversibility*, N.J. Temple and D.P. Burkitt, eds., Humana Press, Totowa, 1994, pp. 119–152.

Capra, F., *The Tao of Physics*, Fontana, London, 1983.

———, *The Turning Point: Science, Society and the Rising Culture*, Bantam, New York, 1982.

———, *The Web of Life: A New Scientific Understanding of Living Systems*, Doubleday, New York, 1996.

Chang, E.C., trans., *Knocking at the Gate of Life*, Rodale Press, Emmaus, 1985.

Checkland, P., *Systems Thinking, Systems Practice*, John Wiley & Sons, Chichester, 1981.

Cheng, Man-ching, and R.W. Smith, *T'ai-Chi: The "Supreme Ultimate" Exercise for Health, Sport, and Self-Defense*, Charles E. Tuttle, Rutland, 1967.

Chia, M., *Taoist Ways to Transform Stress into Vitality*, Healing Tao Books, Huntington, 1985.

———, and M. Chia, *Cultivating Female Sexual Energy*, Healing Tao Books, Huntington, 1990.

———, *Chi Nei Tsang: Internal Organs Massage*, Healing Tao Books, Huntington, 1990.

Coburn, D., et al., eds., *Health and Canadian Society: Sociological Perspectives*, Fitzhenry and Whiteside, Markam, 1987.

Colborn, T., D. Dumanoski, and J.P. Myers, *Our Stolen Future*, Penguin, New York, 1996.

Coleman, E., *The New Organic Grower*, Chelsea Green, Chelsea, 1989.

Conrad, L.I., et al., *The Western Medical Tradition: 800 B.C. to A.D. 1800*, Cambridge University Press, Cambridge, 1995.

Conrad, P., and R. Kern, eds., *The Sociology of Health and Illness: Critical Perspectives*, St. Martin's Press, New York, 1994.

Del Giudice, E., "Coherence in Condensed and Living Matter," *Frontier Perspectives*, Vol. 3, No. 2, 1993, pp. 16–20.

Dobbs, B.J.T., and M.C. Jacob, *Newton and the Culture of Newtonianism*, Humanities Press, New Jersey, 1995.

Dossey, L., *Space, Time, and Medicine*, Shambhala, Boulder, 1982.

————, "Modern Medicine and the Relationship Between Mind and Matter," in *The Interrelationship Between Mind and Matter*, B. Rubik, ed., Temple University, Philadelphia, 1989, pp. 149–168.

Dubos, R., *Man Adapting*, Yale University Press, New Haven, 1965.

Eisenberg, D.M., et al., "Unconventional Medicine in the United States," *NEJM*, Vol. 328, No. 4, 1993, pp. 246–252.

Ellis, A., N. Wiseman, and K. Boss, *Grasping the Wind*, Paradigm, Brookline, 1989.

Fawzy, F.I., et al., "Short-term Psychiatric Intervention for Patients with Malignant Melanoma: Effects on Psychological State, Coping, and the Immune System," in *The Psychoimmunology of Cancer: Mind and Body in the Fight for Survival*, C.E. Lewis, et al., eds., Oxford University Press, Oxford, 1994, pp. 291–319.

Fröhlich, H., ed., *Biological Coherence and Response to External Stimuli*, Springer, Berlin, 1988.

Fröhlich, H., "Coherent Electric Vibrations in Biological Systems and the Cancer Problem," *Institute of Electrical and Electronic Engineers Transactions on Microwave Theory and Techniques*, 1978, Vol. 26, pp. 613–617.

Gibbs, W.W., "Gaining on Fat," *Sci. Am.*, August, 1996.

Golub, E.S., *The Limits of Medicine: How Science Shapes Our Hope for the Cure*, Random House, New York, 1994.

Gopalan, C., "Dietetics and Nutrition: Impact of Scientific Advances and Development," *J. Am. Diet. Assoc.*, Vol. 97, 1997, pp. 737–741.

Graham, G., *Philosophy of Mind*, Blackwell, Oxford, 1993.

Greenwald, P., "Chemoprevention of Cancer," *Sci. Am.*, September, 1996, pp. 96–99.

Hall, J., "Herbs and the Brain," *Toronto Star*, Nov. 1, 1996.

Hammer, L., *Dragon Rises, Red Bird Flies*, Station Hill Press, Barrytown, 1990.

Heisenberg, W., *Physics and Beyond*, Harper and Row, New York, 1971.

Hooker, M., *Descartes: Critical and Interpretive Essays*, Johns Hopkins University Press, Baltimore, 1978.

Ingber, D.E., "The Architecture of Life," *Sci. Am.*, January, 1998, pp. 48–57.

Ishida, H., "Body and Mind: The Chinese Perspective," in *Taoist Meditation and Longevity Techniques*, L. Kohn, ed., University of Michigan Press, Ann Arbor, 1989, pp. 41–71.

Josephson, B.D., "The Elusivity of Nature and the Mind-Matter Problem," in *The Interrelationship Between Mind and Matter*, B. Rubik, ed., Temple University, Philadelphia, 1989, pp. 219–222.

Kabat-Zinn, J., *Full Catastrophe Living*, Bantam, New York, 1990.

Kaptchuk, T.J., *The Web that Has No Weaver*, Congdon and Weed, New York, 1983.

————, "Oriental Medicine: Culture, History and Transformation," in *Introduction to Fundamentals of Chinese Medicine*, by N. Wiseman, A. Ellis, and P. Zmiewski, Paradigm, Brookline, 1985, pp. xvii–xxxvii.

Kawachi, I., B.P. Kennedy, and K. Lochner, "Long Live Community: Social Capital as Public Health," *American Prospect*, Nov., 1997, pp. 56–59.

Kienle, G. and H. Kiene, "The Powerful Placebo Effect: Fact or Fiction?" *Clinical Epidemiology*, Vol. 50, No. 12, 1997, pp. 1311–1318.

Kitson, A., trans., *Sun-do: Taoist Secret Breathing Method*, Won Dang Ahm, Vancouver, 1987.

Krizmanic, J., "Medicine: Holistic in the Heartland," *Vegetarian Times*, November, 1994, p. 22.

Kuhn, T.S., *The Structure of Scientific Revolutions*, University of Chicago Press, Chicago, 1970.

La Mettrie, *Man a Machine*, Open Court, La Salle, 1912.

Larre, C., and E. Rochat de la Vallée, *Rooted in Spirit: The Heart of Chinese Medicine*, Station Hill Press, Barrytown, 1995.

Laszlo, E., *The Systems View of the World*, Hampton Press, Cresskill, 1996.

Lau, D.C., trans., *Lao Tzu: Tao Te Ching*, Penguin, Middlesex, 1981.

Legge, J., trans., *I Ching*, Bantam Books, Toronto, 1964.

Lemley, B., "Why So Many Doctors Hate Andrew Weil," *Discover*, August, 1999, pp. 56–63.

Lewontin, R.C., S. Rose, and L.J. Kamin, *Not in Our Genes: Biology, Ideology, and Human Nature*, Pantheon Books, New York, 1984.

Li, Shi-zhen, *Pulse Diagnosis*, Paradigm, Brookline, 1985.

Lin, A., *A Handbook of TCM Urology and Male Sexual Dysfunction*, Blue Poppy Press, Boulder, CO, 1992.

Lilienfeld, R., *The Rise of Systems Theory*, John Wiley & Sons, New York, 1978.

Lu, G.D., "China's Greatest Naturalist: A Brief Biography of Li Shih-Chen," *American Journal of Chinese Medicine*, Vol. 4, pp. 209–218, 1976.

———, and J. Needham, "A Contribution to the History of Chinese Dietetics," *Isis*, Vol. 42, 1951, pp. 13–20.

Lu, H.C., *Chinese Foods for Longevity*, Sterling, New York, 1990.

———, *Chinese System of Food Cures*, Sterling, New York, 1986.

———, *Legendary Chinese Healing Herbs*, Sterling, New York, 1991.

Maciocia, G., *Tongue Diagnosis in Chinese Medicine*, Eastland Press, Seattle, 1987.

Magner, L.N., *A History of Medicine*, Marcel Dekker, New York, 1992.

———, *A History of the Life Sciences*, 2nd ed., Marcel Dekker, 1994.

Matsumoto, K., and S. Birch, *Five Elements and Ten Stems*, Paradigm, Brookline, 1983.

———, *Hara Diagnosis: Reflections on the Sea*, Paradigm, Brookline, 1988.

McKeown, T., "A Basis for Health Strategies," *BMJ*, Vol. 287, 1983, pp. 594–596.

McKinlay, J.B., and S.M. McKinlay, "Medical Measures and the Decline of Mortality," in *The Sociology of Health and Illness*, P. Conrad and R. Kern, eds., St. Martin's Press, New York, 1994.

McLachlan, G., and T. McKeown, eds., *Medical History and Medical Care: A Symposium of Perspectives*, Oxford University Press, London, 1971.

Milburn, M.P., "Emerging Relationships Between the Paradigm of Oriental Medicine and the Frontiers of Western Biological Science," *Am. J. Acu.*, Vol. 22, No. 2, 1994, pp. 145–157.

———, "Bioelectromagnetics: Implications for Oriental Medicine and Acupuncture," *Am. J. Acu.*, Vol. 23, No. 1, 1995.

———, and M. Oelbermann, *Electromagnetic Fields and Your Health*, New Star Books, Vancouver, 1994.

Mindell, E., *Earl Mindell's Soy Miracle*, Simon and Schuster, New York, 1995.

Mitukuni, Y., "The Chinese Concept of Nature," in *Chinese Science: Explorations of an Ancient Tradition*, S. Nakayama and N. Sivin, eds., The MIT Press, Cambridge, 1973.

Nakayama, S. and N. Sivin, eds., *Chinese Science: Explorations of an Ancient Tradition*, The MIT Press, Cambridge, 1973.

Needham, J., *The Grand Titration: Science and Society in East and West*, University of Toronto Press, Toronto, 1969.

———, *Science and Civilization in China*, Vol. 2, Cambridge University Press, Cambridge, 1956.

———, *Science and Civilization in China*, Vol. 5, Cambridge University Press, Cambridge, 1983.

———, *Time: The Refreshing River*, Macmillan, New York, 1943.

———, and G.D. Lu, "Hygiene and Preventive Medicine in Ancient China," *JHMAS*, Vol. 17, 1962, pp. 429–478.

Ni, Maoshing, *The Tao of Nutrition*, SevenStar Communications, Santa Monica, 1987.

Nordenström, B., "Bioelectrical Circuits in the Body," *Frontier Perspectives*, Vol. 2, No. 2, 1991, pp. 16–18.

Ornish, D., *Dr. Dean Ornish's Program for Reversing Heart Disease*, Random House, New York, 1990.

———, *Eat More, Weigh Less*, Harper, New York, 1993.

Payer, L., *Medicine and Culture: Varieties of Treatment in the United States, England, West Germany, and France*, Penguin Books, New York, 1988.

Pelletier, K., *Mind As Healer, Mind As Slayer*, Dell, New York, 1977.

Perry, D.A., et al., "Bootstrapping in Ecosystems," *Bioscience*, Vol. 39, No. 4, 1989, pp. 230–236.

Popp, F.A., and B. Becker, eds., *Electromagnetic Bioinformation*, 2nd ed., Urban & Schwarzenberg, Munich, 1988.

———, "Biophotons and Their Regulatory Role in Cells," *Frontier Perspectives*, Vol. 7, No. 2, 1998, pp. 13–22.

Porkert, M., *The Theoretical Foundations of Chinese Medicine*, MIT Press, Cambridge, 1974.

———, and C. Ullman, *Chinese Medicine*, M. Howson, trans., Henry Holt, New York, 1988.

Porter, A., *Cybernetics Simplified*, English Universities Press, London, 1969.

Prigogine, I., and I. Stengers, *Order Out of Chaos: Man's New Dialogue with Nature*, Bantam, New York, 1984.

Qiu, Mao-liang, ed., *Chinese Acupuncture and Moxibustion*, Churchill Livingstone, Edinburgh, 1993.

Requena, Y., *Character and Health: The Relationship of Acupuncture and Psychology*, Paradigm, Brookline, 1989.

Schedlowski, M. et al., "The Effects of Psychological Intervention on Cortisol Levels and Leucocyte Numbers in the Peripheral Blood of Breast Cancer Patients," in *The Psychoimmunology of Cancer: Mind and Body in the Fight for Survival*, C.E. Lewis, et al., eds., Oxford University Press, Oxford, 1994, pp. 336–348.

Schilpp, P.A., ed., *The Philosophy of Alfred North Whitehead*, Tudor Publishing, New York, 1951.

Schipper, H., E.A. Turley, and M. Baum, "A New Biological Framework for Cancer Research," *Lancet*, Vol. 348, 1996, pp. 1149–1151.

———, C.R. Hoh, and T.L. Wang, "Shifting the Cancer Paradigm: Must We Kill to Cure?" *Journal of Clinical Oncology*, Vol. 13, No. 4, 1995, pp. 801–807.

Sheldrake, R., *A New Science of Life*, Paladin, London, 1987.

———, *The Presence of the Past*, Collins, London, 1988.

———, "Three Approaches to Biology: Part II. Vitalism," *Theoria to Theory*, Vol. 14, 1981, pp. 227–240.

———, "Three Approaches to Biology: Part III. Organicism," *Theoria to Theory*, Vol. 14, 1981, pp. 301–311.

Shurtleff, W., and A. Aoyagi, *The Book of Tofu*, Ballantine, New York, 1979.

Spence, J.D., *The Search for Modern China*, W.W. Norton, New York, 1990.

Stapp, H.P., "A Quantum Theory of Consciousness," in *The Interrelationship Between Mind and Matter*, B. Rubik, ed., Temple University, Philadelphia, 1989, pp. 207–217.

Steen, R.G., letter to the editors, *Sci. Am.*, May, 1994, p. 10.

Steingraber, S., *Living Downstream: An Ecologist Looks at Cancer and the Environment*, Addison-Wesley, New York, 1997.

Swerdlow, J.L., "Quiet Miracles of the Brain," National *Geographic*, June, 1995, pp. 2–41.

Temple, N., and D.P. Burkitt, eds., *Western Diseases: Their Dietary Prevention and Reversibility*, Humana Press, Totawa, 1994.

Temple, R., *The Genius of China*, Simon & Schuster, New York, 1986.

Thorogood, M., et al., "Risk of Death from Cancer and Ischaemic Heart Disease in Meat and Non-meat Eaters," *BMJ* 1994; 308:1667–1671.

Time Magazine, Electronic Edition, "Alternative Therapies Challenging the Mainstream," December, 1996.

Trichopoulos, D., F. P. Li, and D.J. Hunter, "What Causes Cancer?" *Sci. Am.*, September, 1996, pp. 80–87.

Trowell, H.C., and D.P. Burkitt, *Western Diseases: Their Emergence and Prevention*, Harvard University Press, Cambridge, 1981.

Unschuld, P.U., *Medicine in China*, University of California Press, Berkeley, 1985.

Van Peursen, C.A., *Body, Soul, Spirit: A Survey of the Body-Mind Problem*, Oxford University Press, London, 1966.

Veith, I., trans., *Yellow Emperor's Classic of Internal Medicine*, University of California Press, Berkeley, 1972.

Vendler, Z., "The Ineffable Soul," in *The Mind-Body Problem*, R. Warner and T. Szubka, eds., Blackwell, Oxford, 1994, pp. 317–328.

Vesey, G.N.A., ed., *Body and Mind*, George Allen and Unwin, London, 1964.

Von Bertalanffy, L., "The History and Status of General Systems Theory," in *Trends in General Systems Theory*, G.J. Klir, ed., Wiley & Sons, New York, 1972.

———, *Perspectives On General Systems Theory*, George Braziller, New York, 1975.

———, "The Theory of Open Systems in Physics and Biology," *Science*, Vol. 111, 1950, pp. 23–29.

Whitehead, A.N., *Adventures of Ideas*, Mentor, New York, 1955.

Willett, W.C., G.A. Colditz, and N.E. Mueller, "Strategies for Minimizing Cancer Risk," *Sci. Am.*, September, 1996, pp. 88–95.

Wiseman, N., A. Ellis, and P. Zmiewski, *Fundamentals of Chinese Medicine*, Paradigm, Brookline, 1985.

Wong, K.C., and L.T. Wu, *History of Chinese Medicine*, AMS Press, New York, 1973.

Yang, S.Z., and D.W. Liu, trans., *Fu Qing-zhu's Gynecology*, Blue Poppy Press, Boulder, 1992.

Zhuo, Da-hong, "Comparative Therapeutic Exercise: East and West," *Comp. Med. East and West*, Vol. VI, No. 4, 1982, pp. 263–271.

Index

RELATED BOOKS BY THE CROSSING PRESS

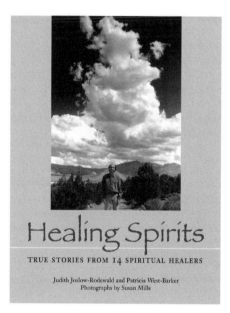

Healing Spirits: True Stories from 14 Spiritual Healers

By Judith Joslow-Rodewald and Patricia West-Barker

Photographs by Susan Mills

Three women traveled across the United States to meet, learn from, and record the stories of fourteen healers. This book brings together their wisdom, wit, and life experiences. They have nothing in common except their commitment to helping others achieve their highest potential. The stories they tell about their lives and practices are as entertaining as they are illuminating, as personal as they are universal, as immediate as they are timeless.

Spiritual growth, life after death, altered states of consciousness, shamanism, mediumship, magic, and miracles are not abstract theories to these people. What they all share is an unshakable belief that everyone is a potential healer with an innate ability to move toward wholeness.

$20.95 • Paper • ISBN 1-58091-064-5

RELATED BOOKS BY THE CROSSING PRESS

The Accidental Vegan
by Devra Gartenstein

Vegetarian and ethnic dishes have made their way into mainstream American kitchens. From Thai noodles to Greek tahini sauce, these recipes are easy to create and require little prep time. Gartenstein offers ideas about low-fat cooking, how to shop for exotic ingredients, how to cook well with a minimum of time, and the all-important substitutions.

$14.95 • Paper • ISBN 1-58091-079-3

The Balanced Diet Cookbook: Easy Menus and Recipes for Combining Carbohydrates, Proteins and Fats
By Bill Taylor

This cookbook provides simple recipes, complete menu plans, and food charts for followers of the Zone plan and others interested in balanced eating for better health.

$16.95 • Paper • ISBN 0-89594-874-5

Essential Reiki: A Complete Guide to an Ancient Healing Art
By Diane Stein

This bestseller includes the history of Reiki, hand positions, giving treatments, and the initiations. While no book can replace directly received attunements, Essential Reiki provides everything else that the practitioner and teacher of this system needs, including all three degrees of Reiki, most of it in print for the first time.

$18.95 • Paper • ISBN 0-89594-736-6

Everyday Tofu: From Pancakes to Pizza
By Gary Landgrebe

This book offers all Americans an opportunity to incorporate tofu into their everyday diets. We are not asking them to change their habits. We say sincerely that Americans who have remained aloof from the tofu craze will honestly be pleased by these recipes which combine tofu with their favorite foods and seasonings to create Western style main dishes, breads, and desserts.

$12.95 • Paper • ISBN 1-58091-047-5

The Healing Energy of Your Hands
By Michael Bradford

Bradford offers techniques so simple that anyone can work with healing energy quickly and easily.

$14.95 • Paper • ISBN 0-89594-781-1

RELATED BOOKS BY THE CROSSING PRESS

The Herbal Medicine-Maker's Handbook: A Home Manual

by James Green

This guide to the kitchen pharmacy discusses the entire process of preparing herbal medicines at home, from methods of growing, gathering, and drying herbs to different ways of extracting their vital essences and making healing balms, lotions, and more. By the author of the best-selling *The Male Herbal* (50,000 copies sold).

$20.95 • Paper • ISBN 0-89594-990-3

Japanese Vegetarian Cooking

By Patricia Richfield

Easy-to-follow directions, information on techniques, plus a glossary of Japanese ingredients make this a must-have cookbook for all Japanese food fans.

$14.95 • Paper • ISBN 0-89594-805-2

The Optimum Nutrition Bible

By Patrick Holford

Optimum nutrition is a revolution in health care. It means giving yourself the best possible intake of nutrients to allow your body to be as healthy as possible. *The Optimum Nutrition Bible* shows you precisely how to achieve this, and gives a step-by-step plan to create your own personal supplement program. The results will speak for themselves.

$16.95 • Paper • ISBN 1-58091-015-7

Pocket Guide to Hatha Yoga

By Michele Picozzi

Hatha yoga is a holistic form of exercise tailor-made for modern Westerners. This guide offers a roadmap for the beginner and a comprehensive resource for the continuing yoga student.

$6.95 • Paper • ISBN 0-89594-911-3

To receive a current catalog from The Crossing Press
please call toll-free, 800-777-1048.
www.crossingpress.com

www.crossingpress.com

BROWSE through the Crossing Press Web site for information on upcoming titles, new releases, and backlist books including summaries, excerpts, author information, reviews, and more.

SHOP our store for all of our books and, coming soon, unusual, interesting, and hard-to-find sideline items related to Crossing's best-selling books!

READ informative articles by Crossing Press authors on all of our major topics of interest.

SIGN UP for our e-mail newsletter to receive late-breaking developments and special promotions from The Crossing Press.

WATCH for a new look coming soon to the Crossing Press Web site!